The Practice of Autonomy

The Practice of Autonomy
Patients, Doctors, and Medical Decisions

Carl E. Schneider

University of Michigan Law School

New York   Oxford
Oxford University Press
1998

Oxford University Press

Oxford   New York
Athens   Auckland   Bangkok   Bogotá   Buenos Aires   Calcutta
Cape Town   Chennai   Dar es Salaam   Delhi   Florence   Hong Kong   Istanbul
Karachi   Kuala Lumpur   Madrid   Melbourne   Mexico City   Mumbai
Nairobi   Paris   São Paulo   Singapore   Taipei   Tokyo   Toronto   Warsaw

and associated companies in
Berlin   Ibadan

Copyright © 1998 by Oxford University Press, Inc.

Published by Oxford University Press, Inc.
198 Madison Avenue, New York, New York 10016

Library of Congress Cataloging-in-Publication Data
Schneider, Carl E., 1948–
The practice of autonomy:
patients, doctors, and medical decisions / Carl E. Schneider.
p. cm. Includes bibliographical references and index.
ISBN 0-19-511397-7
1. Patient participation. 2. Autonomy (Psychology)
3. Medical care—Decision making. 4. Patient satisfaction. I. Title.
R727.42.S36   1998
610.69′ 16—dc21   98-12178

1 3 5 7 9 8 6 4 2

Printed in the United States of America
on acid-free paper

To Joan
Of her choice virtues only gods should speak

Acknowledgments

This book began in an empirical investigation of how patients make medical decisions. It is not a final report on that research, although it is crucially informed by it and although I have drawn from it a number of times. Rather, the book is the fruit of my reflections on some of the normative issues that research raises. I am enormously grateful to the patients, doctors, nurses, social workers, and dieticians I have interviewed during that research. I owe special thanks to the remarkable physician who heads the unit in which I have conducted much of my research, who first allowed me to study his unit, and who has continued to endure my presence and ease my way. I owe similar thanks to the equally remarkable codirector of that unit, who has similarly been generous with his time and intelligence. Likewise, I am grateful to the social worker who has lavished so much time, effort, and insight in helping me study and understand the lives of the chronically ill. I am glad to be able to thank by name Joel Howell, with whom I have for some years taught a course for both law students and medical students and from whom I continue to learn what the calling of medicine at its best can be.

The research from which this book grows was begun (and first publicly sketched) at the annual institute for teachers of law and medicine sponsored by the Cleveland Clinic and the Cleveland–Marshall College of Law. The book began to take form as a paper presented at a conference sponsored by the Poynter Center and the Indiana Law School, where I benefited from the illuminating and incisive responses to my paper from Bernice H. Pescosolido and Peter Cherbas, as well as my host, Roger Dworkin. I presented related papers at the Fifth Annual Bioethics Summer Retreat; the Paris meeting of the European Society for Philosophy of Medicine and Health Care; the Program for Society and Medicine, University of Michigan Medical School; a Keck Foundation Conference on Professional Ethics, University of Michigan Law School; the Robert Wood Johnson Foundation's Clinical Scholars Program, University of Michigan Medical School; the 1996 meeting of the North American section of the International

Society of Family Law, Quebec City, Quebec; the 1996 meeting of the Law and Society Association, Glasgow, Scotland; the Robert Wood Johnson Foundation Scholars in Health Policy Research Program, University of Michigan; the Center for Biomedical Ethics, Case Western Reserve University School of Medicine; the University of Michigan Decision Colloquium; and faculty workshops at the Arizona State University Law School, the University of Tokyo Law School, the Quinnipiac School of Law, the Ritsumeikan University Law School, the Kyoto Sangyo University Law School, the Case Western Reserve University Law School, the University of San Diego School of Law, the Vanderbilt University School of Law, and the University of Michigan Law School.[1] I greatly appreciate the attentive and acute comments of the audiences at all those venues.

I owe many other debts. Gail Agrawal, John Arras, Anne Wolfe Bennett, Alfred F. Conard, Carla Craig, Rebecca Dresser, Nancy Dubler, Mark A. Hall, Rodney A. Hayward, Donald J. Herzog, Joel Howell, Stanton D. Krauss, Hilde Lindemann Nelson, James Lindemann Nelson, Martin Pernick, Richard H. Pildes, Carl J. Schneider, Dorothy Schneider, Joan W. Schneider, Elizabeth Scott, Kenneth W. Simons, A. W. B. Simpson, Sonia Suter, Kent D. Syverud, Carol Weisbrod, Patricia D. White, and Barbara Bennett Woodhouse all made perceptive and penetrating comments on various incarnations of the manuscript. Particularly lavish thanks go to Renée R. Anspach, Richard O. Lempert, and Robert Zussman, fine scholars and exemplary colleagues who commented extensively and acutely on the manuscript and tolerantly tried to steer me away from the shoals of sociology. Penny F. Pierce kindly shared her knowledge of how patients make decisions. Lee E. Teitelbaum and Patricia D. White worked with me on the project to study patients' decisions in which this book began and gave me the benefit of many fruitful conversations from which I am still learning.

I am also pleased to thank several institutions which have helped fund the preparation and presentation of the ideas in this book. They include the University of Michigan Law School William Cook Fund, the Keck Foundation, and the Japan Society for the Promotion of Science.

Finally, I am glad to have the opportunity to thank my fine secretary, Laura Harlow. She has organized all my work so that this book could be written. With patience and persistence she has handled stage after stage of the manuscript. With care and intelligence she has saved me from many errors. And she has brought to all these tasks uncommon good humor, good will, and good sense.

Contents

Introduction

[E]xperience shows that there are times in every one's life when one can be better counseled by others than by one's self. Inability to decide is one of the commonest symptoms of fatigued nerves; friends who see our troubles more broadly, often see them more wisely than we do; so it is frequently an act of excellent virtue to consult and obey a doctor, a partner, or a wife.

William James
The Varieties of Religious Experience

Medical Decisions in the Age of Informed Consent

Every human being of adult years and sound mind has a right to determine what shall be done with his own body; and a surgeon who performs an operation without his patient's consent, commits an assault. Benjamin Cardozo, *Schloendorff v. Society of New York Hospital*

We live in the time of the triumph of autonomy in bioethics. But what should that triumph mean for the way doctors and patients deal with each other and the choices they make? What have the victors and the vanquished contended for? What do autonomists want for patients? What do their opponents want of doctors? What do patients want for themselves? What should they want for themselves? What does "autonomy" mean in the lives of the ill? How should the law try to structure and police the relationship between doctor and patient? These are the questions autonomy's triumph raises and this book addresses. In this section, I want to sketch the path I will take in answering them.

In recent years, bioethicists and lawyers have excoriated traditional medical ethics, saying it scants the patient's interest in autonomy. But these critics have, I think, been less concerned with what patients do want than with what they should want. I wish to develop the latter by exploring the former. That is, I want to investigate how medical ethics should be understood, how medicine should be practiced, and how patients should live by asking these questions from the patient's perspective. This inquiry yields some unexpected results. Much of what autonomists want for patients,[1] many patients want for themselves. At least some patients crave and contend for all that lawyers and bioethicists advocate—the authority and the ability to make their own medical decisions. Yet many patients reject the full burden of decision autonomists would wish upon them.

Because this proposition runs counter to bioethics' assumptions, I will spend a good deal of time proving it. I will do so by investigating several kinds of data, particularly quantitative studies and the memoirs patients have written about their illnesses. One plausible response to these data is that such patients misconceive their own interests and even wishes. This raises the question whether they might have good reasons not to make their own medical decisions. I will propose three: that making decisions of all kinds is hard and that medical decisions can be surpassingly difficult; that for the sick, other enterprises will seem more pressing than medical decisions; and, most problematically, that the sick sometimes wish to be dissuaded from choices they would otherwise make. Furthermore, patients may have cause to worry about how sagely they can make medical decisions, since the evidence suggests that they do not gather information as broadly or evaluate it as systematically as bioethicists and lawyers expect and want. To be sure, physicians reason imperfectly too. But their reason is both better informed and better subject to discipline, and patients thus might reasonably want to confide decisions to them.

I will next examine two responses to my argument that many patients resist making their own medical decisions. The first notes that patients plainly want to be informed about their illness and asks why they seek information if they do not want to make decisions. The second asks how the data I present can be reconciled with the maxim that "control" is a preeminent human desire and a particularly urgent need of the ill. I will try to make the position of the reluctant patient more understandable by disaggregating the broad category "medical decision" to show how different kinds of choices may evoke different attitudes about making medical decisions.

Having studied what patients *do* want, I will consider what they *should* want. One might say of patients who decline to make medical decisions that they have exercised their autonomy in deciding not to decide. There is truth in this reaction, but there is trouble as well. I will explore it by sketching a position I call *mandatory autonomism*. This is the view that patients *should* make their own medical decisions even if they would rather not. I will propose four rationales for that view. First, that it helps subdue overweening medical imperialism. Second, that it is therapeutically beneficial. Third, that it is an antidote to patients' false consciousness. Fourth, that it is a moral duty. I will scrutinize these arguments in turn, finding something to like in each, but also finding much to dispute.

I will close by looking more broadly at autonomy's role in its time of triumph. If some patients want autonomy and others do not, if patients should sometimes make decisions but at other times need not, patients should presumably allocate decisional authority case by case. But while that principle is attractive, it is also problematic. First, it is hard to implement. Second, the bureaucratization of modern medicine seems to be shifting the authority to make medical decisions away from *both* doctor and patient and toward the organizations that increasingly dominate American medical care. Finally, perhaps reformist energies in medicine are no longer best directed at perfecting the exercise of patients' autonomy. Patients want more from doctors than autonomy; they want competence and kindness. I will close by asking how those goals might have a place in our agenda for medicine.

I should warn the reader at the outset that this is a work written against the grain. Of course I rejoice in the bioethical revolution. I detest and resent medical arrogance. I distrust unchecked power. I know the battle against medical autocracy is not won. But today, when all this has been said so often, so passionately, and so convincingly, little is to be gained by rehearsing yet again the conventional bioethical wisdom. I therefore want to take that wisdom as given, to show why it may not be easy to apply, to probe its limits, to see what other wisdom it must accommodate. For surely bioethics has come of age and has achieved the maturity to confront the world in its true and tragic complexity, to go beyond paradigms and politics.

My method has centrally been to try to write from the patient's perspective. I do not mean I have propounded yet another argument for patient autonomy and the power of patients to make their own medical choices. Rather, I have striven to understand how human beings who become sick interpret their fate, how their illness fits the fabric of their lives, what they seek for themselves and want from their doctors. I conclude that patients desire both more and less than autonomy. From the perspective of the sick, the authority to make medical decisions may not loom so large; but in other ways the sick may want more from doctors— particularly more personal concern—than doctors have felt called on to give. I have endeavored, then, to see the law of medicine, the principles of bioethics, and the encounter between doctor and patient from the patient's point of view. This has led me to doubt what the conventional wisdom assumes—that patients want primarily to be "empowered"—and to believe that what patients want, what they reasonably want, is complex, ambiguous, and ambivalent. My goal is to chart that complexity, to plumb that ambiguity, to explain that ambivalence, and thus to take the autonomy paradigm beyond its present pieties and into the bleakly uncertain realities in which patients and doctors work, live, and die.

The arduous path to that goal is made rockier by the fact that patients want different things. The population of the sick is ultimately the population of the world, and its preferences are as many, as contradictory, as labile as human preferences generally are. Bioethics and the law have articulated one of those preferences fervently and persuasively. I want to supplement that accomplishment by bringing to the foreground the uncertainty and the unease patients feel about autonomy and the other ends they value.

I said this book is written against the grain. I meant in part that my point of departure is the substantial number of patients who seem reluctant to make their own medical decisions. This book is organized around these wayward patients not because they have cornered the truth about the place of autonomy in bioethics or because I think they fully represent the universe of patients, but because they are a valuable yet neglected source of insight. Autonomists have cogently made the case for the patient as decider. The patients I describe seem to reject that role. By combining these two perspectives, we may better understand the whole range of views patients take and ought to take toward medical decisions. Through this juxtaposition we may uncover more of the complexity the doctrine of patient autonomy actually presents to patients and their doctors.

I originally began to consider these issues in my capacity as a law professor who teaches and writes about health law and bioethics. I was struck by the characteristically confident assumption of many bioethicists and legal academics that the law can put right what has gone wrong in medicine. The usual instruments of that redemption are three doctrinal expressions of the autonomy principle— informed consent, advance directives, and the constitutional right to make one's own medical decisions. In part, then, this book examines the normative and empirical status of those legal doctrines and the law's ability to shape human behavior through them.

But I have written this book for a wider audience than lawyers and bioethicists. First, I hope its readers will include doctors. In my observation, doctors sometimes slip into the tempting trap of seeing the law of informed consent as stating the whole of the physician's duty to the patient's autonomy interests. They then think that, ethically and practically, what they are required to do is absurdly shallow. In addition, what doctors hear from bioethicists sometimes strikes them as unresponsive to the ambiguity and awkwardness of life in the examining room and on the wards. I hope this book will quickly leave behind the bounds and bonds of the law for a broad and textured discussion of how doctors ought to involve patients in medical decisions, whatever the law may say or fail to say.

As the doctrine of patient autonomy has developed, it has ventured beyond describing how doctors should treat patients toward prescribing how patients should conduct themselves. The new autonomists, I will argue, may want to do more than free patients from medical tyranny; they may be edging toward imposing on patients the duty of freedom, the moral obligation to make their own medical decisions. This book, then, is also written for patients. It asks how far patients ought, as a matter of good sense and moral duty, personally make the medical decisions that affect them. But it addresses them with humility and diffidence. In the years I have spent interviewing the ill and reading their memoirs, I have increasingly come to appreciate the difficulty of patients' lives and to admire the sense, decency, and courage with which they lead them. The most I can hope is that they may find in my reflections some echo of what they have taught me.

This, then, is a book about the ill and those who seek to cure them. But in addressing its subject, it may also raise fundamental questions about some of our core cultural values. It offers, in other words, a case study of the place of the autonomy ideal in American life, a study that allows us to ask how far people want to be, can be, and should be autonomous. Thus, it is not a polemic on the degradation of medicine, nor a prescription for reforming it, but rather a meditation on the lives and duties of the sick and on the cultural and moral lessons they can teach.

Logic and Experience

[T]he rationalist does not neglect experience, but he often appears to do so because . . . of the rapidity with which he reduces the tangle and variety of experience to a set of principles which he will then attack or defend only upon rational grounds. He has no sense of the cumulation of experience, only of the readiness of experience when it has been converted into a formula . . . . Michael Oakeshott, *Rationalism in Politics*

It is no doubt true that you cannot get from *is* to *ought*. But you ought to know what *is* is before you say what *ought* ought to be. Yet we who write about bioethics can hardly know what that *is* is. Most us are not doctors. All of us have been and will be patients, but few of us are unfortunate enough to have wide personal experience with medical care. And all of us—doctors and patients, lawyers and bioethicists—have readily to hand only our own limited and thus misleading experiences. I suppose few bioethicists or lawyers would dispute these observations, but few of them have closely examined the empirical setting of the ethical issues they address. Because I have tried to do so, I am pausing here, before developing my substantive arguments, to explain why. This section, that is, offers some introductory reflections on the methods this book adopts.

Bioethicists, like lawyers, are prone to what I once called "hyper-rationalism."[2] Hyper-rationalism has both a methodological and a substantive aspect. As a method, it "is essentially the substitution of reason for information and analysis. It has two components: first, the belief that reason can reliably be used to infer facts where evidence is unavailable or incomplete, and second, the practice of interpreting facts through a [narrow] set of artificial analytic categories."[3] Hyper-rationalism, in other words, tempts us to believe we can understand how people think and act merely by reasoning and without investigating. It lures us to discuss human behavior without studying how people actually behave. It is the conceptualist's revenge for the world's complexity.

Methodological hyper-rationalism, then, describes a way of understanding so-

cial problems. Substantive hyper-rationalism furnishes the assumptions about
how people think and act that stand in for the information that might be garnered
from empirical inquiry. In bioethics, as in many other areas of thought,[4] these assumptions see people as operating in remarkably rational ways. They hold that
people deliberate explicitly about their situations, that they do so in predomi-
nantly rational terms, that they are autonomy maximizers, and that they have
well-worked-out agendas they need autonomy to implement. These assumptions
see people primarily as makers of decisions who reach out for control over their
lives. Finally, while these assumptions do not entirely abstract people from their
social contexts, they tend to simplify those contexts severely.[5]

Bioethics has too often succumbed to the seductions of hyper-rationalism.
This should be no surprise. The primary work of bioethics is ethics. The primary
training of bioethicists has been in philosophy, theology, and law, all fields distinguished by their concern with abstract principles. The presence and malignity of
bioethics' primary target—medical paternalism—are hardly doubted, and so perhaps its hyper-rationalism has hardly mattered. But as bioethics has moved out of
its childhood, its hyper-rationalism has increasingly hurt. Let me count some of
the ways.

For one thing, hyper-rationalism's assumptions can mislead us into exaggerat-
ing the uniformity of human nature and conduct. As Howard Brody observes,
"Some statements in the medical ethics literature suggest that there is basically
one way to be sick, that sickness affects all sick individuals in this one way, and
that therefore one can usefully generalize, for ethical purposes, among all such
cases without inquiring too finely into the details."[6] Similarly, the law of bioethics works through large categories. The duty of informed consent, for example, applies to all but a few medical decisions (those involving emergencies and
patients who would genuinely be injured by a disclosure). And the ambition of
the Patient Self-Determination Act[7] is to reach every patient who enters a medical institution.

Hyper-rationalism's assumptions also imply that patients make decisions
much more rationally than seems credible. As Daniel Chambliss observes,
"Much of bioethics assumes that people are autonomous decision makers sitting
in a fairly comfortable room trying logically to fit problems to given solution-
making patterns. The whole business is almost deliberately unreal . . . ."[8] Even
some work in medical sociology and social psychology succumbs to this failing.
As Irving Janis writes, "The theoretical concepts that have been dominant in the
literature on decision making for over 25 years are based on cognitive theories,
such as 'game theory' and 'subjective expected utility' (SEU) theory, which assume that people make deliberate choices on a rational basis, taking account of
the values and the probabilities of the consequences to be expected from choosing each of the available alternatives."[9] As empiricists in fields from sociology to
psychology to anthropology have labored to show, this view overstates human ra-

tionality and understates the strength of social and cultural factors in people's lives.[10]

If social scientists may be thus led astray by hyper-rationalism, how can lawyers and bioethicists be far behind?[11] Consider, for instance, how they seem to believe people should and can make decisions. The American Medical Association, for instance, has been able to say that the "decision whether to permit or to perform a transplantation procedure . . . must be a reasoned, intellectual decision, not an emotional decision."[12] One influential bioethicist has been able to write, "Consent must be voluntary and free—the product of deliberative reflection on all possible courses of action."[13] Two other prominent bioethicists have been able to suggest, "Autonomy requires that individuals critically assess their own values and preferences; determine whether they are desirable; affirm, upon reflection, these values as ones that should justify their actions; and then be free to initiate action to realize the values."[14] No wonder Renée Anspach speaks for several sociologists when she concludes that "many ethical discussions rely on what, from a sociological vantage point, appears to be an idealized vision of decision making in which both the medical and social dimensions have been simplified. Many writers assume that moral choice rests exclusively with the individual moral agent, who reaches decisions apart from institutional constraints."[15]

Hyper-rationalism's substantive assumptions could be true. But that has hardly been demonstrated. Indeed, they are surely false. Their picture of human nature is too simple, too disembodied, to be convincing. They present a bloodless, flat, distant, abstract, depersonalized, impoverished view of the way people think, feel, and act, of the social circumstances in which people live, of the ethical lives they lead. And hyper-rationalism's simplifications are particularly implausible in bioethics, a field that treats people in their least rational moments, in their most emotional travails, in their most contextual complexity.

Hyper-rationalism does have its uses. It promotes the generalizations that free courts and commentators to reason logically about the normative problems that are, after all, their central concerns. And some simplification of life's complexity is necessary if human problems are to be handled practically and promptly, if comprehensible rules are to be devised, if useful precedent is to be developed, if institutions are to function smoothly. Nevertheless, we should insinuate as much of that complexity as possible into normative discourse lest we perilously distance norms from the people and circumstances they govern.

This is a peril law knows all too well. One of the most telling bodies of modern legal writing is the scholarship which makes sport of the idea (so natural and right to lawyers) that people know the law's rules, accept them, and respond to them thoughtfully, rationally, and tamely. A classic work in this sobering and reproving genre is Stewart Macaulay's *Non-contractual Relations in Business: A Preliminary Study.*[16] Macaulay interviewed suppliers and purchasers in Wisconsin to see how they used contracts and how the law of contracts shaped their behavior. He found that firms do not think of themselves as using contract law (even when, legally, they are) and that "[d]isputes are frequently settled without reference to the contract or potential or actual legal sanctions." Far from heeding the law, businessmen devise their own system of norms and informal sanctions.[17] As one of them said, "'You don't read legalistic contract clauses at each other if you ever want to do business again. One doesn't run to lawyers if he wants to stay in business because one must behave decently.'"[18]

Another striking study reaching the same kind of conclusion about the relevance of law to people's lives is Robert Ellickson's fascinating investigation of ranchers and farmers in Shasta County, California.[19] Ellickson set out to test the Coase Theorem's principle that people will bargain to reach an economically efficient solution to their disputes whatever the law's allocation of tort liability. Ellickson found that, as the theorem predicts, the allocation of liability does not matter when wandering cattle damage a farmer's crops, but not because people bargain to achieve economic efficiency. Rather, disputes are generally avoided in deference to an informal norm of neighborliness and reciprocity, a norm enforced by the community's own homemade sanctions. In short, a chastening literature[20]

> reveals that, to the lawyer's chagrin, businesses resist using contracts, ranchers do not know what rules of liability govern damage done by wandering cattle, suburbanites do not summon the law to resolve neighborhood disputes, engaged couples do not know the law governing how they will own property when they marry, citizens repeatedly reject the due process protections proffered them, and, what is worse, all these people simply don't care what the law says.[21]

The law regulating medicine abounds in its own examples of this provoking phenomenon. For example, the law's principal bioethical reforms have been used far less than their advocates anticipated. Linda Emanuel notes of the Patient Self-Determination Act that its "measured effects have been small."[22] One study of advance directives concludes that they "are rarely used and perforce have little effect on medical decision-making."[23] Arthur Caplan reports, "No more than 10 percent of the population has either a living will or a durable power of attorney . . . ."[24] He adds, "Similarly dismal statistics are reported for the practices surrounding the issuance of DNR (do-not-resuscitate), DNI (do-not-intubate), and DNT (do-not-treat) orders in hospitals and nursing homes . . . ."[25] For instance, one study found that "the enactment of DNR legislation in the State of New York appears to have had little effect on the frequency of CPR [cardiopulmonary resuscitation] and the degree of patient or family involvement in the DNR decision at our institution."[26] Robert Zussman summarizes this literature as mounting "a powerful case that decisions to terminate treatment do not work in the way envisioned by medical ethicists. In particular, they show that patient self-determination remains an elusive ideal despite the widespread introduction of hospital policies intended to achieve just that."[27] Caplan argues that the experiment of organ-donor cards "has been a failure," since despite the common provision of a donor form on the back of driver's licenses, "no more than 20 percent of all Americans have signed."[28] Likewise, Caplan reviews a number of studies that "indicate that despite the enactment of legislation in forty-four states requiring requests to be made of family members about organ and tissue donation when someone dies in a hospital setting, more than a third of all hospitals never do so, and an even larger number do so only sporadically . . . ."[29] And there is evidence that "the existence of Good Samaritan legislation made no difference to the willingness of physicians to stop and assist."[30]

Similarly, despite the labor that has been poured into it, the law of informed consent seems rarely to result in significant verdicts for plaintiffs, since "few patients sue physicians in general, even fewer sue claiming lack of informed consent, and yet fewer prevail on that theory."[31] Jay Katz concludes glumly that that law "has had little impact on patients' decision-making either in legal theory or medical practice."[32] Some substantiation of this lies in the fact that "the empirical and anecdotal studies of patients who refuse treatment almost never portray the process of obtaining informed consent as playing a causative role."[33] Frequent and menacing though malpractice suits seem to doctors, "for every 8 potentially valid claims, only 1 claim was actually filed." And "even when we narrowed our focus to the more serious and 'valuable' tort claims—iatrogenic injuries to patients under seventy that produced disabilities (including death) lasting six months or more—we still found that for every 3 such events there was only 1 tort payment."[34]

This literature, then, should alert us to the dangers of hyper-rationalism, to the perils of believing ratiocination can ascertain how people will interpret their problems, organize their lives, resolve their disputes, and respond to legal norms. But what is the antidote to hyper-rationalism? There are several. For instance, Howard Brody proposes that the philosophy of medicine can "advance by . . . abstract discussions; but it can advance only so far. At some point we will require a richer context for the discussion to proceed fruitfully. This context can be provided by stories of sickness."[35] This attractive and profitable solution has its formal, well-established, and mainstream counterparts. Casuistry is an ancient and still honorable mode of ethical discourse, and cases lie at the heart of our legal system's common-law and constitutional methods. But necessary though those methods are, they are not by themselves sufficient. Too much depends on how a case is selected for study, on the richness of the problem it presents, and on how much information can be obtained about it. Ultimately, a single case, or even a few cases, cannot represent the sweep of cases the world so prolifically spawns.

We need, then, to inhabit all the mansions in the house of bioethics. And among the least visited of them is empirical research—quantitative and qualitative. It offers a breadth, rigor, and precision of understanding available in no other way. It provides a disciplined means of reviewing our assumptions and a systematic method of identifying neglected issues. It is a fruitful way of obtaining a more detailed, complex, and acute understanding of what patients want, think, and do, one which can deepen—and darken—our understanding of bioethical problems.[36]

All this being said, let me acknowledge the inevitable and substantial difficulty of drawing solid conclusions about the psychological and social reality of bioethical problems from the empirical evidence that is currently available.[37] Empirical work relevant to bioethics has not always been well planned and performed. It has not developed according to any larger vision, but has responded to a smorgasbord of discrete problems in a hodgepodge of fields from law to sociology and psychology to clinical medicine. It has often asked quite narrow questions, and not always the ones most urgent to bioethicists. For example, the literature on medical decisions generally "concentrates on the role of biomedical variables." Only a "much smaller body of literature on decision-making examines the social and cultural influences upon medical decision-making."[38] And given the variety of medical decisions that are made, the variety of contexts in which they occur, and the variety of people who make them, a study of one situation will often be a poor guide to others. Empirical work is also time-bound, a particularly acute problem in an era and in areas as roiled by fulminant change as today's medicine, bioethics, law, and society. Finally, because life is complicated and research is hard, even relevant and skillful studies can produce results that conflict with the conclusions of other competent research.[39]

But I do not want to concede too much. Good empirical research into bioethical issues is being done.[40] And it is better to have some information than none—ultimately, we are wiser to use the best empirical evidence we can muster than idly to rely on unexamined assumptions about an uncertain reality. In any event, in this book I propose to use empirical data not so much as infallible guides to what happens, but to introduce more of the world's complexity into our thinking.

I have been arguing that the law and ethics of medicine need a keener understanding of the social and psychological context in which doctors and patients live. But what sources will I consult that may help provide such an understanding? They are several and draw on several different academic and methodological traditions. Each is limited, from our perspective, since none of the traditions on which they rely systematically asks how patients want medical decisions to be made. However, taken together, they paint a suggestive, if incomplete, picture.

First, I will examine empirical studies of medical care. These tend to be published in medical journals and to be quantitative. They have the advantage that they apply standards of methodological rigor. They have the disadvantage that they generally ask only a few narrow questions, so one is left unsure why the patients studied feel as they do or how they fit into larger patterns. In particular, these studies generally scant the sociology and psychology of patients' decisions. Second, I will recruit the investigations of medical sociologists. These tend to be qualitative, and often ethnographic. They are interested in the very questions the quantitative literature overlooks—the sociological and psychological aspects of a patient's life. Unfortunately, medical sociologists have not been primarily interested in how, or even if, patients make medical decisions.[41] Third, I will consult the work of various kinds of psychologists who have been interested in how people make decisions and in people's desire to control their lives. While relatively little of this work has been explicitly directed toward medical decisions, some of it has, and much of the rest is relevant to us.

Fourth, I will crucially rely on the memoirs of patients and their families. These are an incomparable source of mature and thoughtful reflection on what it means to be ill, and they are now numerous enough to be a fountain of insight.[42] Of course, this source has the defects of its virtues. Exactly because these memoirs are detailed individual accounts, they are unsystematic: They tend to be written by people with truly grim diseases, and some afflictions—especially cancer and AIDS—are represented out of proportion to others—like renal, liver, and even heart disease. Nor are the authors a cross-section of society. People who write books are ordinarily better educated, richer, and more articulate than the population as a whole. As one might expect, people whose business is words— writers,[43] journalists,[44] and professors[45]—are grossly overrepresented. For that matter, so are doctors[46] and even entertainers.[47] Working-class authors rarely appear, and the poor are almost absent. On the other hand, many kinds of people have been moved to tell about their illness, to write the book they wished they could have read when they fell ill. These include a number of people who are demographically quite ordinary (even if the inclination and ability to write a book are not so ordinary).[48]

However, since I will be principally concerned with the limits of autonomy, with the extent to which people decline to exert all their authority over medical decisions, the overrepresentation of the educated, the articulate, and the prosperous among the memoirists is less troublesome than it might seem: The people who tend to write books are probably the people likeliest to want, seek, and exercise autonomy. If they do not want to assert their autonomy to the full, it seems unlikely that most other people do. Furthermore, memoirists and nonmemoirists have not necessarily had such different experiences and reactions that the reports of the former catch nothing in the lives of the latter.

Fifth, I will draw on my own empirical investigations of how patients make medical decisions. For that research I have interviewed and observed renal patients and their families, doctors, nurses, social workers, and dieticians, as well as occasional patients of other kinds. This research speaks directly to the questions this book addresses and is relatively intensive. It has the concomitant disadvantage of narrowness, of examining only a few sorts of patients in a few medical contexts.[49]

In short, this book does not intend to be a definitive empirical investigation of how patients and doctors make medical decisions. (Indeed, I doubt such a book is even possible.) But it does attempt to marshal the available empirical evidence to look critically at the autonomy paradigm in bioethics and law, at the way the sick respond to their illness, and at the way doctors approach their patients.

The Practice of Autonomy

1

The Autonomy Paradigm

My God, my God, how soon wouldst thou have me go to the physician, and how far wouldst thou have me go with the physician?

John Donne
Devotions Upon Emergent Occasions

The Paradigm in Bioethics and Law

To rest upon a formula is a slumber that, prolonged, means death.
Oliver Wendell Holmes, Jr., *Ideals and Doubts*

The law and ethics of medicine are today dominated by one paradigm—the autonomy of the patient. "Paradigms," Thomas Kuhn famously said, "gain their status because they are more successful than their competitors in solving a few problems that the group of practitioners has come to recognize as acute."[1] Bioethics was born out of a crisis of imperialism in biomedical research and medical treatment.[2] It was thus to be expected that, as Renée Fox writes, "from the outset, the conceptual framework of bioethics has accorded paramount status to the value-complex of individualism, underscoring the principles of individual rights, autonomy, self-determination, and their legal expression in the jurisprudential notion of privacy." Even where the question has been the just allocation of scarce resources, "[t]he view of distributive justice underlying it is structured around an individual, rights-oriented conception of the general or common good, in which greater importance is assigned to equity than to equality."[3]

Even in their hour of triumph, paradigms rarely go unchallenged. As I will explain in the next section, the heft and force of the autonomy paradigm have recently been criticized and amendments to it mooted. And even a field dominated by a single paradigm may not be monolithic. Bioethics is complicated by its origin in several diverse fields, and it is divided between "advocates" and "academics."[4] The academics tend to articulate the autonomy paradigm more cautiously, completely, subtly than the advocates,[5] although there is at least a tincture of the advocate in most of the academics. However, "no important thought achieves social power undegraded."[6] The intricate and somber refinement of a Freud is soon debased into the remissive banalities of popular psychology.[7] The cautious balances of constitutional doctrine degenerate into claims that professional baseball players have a constitutional right to chew tobacco on the playing field. Thus the advocate's blunter versions are in some ways the more consequential formulations of the autonomy paradigm. It is they that dominate the world in which medical policies are formulated and social decisions are made and that most beguile the public mind.

In any event, there is little doubt about the triumph of the autonomy paradigm. It is now common to make such strong and categorical assertions as: the fact that the patient "bears rights as a citizen should preclude any form of medical paternalism."[8] As Caplan observes, "there are relatively few bioethicists who argue that respect for autonomy is not the preeminent value governing the actions of health-care providers."[9] He continues colorfully, "The Freddy Kruger of bioethics for the better part of two decades has been the doctor who pushes his or her values onto the patient . . . . This devil has been completely exorcised and a large part of contemporary bioethics scholarship seems to be devoted to the task of assuring that the paternalistic doctor stays dead and buried . . . ."[10]

It is perfectly true that in the most canonical expressions of bioethics' truths other considerations are recited and esteemed.[11] However, in the great mass of bioethical work it is abundantly plain which principle predominates: And now abideth beneficence, social justice, and autonomy, these three; but the greatest of these is autonomy. Thus Fox observes that even the "benefiting of others advocated in bioethical thought is circumscribed by respectful deference to individual rights, interests, and autonomy; and minimizing the harm done to individuals is more greatly accentuated than the maximization of either personal or collective good."[12]

I have been discussing what bioethicists say, not what doctors do. What doctors have historically done is not what bioethicists would now have them do. Yet the world's astir, and doctors are changing. Doubtless many doctors still practice medicine the old-fashioned way, but we must recognize how much medical attitudes have changed, even while regretting they have not changed more. These changes are most obviously represented in the profession's official pronouncements. Thus the AMA—hardly a cadre of Maoist radicals—could say even some years ago that "the patient's right of self-decision can be effectively exercised only if the patient possesses enough information to enable an intelligent choice. The patient should make his own determination of treatment."[13] And the workaday success of the autonomy paradigm cuts deeper than professional piety. Robert Zussman, for instance, reports that "the notion of rights in medicine . . . has . . . become part of the culture of medicine itself."[14] He concludes that the "notion of rights as a broad cultural concept (the acceptance of which is among the indirect effects of the legal doctrine) has had far-reaching consequences, including, most important, an empowerment of the patient . . . ."[15] That notion of rights is enhanced by physicians' (often alarmist) convictions about the extent to which the law gives teeth to patient's claims of authority. In short, "bioethics has become an established presence in medicine . . . . [B]oth patients and physicians are very conscious of patients' right to refuse treatment, of the need for informed consent, and increasingly, of the importance of the patients' participation in their own care."[16]

Further indicia of change abound. For instance, medical training now seems to nudge students toward autonomism: "Although on the average all students at the beginning of their medical school careers leaned toward less physician authority and more patient rights . . . , by the end of their first internship year their mean scores had moved even more strongly in this direction."[17] In the crucial area of informed consent, Norio Higuchi comments, "According to a 1961 survey, 90 percent of the physician-respondents answered that they would not tell their patients they had cancer. In 1977, however, another survey showed that 97 percent of the doctors said they would tell a cancer patient of a cancer diagnosis."[18] Troyen Brennan (a doctor himself) believes "informed consent is now enshrined in . . . the mind-set of physicians."[19] Debra Roter and Judith Hall see evidence "that physicians may be accommodating their patients with a more egalitarian relationship and tolerance for patient participation in decision making."[20] To take a final example, Arthur Caplan notes that "[d]octors and nurses report in survey after survey that they support the concept of advance directives . . . ."[21]

The autonomy paradigm can appeal to doctors for several reasons. To paraphrase Cardozo, "The great tides and currents which engulf the rest of men, do not turn aside in their course, and pass the doctors by."[22] Doctors are swayed by the same influences that move the rest of American society, and those influences impel them toward patient autonomy. Some doctors like a practice that cultivates a closer and more collegial relationship with the patient. Less admirably, but not less significantly, doctors can make the autonomy paradigm a welcome and acceptable way of passing on burdensome problems to patients. Zussman puts perceptively what I have observed in my own research:

> Whether because of fear or because of indifference, overwork, or diffidence, physicians may be prepared to abdicate responsibility for some decisions to patients. Giving patients information, they have discovered, may be easier than withholding it. While a number of observers of the medical scene have argued that patients and patient advocates may demand rights in response to the impersonality of relations with physicians, few have noted that physicians may also become advocates of patients rights in response to the impersonality of their relations with patients.[23]

Thus one study noted that doctors "often seemed too ready to concede patients' 'right to refuse' rather than to recognize the clinical problems that lay at the bottom of the refusal (e.g., poor or inconsistent communication) and to take steps to remedy them."[24]

This change in medical attitudes is beginning to filter into patients' accounts of their illness. Tim Brookes observes that "[t]he goal of the latest asthma treatment is what is usually called (with the usual medical tin ear for the subtleties of language) 'patient empowerment' or 'patient education'—in other words, gentling the patient along towards becoming more of her own doctor, monitoring her own symptoms, understanding her own medication, using the physician as a resource."[25] Another kind of example comes from Kenneth Shapiro, a cancer patient of many years standing. He begins his account of his innumerable encounters with doctors by saying that he has "taken upon myself more of the therapeutic decision-making responsibilities than most physicians are accustomed to . . . ."[26] Yet by and large the problem he had with doctors was not that they objected to his making decisions or to the decisions he reached. Rather it was with doctors who were unavailable in times of need.

In my own field—the law governing medicine—the autonomy paradigm's prominence is plain. It is now a weary commonplace that "Anglo-American law starts with the premise of thorough-going self-determination."[27] Certainly autonomy has enjoyed an expansive role in that law during the life span of bioethics: The doctrine of informed consent has become solidly entrenched.[28] State legislatures have labored to enhance patients' autonomy by authorizing various kinds of advance directives. Congress has enacted the Patient Self Determination Act, which essentially requires hospitals and nursing homes to give their clients an opportunity to make advance directives.[29] And in a long series of cases posing the question when medical treatment may be withdrawn, state courts have generally striven to effectuate the supposed desires of the patient.

Two recent constitutional cases are not to the contrary. *Cruzan v. Director, Missouri Department of Health,*[30] which has been assailed as curtailing rights of autonomy, can be understood as at least compatible with them. In it, the Supreme Court unanimously endorsed the proposition that patients have some kind of constitutional status in making medical decisions. The majority's holding was essentially based not on a denial of Cruzan's autonomy rights but on the presence of reasonable doubts about how she might have wished to exercise them. *Washington v. Glucksberg*[31] does hold there is no constitutional right to the help of a doctor in committing suicide. But a contrary holding would have been remarkable. To reach, it the Court would have had "to reverse centuries of legal doctrine and practice, and strike down the considered policy choice of almost every state."[32] Furthermore, all the opinions in *Glucksberg* affirmed more or less directly the patient's claim to constitutional protection in refusing medical treatment.[33]

In sum, patient autonomy has achieved paradigmatic status in both the ethics and the law of medicine. But "autonomy" is too general an idea to have real meaning in and of itself. Rather, its meaning must be found in its application. And its application is most crucial in the problem this book principally addresses—medical decisions. When ethicists and lawyers discuss medical decisions, they agree that patient autonomy should be the governing principle: "[I]n recent decades there has been a call for greater patient autonomy or, as some have called it, 'patient sovereignty,' conceived as patient *choice* and *control* over medical decisions."[34] This call has been answered, so that in "contemporary medical ethics, . . . engaging the patient as an active participant in medical decision making is seen as particularly important."[35] The standard view broadly makes the physician the proposer and the patient the disposer. Dan Brock advances a particularly lucid, measured, and moderate statement of that view:

> Most simply put, the physician's role is to use his or her training, knowledge, and experience to provide the patient with facts about the diagnosis and about the prognoses without treatment and with alternative treatments. The patient's role in this division of labor is to provide the values—his or her own conception of the good—with which to evaluate these alternatives, and to select the one that is best for himself or herself.[36]

This is the standard view. Nevertheless, most bioethicists have been understandably vague about the nature and scope of patients' autonomy, about how it should be used, and about how doctor and patient are to make principle practice.[37] When Brock says the patient should select the best alternative, just what does he mean? What does he expect patients will actually do in their encounters with doctors? Does he really mean patients should select the best course for *every* medical decision their doctor makes? Does he envision as formal a process as he seems to describe? How far does he think patients can truly articulate their "values" or make choices by applying them?

The vagueness of bioethicists' expectations for patients may be gauged by considering the frequent admonition that patients should "participate" in medical decisions. What does this mean? The term is strong enough to include the two-part procedure Brock describes, a procedure that seems to give patients considerable authority. But it is also weak enough to subsume a process in which the doctor simply solicits the patient's preferences (or even "values") and then decides for the patient. In short, it is simultaneously strong and weak enough to be essentially meaningless, to describe both the potential revolution of tomorrow and the rejected regime of yesterday.

The vagueness of the bioethical prescription is also revealed when autonomists assert—or simply assume—that patients should make *all* the medical decisions that affect them. Autonomists cannot mean this. So many medical decisions may be made during even a single encounter between doctor and patient that that goal is, as stated, impossible. Every time a doctor listens to a heart, palpates a liver, or reads an EEG, a decision follows about whether there is a problem worth pursuing. Patients cannot make an informed choice about each such issue. But then which choices should they make?

Bioethicists have not had to think meticulously about these problems, since they have regarded it as their principal mission to vanquish paternalism and establish broad principles of patient authority. Nor have courts and lawyers had to struggle to be exact, since they have contentedly assumed that once patients are properly informed, their "participation" in medical decisions must naturally follow. Hence the very indefinite use of very vague terms. For instance, the authors of the ethics chapter in a standard internal-medicine textbook begin by invoking "a more equal relationship of shared decision making in which physicians provide information and counseling that allows competent adult patients to make their own choices." In the next sentence they say that "[t]he process by which physicians and patients make decisions together" is "summarized by the phrase 'informed consent.'" In the next paragraph they advise physicians to "involve patients in their own medical care decisions." Shortly thereafter they praise "[e]mpowering patients to participate in decision making."[38] None of these specifications of the patient's role is precise, and each differs in some degree from the others. One is thus left uncertain just what decisional process the authors contemplate (and their student readers will understand them to urge).

The point is that one can imagine a long and elaborate continuum of patient participation in medical decisions. At one end fall patients who insist on delegating every decision to their doctors. At the other are patients who acquire all the information they humanly can, monitor their physicians closely so they know when a decision is called for, and then make each decision on the basis of their appraisal of the medical data, seen through the lens of their own considered beliefs. The problem is that between these two extremes lies a wide and delicately shaded range of possibilities.

Nevertheless, many bioethicists seem to intend that patients' choices should be autonomous in quite a strong sense. For example, Beauchamp and Childress want a decision in which "a patient or subject with substantial *understanding* and in substantial *absence of control* by others *intentionally authorizes* a professional to do something."[39] The standard view of patient predominance is enacted into law in the doctrine of informed consent.[40] That doctrine makes it the "the prerogative of the patient, not the physician, to determine for himself the direction in which his interests seem to lie."[41] Medical decisions may only be made with the patient's consent, and again consent is often intended strongly. As one leading case avers: "True consent to what happens to one's self is the informed exercise of a choice, and that entails an opportunity to evaluate knowledgeably the options available and the risks attendant upon each."[42] The opinion insists informed consent must secure "the patient's right of self-determination on [a] particular therapy"[43] and "enable the patient to chart his course understandably" by assuring some "familiarity with therapeutic alternatives and their hazards."[44]

The reaction of commentators to the law of informed consent confirms the elevated status of the autonomy paradigm and the ambitious hopes they hold for decisions made under its aegis. They widely feel that that law is wretchedly inadequate to its vocation of promoting patients' autonomy, a reaction which suggests how lofty their aspirations for patient autonomy are. Jay Katz, for instance, derides that law as "largely a charade,"[45] as "substantially mythic and fairy tale-like as far as advancing patients' rights to self-decisionmaking is concerned," as only making "a bow toward a commitment to patients' self determination."[46] Appelbaum, Lidz, and Meisel call informed consent "a doctrine and a set of practices that compromise all values and satisfy none in their entirety."[47] Shultz advocates broadening its scope grandly. (She would require doctors to tell patients not just about proposed treatments, but also about inquiries the physician decides not to pursue.)[48] More generally, commentators say that "[t]he rise of patients' rights, both in law and ethics, instigated a revolution not yet completed,"[49] a "revolution in medical relationships [which] remains incomplete and embattled,"[50] a revolution in which "[t]he struggle is to recognize patients' rights."[51]

In sum, the overwhelming weight of bioethical opinion endorses not just the autonomy principle, but a potent version of it. The autonomy paradigm continues to flourish, planted as it is in the fertile soil of American rights thinking, anchored as it is by roots that run deep in the structure of American law, tended as it is by legions of the faithful.[52] That paradigm is sustained by the methodologically and substantively hyper-rationalistic assumption that autonomy is what people primarily and pervasively want and need. Correspondingly and crucially, the law of bioethics assumes its principal task is to remove impediments to the exercise of autonomy, that once those impediments are gone, people will naturally gather evidence about the risks and benefits of each medical choice, apply their values to that evidence, and reach a considered decision.

The Paradigm in Excelsis

You grabbed my hand in that cold white room Mr. Dantio and you said I'm a fighter but only if there's a chance all these doctors want to cut me stick tubes in me I don't really understand I'm just a salesman now cake decorations, that's something I understand, you tell me what should I do. And I said I can't tell you that Mr Dantio, Salvadore, I'm not you.
                                                    Susan Onthank Mates, *The Good Doctor*

Paradigms are not stable; they are defined and refined, elaborated and enlarged as work under them continues. The autonomy paradigm is no exception: Autonomy is in some circles attaining a new potence. I detect signs in teaching my classes, talking with my colleagues, conducting my empirical research among doctors and patients, studying the relevant professional literatures, reading the memoirs of patients, and even visiting my medical attendants that autonomy is coming to be viewed not just as something to which patients are entitled, but as something they ought to want and even should be taught—compelled?—to exercise.

It is impossible to say just how widespread this view is. But even had it not yet surfaced, it would be helpful to invent it because it is the natural extension of much autonomist thought. To put the point differently, it represents one logical pole of the autonomist geography. As such, it is a rewarding vantage point for exploring the structure and principles of the autonomy paradigm. For that reason, we shall examine it at length.

Two Models of Autonomy

I propose that we distinguish two models, two ideal types, of autonomy. The first is the "optional" model. An optional autonomist embraces the view Brock states lucidly: "The moral doctrine of informed consent as interpreted here *entitles,* but *does not require,* a patient to take an active role in decision making regarding treatment."[53] The optional autonomist (as an ideal type) believes that patients typically face individual and structural barriers that discourage them from exercising their autonomy, that those barriers should be razed where possible, and that patients should be helped over any remaining barriers if they want assistance. But the distinguishing feature of the optional model is a reluctance to say people *should* exercise autonomy. An optional autonomist accepts that people may not want to exercise their autonomy in medical matters to the full and that they have their reasons.

The "mandatory" model, on the other hand, holds that patients need to exercise their autonomy and should do so. A mandatory autonomist (again as an ideal type) doubts people truly want to abjure their autonomy, believes patients' decisions are better than doctors', and, what is more, subscribes to an ideal that obliges people to make their own decisions. As Brock writes, that ideal exalts "the self-governing person who makes decisions for him- or herself, after personally weighing alternatives against reflectively adopted values. In turning over a major health care decision to another, a patient does *not* meet that ideal of self-determination."[54] In short, unlike the optional autonomist, the mandatory autonomist favors a view of autonomy that makes it practically unwise and morally objectionable for the patient to forswear making medical choices personally.

I have described two models of autonomy. "In their extreme forms," as William James wrote in a different context, "the two types are violently contrasted; though here, as in most other current classifications, the radical extremes are somewhat ideal abstractions, and the concrete human beings whom we oftenest meet are intermediate varieties and mixtures."[55] Because mandatory and optional autonomy are not categories that have fully emerged in bioethical debate, many autonomists have not specified where on the continuum between them they fall. I suspect many autonomists would, if asked, endorse the optional principle. I have already quoted Brock to that effect, and Beauchamp and Childress expressly say "[t]he patient may delegate decision-making authority to the physician or request not to be informed. In effect, the patient makes a decision not to make an informed decision."[56] However, I also suspect that many autonomists are so devoted to a strong version of autonomy and its entourage of ideals and are so sensitive to the ways people yield to pressures to surrender their autonomy that they cannot easily credit that many patients truly want to waive their authority. Thus while Brock acknowledges that "[p]atients often do not take an active role in decision making . . . ," his ensuing discussion leads one to infer that he would doubt that patients often have "good reasons for avoiding an active role in particular decisions about their health care."[57] Likewise, the President's Commission expressly favors a flexible approach to dividing authority between doctor and patient, but its discussion of autonomy has a different cast and radiates a special warmth. The Commission says, "Respect for self-determination thus promotes personal integration within a chosen life-style." It admonishes us, "This is an especially important goal to be nourished regarding health care. If it is not fostered regarding such personal matters, it may not arise generally regarding public matters. The sense of personal responsibility for decisionmaking is one of the wellsprings of a democracy."[58]

Statements more expressly advocating some version of mandatory autonomy are increasingly evident. Mandatory autonomism is espoused in terms by, for example, Haavi Morreim, who writes, "In matters of health, and of health care, it is time to expect competent patients to assume substantially greater responsibility. In the first place, they should generally make their own decisions. Not only is the patient entitled to decide these issues that affect his life so fundamentally; he has a presumptive obligation to do so."[59] Morreim sees the patient's duty expansively: "The patient's obligation to make his own decisions includes not just medical choices, but also other important matters such as health care coverage."[60] She fears an exception for incompetent patients could become a means of defeating patients' obligations to make their own decisions, and she would construe that exception narrowly: "Where the patient has only a partial impairment of his capacity, he can still be involved in decision-making and, to that degree, can be expected to be accountable."[61] Where the patient is wholly incompetent, decisions should be made by a surrogate other than (Morreim intimates) the physician. Indeed, "competent persons arguably have some obligation to consider whom they would like to invest with decision-making authority when they are unable themselves to fulfill this responsibility."[62]

To Morreim, patients' duty to make medical decisions has two primary sources. First, people ought not burden others with their decisions: "[E]ach person has at least a *prima facie* responsibility to make his own life decisions and not presumptively to impose on someone else the burden of making them."[63] In particular, "physicians are not obligated to . . . take upon themselves all their patients' difficult decisions with all the attendant guilt."[64] Second, people owe it to themselves to make their own choices: "It is this capacity to be an agent, to bear responsibility for decisions and actions that are truly one's own, that renders a person worthy of moral respect, dignity, as beyond merely considerate treatment."[65] Morreim warns, "On the most basic level, the failure to treat a competent patient as being responsible to make his own decisions and be accountable for them is a profound moral insult."[66]

Morreim's is a particularly stark statement of mandatory autonomism. However, other versions of it now scatter the landscape. For example, it is hard to understand Katz's esteemed and influential *The Silent World of Doctor and Patient* except in terms of one kind of mandatory autonomism. Katz postulates that patients have "a duty to reflection that cannot easily be waived."[67] They "are obligated to participate in the process of thinking about choices."[68] Doctors have a role in enforcing that duty, for they are "obligated to facilitate patients' opportunities for reflection to prevent ill-considered rational and irrational influences on choice."[69] Katz summons up the avatar of anti-paternalism—John Stuart Mill—to argue that the principle of " 'liberty of action' . . . is misunderstood if it is interpreted to require 'selfish indifference, which pretends that human beings have no business with each other's conduct of life.' "[70] Thus Katz can write, "A patient's waiver of the physician's obligation to disclose and obtain the patient's consent should be accepted only after a committed effort has been made to explore the underlying reasons for the patient's abdication of decision-making responsibility."[71] More specifically, Katz criticizes Christian Barnard's failure to compel his early heart-transplant patients to make satisfactorily autonomous decisions:

> Even if his patients had initially resisted his invitation to converse and think together, Barnard should have insisted that they talk for a while. The inevitable conflict that such insistence creates between the values of autonomy and privacy should be resolved in favor of autonomy. Such invasions of privacy must be tolerated in order to enhance patients' psychological autonomy through insight and not allow it to be further undermined by too hopeful promises, blind misconceptions, and false certainties.[72]

Katz says that if a heart-transplant patient "wanted a new heart, he also had to have the heart to learn more about the procedure."[73] Only by participating in decisions, Katz appears to believe, can patients assume—as they must—responsibility for their own care and conduct.[74] Katz reproves patients who shirk decisions. They are people "who wish to be confirmed as patients, who wish to escape from the painful and overwhelming vicissitudes of their lives by viewing themselves as incapacitated by physical illness."[75] They "have an inordinate need for reassurance that everything can and will be set right."[76] They have succumbed to their "regressive manifestations"[77] and to their "childlike wishes and needs to be relieved of all responsibility for their care."[78]

Another commentator, William Bartholome, acknowledges that some patients may wish to delegate medical decisions and responds, "Clearly there are many patients, particularly elderly ones, for whom this new model [of medical decisions] is both threatening and foreign." Having deployed that condescending device of our therapeutic society—the substitution of psychological accusation for intellectual argument—Bartholome warns that "[m]any providers may be tempted to argue that we ought to be willing to take care of such patients . . . ." After rejecting this suggestion, Bartholome says "the appropriate response to such patients is one in which the provider expresses an understanding of the patient's wishful, albeit 'magical,' thinking, but also gently explains that such a charade is not desirable for either provider or patient, that the provider simply cannot know what is best, and that a dialogue is necessary."[79]

Yet another autonomist forthrightly says, "If we are serious about patient autonomy and decisionmaking, we must render a patient's shifting of responsibility to the physician unacceptable, and we must insist that patients take primary responsibility for making decisions related to their health care."[80] Doctors should inform patients, "test the patients' comprehension of that information[,] and then at least encourage and preferably require that patients make those diagnostic or treatment decisions."[81]

Another version of the view that patients must make their own decisions seems implicit in the argument of the prominent bioethicist Robert Veatch. He believes "it makes no sense to continue to rely on consent as the mode of transaction between professionals and their clients,"[82] since "there is no reason to believe that the process of consent will significantly advance the lay person's role in the medical decisionmaking process."[83] The trouble with consent is that it requires the patient to assent to a course of treatment proposed by a doctor who cannot accurately assess the patient's interests. Even having the patient choose between alternatives presented by the doctor (instead of consenting to the doctor's proposed treatment) "faces serious, probably insurmountable problems,"[84] principally because the doctor cannot adequately understand the patient's preferences or present alternatives neutrally. The only hope Veatch can see is to pair patients with doctors who share their "most fundamental worldviews." Only then would there be "some reason that the technically competent clinician could guess fairly well what would serve the patient's interest."[85]

The belief that patients should seize control of their medical decisions reflects broader cultural developments and thus is not confined to bioethicists and lawyers. As David Mechanic observes,

> [s]ome economists and sociologists . . . believe that patients should be active and aggressive seekers of information rather than depend on physicians and hospitals to provide it. Their ideal is an active patient who shops among possible providers,

14 THE PRACTICE OF AUTONOMY

who defines her treatment needs and participates actively in treatment, and who is willing to challenge the doctor and take responsibility for her own treatment decisions.[86]

The sociologist Eliot Freidson speaks of the "essential right, indeed obligation, of the patient to serve as an active participant in the process of shaping the services that are supposed to exist for his benefit."[87] And two social scientists write, "Patients and their parents who conform to dominant medical norms by taking on the compliant and passive role of 'good patients' and 'good families,' may relinquish self-control and responsibility for their own welfare—inside and outside of the treatment center."[88]

Movement toward some form of mandatory autonomy is visible even among doctors. For example, the attending physicians in the dialysis unit where I conduct my research ardently believe patients should make their own decisions, and they press their patients to do so. As one of them put it, "I think that people need to make their own choices about things." Or as he later put it, "My philosophy and mode of operating is to let the people make decisions. I don't want to be more authoritarian, parental or directive than I need to be and I would like to see all the staff do that." Accordingly, the attendings want patients to be informed: "I tell them as much as I think I can get in . . . ."[89] Patients who do not welcome information are often said to be "in denial." This is not a compliment.

Quill and Brody even observe that "[s]ome 'patient-centered' physicians have gone beyond encouraging patients to participate in medical decisions, forcing them to make decisions almost independently."[90] Quill and Brody believe that "[t]oo often, 'autonomous' patients and families are asked to make critical medical decisions on the basis of neutrally presented statistics, as free as possible from the contaminating influences of physicians."[91] Quill and Brody describe this as the "independent choice model," which wants patients "to make choices unencumbered by the contaminating influence of the physician's experience or other social forces. The independent choice model is literally 'patient-centered' and requires that physicians withhold their recommendations because they might bias the patient."[92]

A number of doctors who write advice books seem particularly taken by mandatory-autonomist ideas. One of the most popular, Bernie Siegel, writes that "about 15 to 20 percent of [seriously ill] patients, either consciously or unconsciously, wanted to die. Another, much larger group seemed most interested in pleasing the doctor." But a "third group, another 15 to 20 percent, consisted of patients whom I call 'exceptional.' These people refuse to be victims. They educate themselves and become specialists in their own care. They don't hesitate to question their doctors, whom they regard as partners rather than authority figures. The key thing about exceptional patients is that they keep their power." And they keep their power because "they make their own decisions."[93]

One medical field—genetic counseling—has considered these problems with particular care. Its ethos favors an aggressively "nondirective" approach which compels patients to make their own decisions.[94] One work in that field, for example, commends this dialogue:

> Mrs. Brothers: what would *you* do about another pregnancy?
> G[enetic] C[ounselor]: It really wouldn't be helpful for me to answer that question for you because I won't have to live with the consequences of the decision. I believe I *can* be of assistance by helping you to discuss your feelings, to consider all options, and to understand the facts upon which your decision should be based.[95]

Patients' memoirs increasingly recount stories manifesting principles of mandatory autonomy. Daniel Cohodes, for example, described the "ideal relationship" he had with his doctor, who invariably "laid out the facts, shared the research literature, conducted computer searches on my behalf, and made certain that I sought appropriate outside expertise when necessary. It was painful at times, both for me and for him. The result is that I feel and believe that I am a full partner in any and all treatment decisions."[96] Writing in response to Cohodes, a physician said that "patients are inherently in a dependent position, and it is primarily the responsibility of the health care provider to encourage and require increased patient participation."[97] One occasionally finds even clearer, sterner examples of mandatory autonomism. One polio patient, for example, asked her doctor what to do about one of her medical problems. "Without hesitation, he refused to tell me. He said it must be my decision and mine alone. He then carefully set out my choices, gave me lots to think about, and left me alone to decide."[98]

Versions of mandatory autonomism have also begun to percolate among patients. As one analysis of patients' memoirs observes,

> The ethic of taking responsibility for one's treatment has by now permeated the milieu in which most of our protagonists experience patienthood. Becoming informed about the disease, questioning doctors, inviting second opinions, and intentionally selecting particular hospitals and individual doctors: all of these strategies appear frequently . . . . Many recognize how a patient's own passivity and denial aids and abets the medical arrogance so often criticized.[99]

So one patient advises others:

> This is your life. Take as much charge of your illness as you can. Be an active participant, rather than a passive victim. Do research into both the traditional and alternative options available to you, and then choose the treatments that you believe in, and the doctors you feel trust in, because both are essential to your healing.[100]

Two recent memoirists who espouse versions of mandatory autonomism are Andy Grove, the CEO of Intel, and Michael Korda, the editor in chief of Simon & Schuster and the author of several popular books. Facing a choice of treatments for prostate cancer reminded Grove "of the uncomfortable feeling I experienced when I first sought out investment advice." He had then concluded that "financial advisers, well intentioned and competent as they might have been, were all favoring their own financial instruments." So he decided "to undertake the generalist's job myself; . . . to take the high-level management of my investments into my own hands." To Grove, "that's the only viable choice any patient has. If you look after your investments, I think you should look after your life as well. Investigate things, come to your own conclusions, don't take any one recommendation as gospel."[101] In the service of these principles, Grove met with 15 doctors and six patients. He read journal articles, which he initially found "overwhelmingly confusing." But the more he read, "the clearer they got, just as had been the case when I was studying silicon device physics 30 years ago."[102] Grove then plotted his data and made his decision.

Similarly, Korda admonishes patients: "Above all, remember that your life and your well-being depend on the informed choices *you* make. Your doctor can *present* you with those choices (and ought to do so objectively, and in layman's terms), but he cannot *decide* for you, nor should you expect him to."[103] You should not expect him to because "in the final analysis, we are all responsible for our own well-being, however tempting it is to blame our misfortunes on doctors."[104] In proffering this counsel, Korda is partly reciting the catechism of his support group. It gave him a leaflet from Patient Advocates for Advanced Cancer Treatments which said, "You are in charge of your own destiny. Throughout your treatment, you will enlist the services of a team of physicians, but remember: it is your life that is at stake. The decisions to be made are yours!"[105] Decisions are yours partly because you cannot count on doctors to keep well informed. Doctors, Korda learned from his group, have

> tunnel vision. If they did radical prostatectomies, then that was what they knew about and recommended, ditto the radiologists. Besides which, they were busy men[,] . . . and they were inclined to dismiss anything new or unfamiliar as dangerous hogwash. They didn't know what was happening in Europe, they weren't following the latest studies—in short, you, the patient, had to tell *them,* the doctors, what was going on out there in the world beyond their own offices or operating rooms, and then overcome their hostility and resistance.[106]

His support group taught Korda "that in some respects my fate *was* now in my own hands, like it or not. Dr. Walsh had given me the best operation he could—probably the best operation *anybody* could—but future choices and decisions I would have to make on my own . . . ."[107]

Perhaps I may close this survey of the emergence of mandatory autonomy with a small illustration from my own experience. A few years ago, my dentist thought I was a candidate for the delights of a root canal. The endodontist did what endodontists do and then presented me with the facts of my case. I said that that was interesting, but did I need a root canal? He told me that was my decision. I replied that I understood that, but that I would be glad of a recommendation. He made it clear that he could not and should not decide this medical issue for me. I asked what he would do if it were his tooth. He told me that his values might not be my values, so that what he might do could not be relevant for me. I was baffled (even after hearing all his information, I had no idea how to think about the question), morally reproved (why was I so debased as to refuse responsibility for this important decision?), irritated (why was I being required to make a basically technical decision?), and even bored (this was not the kind of issue about which I could work up any interesting or even useful ideas). But the endodontist was adamant, sturdy in the righteousness of his cause.

Understanding Mandatory Autonomy

Why might mandatory autonomists believe patients not just may, but should, make their own decisions? This is a question worth asking for two reasons. First, we need to understand the mandatory-autonomy argument because it is a rising and intriguing, if nascent and inchoate, position in bioethical thought. To be sure, no school of bioethical thought self-consciously represents itself as "mandatory autonomist." However, enough bioethicists, doctors, and patients have expressed mandatory-autonomist ideas to justify investigating them. Furthermore, those ideas seem likely to find gathering favor. This is partly because the politics of the autonomist argument promote mandatory autonomy. Reformist politics tend to begin with modest proposals and, bolstered by partial success and frustrated by partial failure, to move toward more exigent demands and a more expansive ideology.

The second reason to examine mandatory autonomism—and another reason it seems likely to prosper—is that the conventional arguments against medical paternalism lead plausibly to, though they do not require, mandatory autonomism. That is, the rationales for autonomism may be read as obliging patients to be autonomous in a strong sense as well as obliging doctors to accommodate that autonomy. Autonomists of all sorts believe people have an interest in making their own decisions. But even the mildest of optional autonomists is likely to think autonomy has merits beyond this basic one. Investigating mandatory autonomism helps us identify those merits, since the mandatory autonomist, having to make a stronger claim, is more urgently pressed to identify all autonomy's virtues. Thus, understanding mandatory autonomy promotes insights into the roles doctors and patients should play in making medical choices and the best ways of structuring those decisions.

Let me put the point somewhat differently. If we ask why some autonomists believe patients not only may, but should, or even must, make "autonomous" decisions we will be led to specify more accurately and analyze more keenly the structure of the autonomist argument. In what follows, then, I propose and sketch four central justifications for mandatory autonomy. These justifications fall into two categories, the first three loosely prudential, the last moral.

The prophylaxis argument. The first justification for mandatory autonomy is the "prophylaxis" argument. In its baldest version, it holds that doctors cannot be trusted to overcome their guild interests and their habits of authority and that therefore patients should want as a matter of prudence and should be urged as a matter of policy to make their own medical decisions. At the core of bioethics is an enduring suspicion that if doctors are allowed any room to be paternalistic, they will exploit it. As Troyen Brennan writes, "Most patient-rights advocates are unconvinced even by [a] compromised beneficence model . . . . Their major objection is that the role of physician in this model has great potential for abuse."[108] This skepticism has its roots in the doubts professions have long provoked in the laity, doubts that persist in patients' memoirs. For instance, some patients, like Andy Grove and Michael Korda,[109] urge patients to make their own decisions because no one but the patient will adequately represent the patient's interests. Thus a cancer patient warned the afflicted "[n]ot to accept passively the recommendations of the first doctor that you see, but to make an energetic and wholehearted effort to investigate all available treatments, to educate yourself, and to become your own most impassioned and informed advocate."[110]

The prophylaxis argument, then, holds that if doctors can decide patient by patient how much decisional weight to exert, it is seductively easy for them to assert authority where they should not, since patients are poorly situated to resist their power. Rules automatically assigning authority to patients are a necessary prophylactic against inevitable abuses of doctoral discretion. As Brennan writes, "Given the psychodynamics of the doctor–patient relationship, it seems that medical ethics must first guarantee autonomy."[111] To put the prophylaxis argument somewhat differently, making autonomy mandatory is a kind of immunization against overweening physicians who seize authority beyond their training, capacity, and right. Any attempt to deprecate the autonomy paradigm will promptly be met with reminders of what things were like in the bad old days, and too often still are like.[112] Eternal vigilance is the price of liberty.

The prophylaxis principle justifies mandatory autonomy partly on the grounds that it serves the specific interests of specific patients. It encourages everyone to be alert to medical imperialism; it protects people who wish to make their own decisions by giving them a spur to assert themselves and a shield against their doctors' impositions. The prophylaxis principle is also an argument from general public policy. It justifies mandatory autonomy by suggesting that the preferences of individual patients who would rather not make their own medical decisions should yield to the larger public need to cabin, crib, and confine the overreaching of physicians.

The therapeutic argument. The "therapeutic" argument for mandatory autonomy rests on the belief that patients who control their treatment will more surely and quickly be restored to health. The therapeutic argument has found favor among several kinds of scholars and some patients. For example, a woman with cancer wrote, "Some studies of newly diagnosed breast cancer patients followed over time have . . . suggested that those women who are the most demanding, assertive and participatory with regard to their treatment tend to live longer."[113] A man with AIDS thought that

> the patient who had a certain reputation for stubbornness and was cited by the doctors and nurses as a difficult patient, tended to be among those that survived. These were patients who refused to blindly accept treatment or medication. Instead they wanted to know both the benefits and the drawbacks involved in any therapies they were to be given. They insisted on participating with their doctors in their own treatment. They refused to turn themselves over totally to the doctor to be fixed. Instead they questioned and researched the doctor's proposals and in the end would accept no treatment that went against their own inner guidance.[114]

A man with cancer insisted, "Patients who take control of their lives, patients who *keep* control of their lives, patients who fight the urge to surrender their fates to strangers in white lab coats, those are the patients who stand the best chance of beating the odds."[115]

The therapeutic argument comes in several forms. First, there are faint hints that "control"—a royally ambiguous term, as we will see—may enhance health by strengthening the immune system. Robert Kaplan writes, "The predominant psychoneuroimmunologic theory connects control with health outcomes through several complex links. Control is presumed to reduce stress, lessened stress is presumed to enhance immune function, and immune function, in turn, is presumed to affect health outcome."[116] Versions of this theory have even begun to flower in the popular mind: "I think we can best ask medicine to help us understand ourselves, for if I've learned one thing in the last two years it's this paradox: that although our immune systems work almost entirely independently of our conscious minds, there is no substantial, long-term healing without self-understanding."[117]

Second, there is a literature which suggests patients benefit for social and psychological reasons from controlling their treatment.[118] For example, patients who make medical decisions may think a treatment theirs by choice, while other patients see treatments as imposed on them. The former may thus be committed to their regimen, while the latter may resist it. Regimens are often tiresome and trying, and patients massively flout them. Incorporating patients in medical decisions may recruit them to their own cause: "Just as patients have learned for years to assume a passive role, it may be important for improved clinical outcomes to help patients learn a more active role."[119]

This recruitment is not just to faithfulness in taking medicine, but to a full devotion of all one's resources to fighting illness. This seems to be what Max Lerner means in writing: "The let-the-doctor-do-it model relieves the patient of incentive and responsibility. When we leave all the decisions to the doctor we surrender part of our fighting faith in our survival and healing."[120] Helped by writers like Norman Cousins, this argument has now penetrated popular culture. Anne Hawkins thus speaks of "the recent discovery, popularized by media channels and legitimized in the claim that it is 'scientific,' that passive, compliant patients fare less well in surviving a serious illness than their aggressive and noncompliant counterparts," and she observes that this faith, "often legitimized by referring to scientific statistics and studies, is pervasive in pathography."[121] As one cancer patient remarks, "[W]e've read the scientific evidence that research shows that cancer patients who have a fighting spirit and who don't accept a negative verdict are far more likely to improve than those who stoically accept feelings of helplessness and hopelessness."[122]

Third, the therapeutic argument rests on the proposition that autonomous decisions will be wiser decisions. A standard bioethical definition of autonomy is the "personal rule of the self while remaining free from both controlling interferences by others and personal limitations, such as inadequate understanding, that prevent meaningful choice."[123] A decision free from "inadequate understanding" should be an informed and thus more rational decision. A decision free from "controlling interferences by others" should be a decision made in the best interests of the person who knows the patient's interests best—the patient. The more you know, the better your choices. The more you know, the better you can protect yourself from exploitation by other people, particularly people with interests of their own, like doctors. When you decide, you are driven to ponder what you truly want and what will actually get it. And only you feel the spur of self-interest to do what is best for you. Moreover, even if other people cared solely for you, they still could not fully appreciate your beliefs and preferences, could not fully put themselves in your place, and therefore could not make optimal decisions for you.

Kaplan argues, for instance, that "patients are rational and they attempt to achieve better health outcomes by exercising personal control"[124] and thus that maximizing patient control maximizes health. The literature substantiating this argument speaks primarily about control other than participation in medical decisions. However, the argument that control of all kinds enhances health has a logical appeal. For example, Schneider and Conrad demonstrate that epileptics try to manipulate the dosages of medicines their doctors prescribe in order to locate the optimal balance between benefits and side effects.[125] Patients are well placed to observe and, to some extent, evaluate the effects of such experiments. Brookes echoes this view when he suggests that a patient who has become "more of her own doctor" is "less likely to use medication erratically and irrationally, suffering periodic collapses, alternately avoiding and clinging to the physician, and dashing between the ER and the latest New Age guru."[126] For another example, many patients today have long been chronically ill, have impenetrable charts, are treated by many people (physicians and otherwise) in any one institution, and are clients of several institutions. Such patients may be the only people with a thorough experience of the history of their diseases and treatments, experience which may be indispensable for making sound decisions. Furthermore, such patients can have an acutely developed sense of how their own bodies and diseases react to treatments (for of course not all people and diseases respond similarly to a given approach). And for a final example, patients are sometimes situated—and may be the only people situated—to catch medical errors. The memoirs of the ill are rife with stories of patients wisely refusing medications prescribed or provided in error and of patients noticing problems no one else was there to see.

In addition, the patient's perspective differs usefully from the doctor's. It is the patient who feels what doctors like to call "discomfort" and thus asks sooner if what patients usually call "pain" is really necessary.[127] (One man I know, for instance, talked his way out of a spinal tap by asking whether its results would matter in choosing a treatment.) Patients may be more anxious than doctors about a medication's long-term consequences or about whether an ambiguous test heralds a serious illness and thus may at least press the doctor to think harder. Further, patients may have a more realistic sense than a physician about their capacity to manage a treatment and about their practical needs.

One doctor-turned-patient sums up the case for the patient's competence and even superiority as a maker of medical decisions. She suggests patients know more than doctors "about what disease symptoms are like, how to live with chronic illness or medical treatments, how to survive acute life-threatening illnesses or injuries, how disease affects work and families, what values patients weigh in making choices, and many other aspects of living with illness and acute chronic conditions."[128] If this is true, it is therapeutically desirable for patients to make, or at least share in, medical decisions.

Another version of the therapeutic argument holds that if patients make their own decisions, they can escape decisions doctors make against the interests of patients, decisions that are more than just "errors." Some of these decisions arise where patients' preferences differ from doctors'. In the worst case, they arise where a doctor's interest conflicts with the patient's. Other undesirable decisions are caused by errors medicine generally has fallen into, often out of its fascination with high technology or its do-something approach. At least some of the sentiment for patients making decisions probably grows less out of enthusiasm for autonomy and more out of a belief that doctors have been making substantively wrong decisions and that patients would be likelier to make right ones. This may well be true, for example, of much of the discussion about termination of treatment, therapies for prostate and breast cancer, caesarean sections, home births, and hysterectomies. In other words, criticism of decision-making at the end of life may be motivated not just by the sense that the dying have had too little authority, but that they have been kept alive beyond reason; criticism of breast-cancer therapy has not just been that patients are inadequately consulted about therapies, but that radical mastectomies have been needlessly performed; the criticism regarding caesarean sections is not just that patients are too rarely given a choice about them, but that by any wise standard they are performed too routinely; and so on. In other words, autonomy arguments are adduced partly, I suspect, as an indirect way of promoting what seem to the critics better medical results.[129]

In sum, proponents of the "therapeutic" argument can believe that making medical decisions inspires patients to learn about their disease, to participate more intelligently and actively in their own care, to adhere better to courses of treatment, and to push their doctors to think more carefully and wisely about their recommendations. If this is true, patients should want to make their own medical decisions. And if it is true, there is something to be said for the perversely paternalistic tactic of pressuring patients into making decisions for their own good even if they do not want to.

The false-consciousness argument. The third justification for mandatory autonomy is the "false consciousness" argument. It holds that patients want to make their own medical decisions but have been blinded to that preference because doctors—who, "for the most part, believe that they are the appropriate ones to be making medical decisions"[130]—have prevented them from taking control. Patients acquiesce in their own defeat by succumbing to their fears and their subconscious desires to revert to childlike submission and need.[131] Once patients are not just permitted to make their own decisions, but are taught, cajoled, or perhaps even made to do so, they will realize they truly want authority and can exercise it judiciously.

The patient's false consciousness has yet deeper roots, for it grows out of deep-seated social attitudes and the cultural and economic power of medicine. Thus Sue Fisher writes that patients

> defer to the physician's superior education and social status—the authority of his/her medical role—and act as if they expect the physician to take responsibility for them. This should not be surprising. The perception that the doctor knows best and will act in the patient's best interest is a socially acquired, taken for granted feature of our common stock of knowledge.[132]

This stock of social knowledge is fostered by "the dominant" who benefit from it. Fisher quotes Mary Daly to argue that " 'Mind Managers are able to penetrate their victims' minds/imaginations only by seeing to it that their deceptive myths are acted out over and over again in performances that draw participants into emotional complicity. Such re-enactments train both victims and victimizers to perform uncritically their preordained roles.' "[133] Thus led, "most of us act out socialized complicity, performing uncritically our 'preordained roles.' "[134]

Mandatory autonomy is the sovereign remedy for false consciousness. It seduces or jars or commands the victims of deception out of complicity with the dominant people and institutions who have inveigled them into serving interests that are not their own. It restores to the blinded the sight to perceive their own capacity to make wise decisions, and it infuses them with the strength and will to do so. Regina Woods, for example, began to be transformed when she found a doctor who, "[e]ven when I did not want to make a decision, . . . refused to allow me to wriggle off the hook."[135] She concluded,

> Such incidents built confidence and at the same time created in me a desire for more control. Dr. Rogers never allowed me to make a coin-toss decision but insisted that I learn enough to make an intelligent one. For my part, I welcomed the chance to make such decisions when I felt sufficiently knowledgeable to do so. After all, the people in white go through a learning process and often make an educated guess at best, so why shouldn't I engage in some of that reasoning?[136]

The moral argument. Finally, mandatory autonomism can be defended in moral terms. This might be done on two grounds. The first begins with the premise that patients have a duty of the sort classically described by Talcott Parsons as part of the sick role—the duty to get well. If for all the reasons we just catalogued patients will make better decisions for themselves than anyone else can make for them and thus get better sooner, patients have *pro tanto* a duty to make their own decisions. This is a plausible suggestion, but since that duty is parasitic on the therapeutic justification for mandatory autonomy, we need not pursue it further here.

The second version of the moral argument does demand our attention, since it is both less obvious than the first and a richer source of the appeal of mandatory autonomy. It contends patients should make their own medical decisions because people have a moral duty to make personally the choices that shape their lives. This argument takes many forms, but one particularly influential and resonant expression of it draws on what Charles Taylor calls a "powerful moral ideal that has come down to us"[137] that grows out of "the massive subjective turn of modern culture."[138] This is the ideal of authenticity. It sees people as endowed with the power to reason and to choose. This is what makes them human. Through their reason, they discover their own true nature. Their overriding duty is fidelity to that nature, to be, in short, authentic. As in earlier moral traditions, one listens to one's inner voice. But where once that voice was a guide to what was right, now "being in touch [with it] takes on independent and crucial moral significance. It comes to be something we have to attain to be true and full human beings."[139] Flouting this duty is wrong because it leads to an inauthentic, a dishonest, life. It is also foolish, since it dooms you to trying to be what you are not.

Authenticity depends on choice. In making choices we probe, we define, we express our natures. As Lawrence Friedman writes, choice is "vital, fundamental: the right to develop oneself, to build up a life suited to oneself uniquely, to realize and aggrandize the self, through free, open selection among forms, models, and ways of living."[140] Only when we make our own decisions on the basis of our own truth are we free. Taylor calls this "self-determining freedom. It is the idea that I am free when I decide for myself what concerns me, rather than being shaped by external influences. . . . Self-determining freedom demands that I break the hold of all such external impositions, and decide for myself alone."[141] Thus one patient quotes a physician who deplores the way most people "*live by habit*," without consciously making "*the choices that shape our lives.*" Illness gives people "*both the chance to become aware of these choices and the motivation to act and make change where and when it is needed. Through a process like this, we may directly experience, for the first time, the effect of our choices on our lives.*"[142]

But in freedom begins responsibility. To be free is to be obliged to exercise your freedom. As a therapist interviewed in *Habits of the Heart* said, "'I do think it's important for you to take responsibility for yourself, I mean, nobody else is going to really do it. . . . In the end you're really alone and you really have to answer to yourself . . . .'"[143] This responsibility is well captured by George Kateb, who writes that

> the aspiration to greater expressiveness, resistance, and responsiveness is the theory of democratic individuality. The theorized aim of greater expressiveness is to come to know oneself, to get to know who one is; but especially to know who one isn't, to know that one is not merely a role or function or ascribed identity, while leaving perpetually unmeasured the possibilities of self-expression. The aim is not necessarily to live more fully or more intensely, but rather to live more honestly, as oneself rather than in "endless imitation."[144]

Freedom, then, must be actively exercised because expressing one's inner self is what makes life satisfying and healthy, because "the meaning of one's life for most Americans is to become one's own person, almost to give birth to oneself."[145] That birth is achieved by making choices. And since medical choices are particularly consequential, people have a particular duty to make them: "I have more at stake than anyone else and will not permit others to make decisions of this magnitude for me."[146] The doctrine of informed consent seeks to make autonomous decisions possible. But what shall it profit a man if he is protected from making decisions under the sway of false ideas or under pressure from other people but does not make a decision at all? As the Emanuels put the point,

> It is an oversimplification and distortion of the Western tradition to view respecting autonomy as simply permitting a person to select, unrestricted by coercion, ignorance, physical interference, and the like, his or her preferred course of action from a comprehensive list of available options. Freedom and control over medical decisions alone do not constitute patient autonomy. Autonomy requires that individuals critically assess their own values and preferences; determine whether they are desirable; affirm, upon reflection, these values as ones that should justify their actions; and then be free to initiate action to realize the values. The process of deliberation . . . is essential for realizing patient autonomy . . . .[147]

At its most persuasive, the moral argument for mandatory autonomy rests on a complex of moral views about how people should live their lives, a complex that draws from or resonates with many of our ideas about dependence and independence, about power and exploitation, about tradition and habit, about authority and subordination, about rights and duties, about altruism and self-regard. In its strong form, and as an ideal type, this complex despises dependence. It makes independence obligatory. It values human choice so urgently as to require that everyone choose to choose.

In espousing this complex of ideas, autonomists evoke a long-standing and deep-seated faith. William James wrote at the beginning of the century now ending:

> The duty of the individual to determine his own conduct and profit or suffer by the consequences seems . . . to be one of our best rooted contemporary Protestant social ideals. So much so that it is difficult even imaginatively to comprehend how men possessed of an inner life of their own could ever have come to think the subjection of its will to that of other finite creatures recommendable.[148]

An often-quoted passage from Isaiah Berlin so well states the contemporary understanding of this "duty of the individual" that it is worth reciting at length. Berlin affirms

> the wish on the part of the individual to be his own master. I wish my life and decisions to depend on myself, not on external forces of whatever kind. I wish to be the instrument of my own, not of other men's, acts of will. I wish to be a subject, not an object; to be moved by reasons, by conscious purposes, which are my own, not by causes which affect me, as it were, from outside. I wish to be somebody, not nobody; a doer—deciding, not being decided for, self directed and not acted upon by external nature or by other men as if I were a thing, or an animal, or a slave incapable of playing a human role, that is, of conceiving goals and policies of my own and realizing them. This is at least part of what I mean when I say that I am rational, and that it is my reason that distinguishes me as a human being from the rest of the world. I wish, above all, to be conscious of myself as a thinking, willing, active being, bearing responsibility for my choices and able to explain them by references to my own ideas.[149]

Were we to trace this view back in time, we would soon encounter Mill's *On Liberty,* which is to autonomism what the rain forest is to oxygen. Its

> rhetoric is revealing, individuality being associated with such positive words as "independence," "originality," "spontaneity," "genius," "variety," "diversity," "experiment," "choice," "vigor," "development," "desire," "feeling"; and the threat to individuality with such negative words as "conformity," "mediocrity," "restraint," the "yoke" of opinion, the "tyranny" of society, the "despotism" of custom.[150]

Mill shares with his principal antagonist—James Fitzjames Stephen—a muscular view of human well-being. For Mill, that view requires people to think their own thoughts, make their own decisions, and follow their own course: "He who lets the world, or his own portion of it, choose his plan of life for him, has no need of any other faculty than the ape-like one of imitation. He who chooses his plan for himself, employs all his faculties. He must use observation to see, reasoning and judgment to foresee, activity to gather materials for decision, discrimination to decide, and when he has decided, firmness and self-control to hold to his deliberate decision."[151] It is perhaps consonant with the letter of this rule to confide one's medical decisions to another person, but doing so flouts its sturdy, striding spirit. Doing so betrays the "indolent and impassive" nature Mill deplored.[152] It acquiesces shamefully in the tendency of these weak piping times of peace to ask not "what do I prefer?" but "what is usually done . . . ? . . . until by dint of not following their own nature, they have no nature to follow . . . ."[153]

These ideas influence doctors and patients not only because they have an estimable lineage in high culture, but also because they have achieved an exalted place—even if in vulgarized form—in popular thought. As Anne Hawkins notes, "Self-assertion in the United States has become itself a bona fide virtue: hence our marked aversion both to passivity in all its forms and to victimization of any kind."[154] Such ideas reflect proud and venerable elements of the American ethos. That ethos is famously individualistic, and that individualism is remarkable for the special homage it has paid to self-reliance. Tocqueville thought the principal characteristic of the American philosophical method was "that in most of the operations of the mind each American appeals only to the individual effort of his own understanding."[155] Tocqueville believed American democracy reared men "intoxicated with their new power. They entertain a presumptuous confidence in their own strength, and as they do not suppose that they can henceforward ever have occasion to claim the assistance of their fellow creatures, they do not scruple to show that they care for nobody but themselves."[156] Emerson exulted even in those strains of American individualism that troubled Tocqueville. Emerson scorned the conformist and rhapsodized that "it demands something godlike in him who has cast off the common motives of humanity and has ventured to trust himself for a taskmaster. High be his heart, faithful his will, clear his sight, that he may in good earnest be doctrine, society, law, to himself, that a simple purpose may be to him as strong as iron necessity is to others!"[157]

As the nineteenth century progressed, two cultural prototypes—the pioneer and the entrepreneur—exemplified this strong version of individualism. That version found particularly marked expression in the economic sphere. The sturdy individualist was responsible for all his choices. But he was centrally responsible for making wise and serious choices about his calling and his living.

As the nineteenth century gave way to the twentieth, this strong version of individualism took on fresh vigor from the gathering power of a vision of the liberated and fulfilled self. That vision has assumed many forms, but at its core is a therapeutic ethos that has flourished in a prosperous, consumer society. The vision, as Peter Clecak writes, looks to the hope "of a more 'abundant life' characterized by an individual's opportunity to define and enact possibilities of feeling and mind as freely and as fully as possible. In the sixties and seventies, this pervasive desire to realize individual 'potential' dominated what remained an essentially individualistic culture."[158] That individual potential cannot be achieved without freedom. To be free, in this understanding, is "somehow to be your own person in the sense that you have defined who you are, decided for yourself what you want out of life, free as much as possible from the demands of conformity to family, friends, or community."[159] As one popular writer urged her readers: "The inner custodian must be unseated from the controls. No foreign power can direct our journey from now on. It is for each of us to find a course that is valid by our own reckoning."[160] It is, in short, an idea particularly satisfying to our psychologized society that people ought to live lives of independence, that their goal should be "the search for personal well-being, adjustment, and contentment—in short, for 'health'"[161]—a search that requires people to peel off the false social constraints that keep them from discovering their own true natures and living their own lives. People can follow their own natures only if they probe their own minds and motives, free themselves from the neuroses that bind them, and, in short, think their own thoughts and make their own decisions.

These ideas have been much enhanced by the social movements of recent decades, for, as Clecak observes, "the search for self-fulfillment was tied increasingly to a second dimension: the idea of social justice."[162] Those movements, paradigmatically the civil rights and women's movements, have brought the problem of systematic dependence to the forefront of contemporary thought. They have attacked dependence as the product of oppressive social structures, and they have advocated autonomy and independence as the only adequate curb on the urge of the powerful to enslave the weak. To languish in dependence can thus be not only to betray oneself but also the oppressed community to which one belongs and to which one owes a duty of independence.

Other social movements have contributed to the ethos that good people make their own decisions, not least medical decisions. For example, the flowering of consumerism has spread to medicine and made patients more skeptical, aggressive, and self-reliant. The general decline in esteem for American institutions and professions has accentuated this effect, while the rise in support groups has given these attitudes an institutional basis. Changing experience with and beliefs about illness and health likewise contribute to the ethos whose genealogy I have been tracing. Herzlich and Pierret write that "as chronic illnesses are becoming increasingly frequent, we witness the emergence of the 'new sick,'" who behave differently from earlier patients.[163] They can survive only if they themselves manage their illness:

> Paradoxically, then, the chronically ill, obliged though they are to follow an uninterrupted course of treatment, are able to escape the absolute authority of the physician and to recover a certain independence. . . . "One can't go to see the doctor

> every time one has to have a dose of insulin, we have to adapt to this ourselves, and they have to delegate their responsibilities to us . . . . [T]his treatment is in my hands, and I am treating myself," says the oldest of the diabetic women. In this manner the sick cease to be "receivers of care" and become "providers of care"; by providing treatments for themselves, they engage in "self-help."[164]

These "self-treating patients assert their right to adopt a specific discourse about their sick body and proclaim the effectiveness of taking autonomous charge of their condition."[165]

Herzlich and Pierret relate this development to another change in attitudes toward health—the elevation of health to a "supreme value . . . 'taken as a primary moral value of our civilization.' . . . This attitude was expressed, for instance, by the young traveling salesman who frequents a fitness center, and who said: 'Health is everything for me, it is primordial, and I live for it.' Participation in the fitness center, he continued, 'has to do with responsibility, responsibility for oneself.'"[166] If health is a "supreme value," you cannot escape making medical decisions by claiming they are too peripheral to address personally.

Herzlich and Pierret are writing about France, but their observations fit America. For us, as Annandale notes, "the general ideology of individual self-responsibility for health and health outcomes . . . has become increasingly marked over the last decade."[167] Americans are charged with responsibility for tending their own health and reminded that the wages of sin is death. They are admonished that they can do more for themselves than any doctor can do for them. In our secularized and multicultural society, health is one of the few uncontroversial moral imperatives and personal responsibility for health one of the most sternly taught moral lessons.[168] Thus one AIDS patient said "there would be a special feeling if the effective treatment or cure [for AIDS] emerged from the treatment activists. It would be a complete affirmation of taking personal responsibility for one's own health."[169]

One more cultural development has added credibility to the argument against delegating important decisions. This development is a sharpening sense of individual uniqueness and a consequent doubt that one person can ever truly understand another person's mind or even interests. This sense has several sources. The rise of psychological thinking has offered reasons to believe humans act in ways whose origins are obscure even to themselves and opaque to anyone else. But the sense that one person is unknowable to another has further cultural roots. Americans increasingly believe people are crucially shaped by their race, their ethnicity, their gender, their religion, their sexual preference, and by all their other traditions, affiliations, and allegiances. So forcefully and differently do such forces mold people that members of one community will be hard pressed to comprehend members of another. Indeed, on extreme versions of this view an attempt to do so is an act of aggression, an effort to deprive a group of the power to define itself.[170]

If people shared a common moral language, some of the mutual incomprehension arising from the uniqueness of individuals and groups might be overcome. But the uniqueness of people extends to their moral principles. Furthermore, this route to mutual understanding is barred by what Taylor calls "the hold of moral subjectivism in our culture. By this I mean the view that moral positions are not in any way grounded in reason or the nature of things but are ultimately just adopted. . . . On this view, reason can't adjudicate moral disputes."[171]

This sense of the uniqueness of individuals and the impenetrability of your mind to my mind gives added depth and force to the principle of mandatory autonomy. If you can't understand me, you have no business making decisions for me. And I have no business letting you try. You owe it to me to let me make my own decisions. And I owe it to myself to do so.

The ideas I have been describing about the virtues of independence have achieved a starring role in the way patients are asked to think about their situation. Hawkins suggests that "the ancient Hippocratic idea of the healing power of nature" has merged "with contemporary (and quintessentially American) emphases on the values of self-reliance, individualism, and perhaps most important, activism" to animate our thinking about how patients should approach their illness.[172] Hawkins observes, for example, that patients' memoirs often interpret the encounter with illness through the metaphors of war and of games: "Both paradigms celebrate courage and self-reliance, both disallow dependency, passivity, and self-pity, and both share the sense that recovering from an illness is like winning a battle or an athletic contest—'beating' an adversary, or the odds, or both."[173] One patient puts the point explicitly: "Our view of dependency is generally that it is a weakness and a flaw. There is a special pride one derives from feeling independent. It is a position that we have valued and taught."[174]

For many, this personal responsibility encompasses an obligation to make, or at least "participate in," medical decisions. For instance, Brookes concluded that if he had

> become a success story it's because I have become *engaged in the process of healing.* This is more than merely taking on a greater responsibility for my own wellbeing—it's an entirely new way of looking at health, illness, and medicine. In particular, I've realized two things: that all illness presents an opportunity to learn about ourselves and the world we inhabit and create, and that chronic illness in particular challenges us to ask if it is possible to be *successfully ill.*[175]

A cancer patient argued that the "*right* to know as much as possible about what is happening to one's bodily functions becomes an *obligation* when there is dysfunction."[176] Max Lerner reflected, "The tumult of choice was confusing, but the necessity of choice was none the less real. It was a self-discipline I had to traverse, that no gravely sick person can escape by placing it on the shoulders of others."[177] Thus Lerner deprecated "people who spend more energy and intelligence finding an apartment or buying a car than on weighing life-and-death decisions."[178] A lupus sufferer felt "the patient with a chronic illness must recognize that while he is not responsible for his disease, he is responsible, and must take responsibility, for its management. In a sense, this makes living with a chronic illness not very different from living without one: For everyone, healthy or sick, living competently requires assuming maximum responsibility for one's own life."[179] Michael Korda teaches a similar lesson, that

> in the final analysis, we are all responsible for our own well-being, however tempting it is to blame our misfortunes on doctors. I *should* have been, at my age, more aware of the dangers of prostate cancer, more concerned when I learned that my PSA was 15, instead of waiting eighteen months for it to go up to 22.
>
> I had taken personal responsibility for my cardiovascular fitness, but such was my fear of cancer that I had simply abdicated any responsibility whatsoever the moment the subject came up. Why hadn't I bought the books and started reading about prostate cancer eighteen months before, I asked myself, and made myself a nuisance with questions? I had done nothing of the kind. Cancer is the Big One, and facing the mere *possibility* of it, I simply went on autopilot and put my fate in the hands of my doctors unquestioningly—something I would not have done if the problem had been a torn rotator cuff, or a disk injury, or some irregularity of the heart.[180]

In sum, the idea that patients are morally obliged to exercise their autonomy flows naturally from many currents in American culture. But it has yet other sources. In part, I suspect it arises from the easy transition from the observation that you have a right do something to the idea that you ought to do it. This is a dynamic that has become familiar in American life. As Fox writes, "[T]he affirmation that patients have the right to know the truth veers toward insistence that they ideally ought to face the truth consciously and deal with it rationally (in keeping with the particular definitions of 'truth' and of 'rationality' inherent to bioethics)."[181]

I earlier quoted doctors who believe patients owe it to themselves to make their own decisions. Many doctors make a different argument that leads to the same conclusion. They believe patients owe it not just to themselves but also to their doctors to participate in medical decisions. Such physicians argue that patients who abdicate decisions to doctors leave doctors with a responsibility they cannot perform well and should not have to bear. In part, this argument reflects contemporary individualism and cultural relativism. As I remarked a moment ago, one strain of American thought holds that each person is so thoroughly unique that no one can entirely understand anyone else. Evidence that physicians' personal preferences about medical care influence their perceptions of what patients want may substantiate that concern.[182] Thus doctors can argue that if they cannot understand patients well enough to make decisions that would serve their wants and beliefs, patients have a duty to physicians to make their own decisions.

This view is also partly a reaction, even a petulant reaction, to the bioethics movement. In its extreme form, it says, "All right. If you don't trust us doctors, if you think we have been paternalists, make your own decisions and don't come bothering us with them. We'll see how well you do on your own." This reaction is reinforced by what I can only call doctors' paranoia about malpractice suits[183] and the hope that if the patient and not the doctor makes the foolish decision, the doctor will be insulated from malpractice liability. As two doctors report, "Many physicians feel that giving patients the full range of choices and withholding their own recommendations are safeguards against lawsuits."[184]

Finally, physicians may want patients to make decisions for a happier reason. Some doctors find that "a knowledgeable participating patient is, in reality, the easiest one to care for. In successive stages of the patient's health care, I see myself as diagnosing, supporting, educating, advising, and assisting as they grow in knowledge and skill. It seems in my interest to do this if I wish to reduce the anxiety that comes with caring for those who require frequent attention."[185]

In sum, there is within the logic of autonomism and the stock of American culture the material to construct a moral justification for mandatory autonomism. That justification finds one of its sturdiest elements in an ideal so compelling that, as Taylor gently observes, even its critics act on its teachings—the ideal of authenticity. That ideal summons people to make their own decisions as part of their duty to find and develop and express their own true selves. It has been ever more firmly buttressed by trends in American society and attitudes. It has readily been applied to medical decisions, and once applied, it has been reinforced by contemporary cultural ideas about health and by the attitudes of some doctors.

The arguments for mandatory autonomy. In this review of the arguments for mandatory autonomy, I have proposed that autonomists may build a multilayered case that patients should want to make the medical decisions that affect them. They should want to protect themselves from medical imperialism. They should want to because, whether they realize it or not, they *do* want to. They should want to because making their medical decisions will be good for them: It will give them a sense and thus the reality of control, and that in turn will have therapeutic value. They should want to because, properly informed, they will make better decisions for themselves than anyone else can make for them. They should want to because making one's own decisions is a moral duty.

The obvious response to the suggestion that one must act autonomously is that deciding not to decide is itself an act of autonomy. This is true enough, but it does not fully respond to the arguments for mandatory autonomy. The first three of those arguments essentially propose that there are prudential reasons to make one's own medical decisions even if one acts autonomously in delegating them. The last argument—the moral argument—is forthrightly directed to showing that, at least in the context of medical decisions, a delegated decision is not properly an autonomous decision. In addition, all four arguments, and particularly the moral argument, embody a character ideal. Those who espouse this ideal will treasure the power to shape their own lives and will scorn to hand over that power to anyone else.

Seen in this light, the autonomy paradigm is not directed just at the doctor. It is also directed at the patient and states a practical and moral imperative. Of course, the paradigm imposes corresponding duties on physicians. They have at least an obligation not to impede such decisions and probably a duty to "facilitate" them. Perhaps they owe patients the benefit of teaching them how to make such decisions. Perhaps, on a strong view of the duty, they should coax and cajole patients into doing so. And possibly they should even structure medical services so patients *must* make them.

I have tried to show why autonomy might in some sense be considered a duty. But a word of caution is in order. Even if autonomy is a duty, it does not necessarily follow that a patient must be autonomous all the time. Few duties are so exigent that they always override all other duties. Nor does it necessarily follow that autonomy is a duty that should be imposed on an unwilling patient. Some duties are duties one owes oneself and enforces against oneself.

The Paradigm in Crisis

It seemed to me kind of a hard choice, so I wanted him to make it.   A patient

The practice of what Kuhn called "normal science" has produced a potent version of the autonomy paradigm in bioethics and the law of medicine. Now we may have reached a late period in that practice, for the normal science of working out what "autonomy" means has produced the expected unexpected: "Normal science does not aim at novelties of fact or theory and, when successful, finds none. New and unsuspected phenomena are, however, repeatedly uncovered by scientific research . . . ."[186] This has now occurred often enough that dissatisfaction with the autonomy paradigm is expressed with growing conviction and feeling. There is frustration that the reforms effected under autonomy's banner have not borne lovelier fruit. There is discomfort with the limits and costs of the autonomy principle.[187] And there are gathering efforts to explore new approaches and new paradigms, both methodological and substantive.[188] Casuistry and narrative, empiricism and feminism, beneficence and social justice have all found their faithful. We may thus be reaching the stage when "the proliferation of competing articulations, the willingness to try anything, the expression of explicit discontent, the recourse to philosophy and to debate over fundamentals" mark "a transition from normal to extraordinary research."[189]

My purpose is to contribute to that debate by reexamining the principle of patient autonomy. I propose no new universal principle, for if we are moving toward a new paradigm, I believe it will not be dominated by any single idea. I will argue, however, that the world is too complex for the wooden versions of the autonomy principle that dominate the law and ethics of medicine. That principle has been too monolithic to accommodate the different kinds of patients, doctors, illnesses, and contexts that characterize the world of medical decisions. And it has been asked to bear too great a weight, too great a share of the burden of thinking about how to structure such decisions.

This does not mean autonomy should be discarded from the tool chest of bioethics. The standard justifications for autonomy have been too often and too ardently recited to need reiteration, but I am happy to acknowledge their force. Further, many patients want some kind of autonomy, and although it is hard to tell, their numbers may be swelling as social attitudes about medical decisions change. There are hints of this in the empirical evidence, since younger people are likelier than their elders to want to make those decisions (although it is unclear whether this represents a change in the direction of social attitudes or a stable difference between the young and the old).[190] Finally, as I have already said, there are legitimate reasons to be alert to the ways autonomy may be wrongly denied and diminished.

Nevertheless, I distrust the simplistic and extravagant versions of the autonomy paradigm that surface too frequently in bioethical and legal discourse. I prefer a less absolutist, better modulated, and more proportional version of autonomy. I also distrust the impulse to promote the autonomy paradigm by every conceivable means, on every conceivable front, and at every conceivable occasion. There are values other than autonomy, and autonomy exacts its costs. So in this book I want to save autonomy from its friends.

In sum, I neither want nor expect autonomy to lose its status in the centerpiece of bioethics.[191] But that centerpiece should be a whole bouquet of concepts, and not just the single flower of autonomy, however beguiling it may be. I think that we should find the evidence I will soon adduce chastening and that we should take it and the kinds of considerations I will soon propound into account in thinking about how doctors and patients should approach medical decisions. We should do so to avoid the

> intellectual error that threatens to arise whenever autonomy has been defended as crucial or fundamental: This is that the notion is elevated to a higher status than it deserves. Autonomy *is* important, but so is the capacity for sympathetic identification with others, or the capacity to reason prudentially, or the virtue of integrity. Similarly, although it is important to respect the autonomy of others, it is also important to respect their welfare, or their liberty, or their rationality.[192]

But where lies the path to the more complex view of autonomy I have urged? What kinds of issues must be better analyzed if we are to set foot on that path? To those questions we now turn.

2

Patients' Preferences About Autonomy
The Empirical Evidence

To history has been assigned the office of judging the past, of instructing the present for the benefit of future ages. To such high offices this work does not aspire: It wants only to show what actually happened.

Leopold von Ranke
Histories of the Latin and Germanic Nations from 1494–1514

Given bioethics' autonomy paradigm and its hyper-rational premises—that people behave predictably, that they are autonomy-maximizers, and that they make decisions by assembling all the relevant data and selecting the course that best promotes their beliefs—it is natural that lawyers and bioethicists commonly take it for granted that patients want to make their own medical decisions. Jay Katz, for example, writes, "I said more, although still not enough, about the prevalent assertion that patients generally do not wish to share the burdens of decision and that they prefer instead to trust their doctors' recommendations blindly. I doubt this assertion."[1] Similarly, the President's Commission comfortably concluded that "the vast majority of people surveyed by the Commission felt that patients . . . ought to participate in decisions regarding their health care."[2]

If, however, we cast aside our hyper-rationalist assumptions we encounter a considerable empirical literature which reaches an arresting conclusion—a significant number of patients say they do not want to make their own medical decisions. Because this literature is complex and, to hyper-rationalists, counterintuitive, I will review a number of quantitative studies. I will then examine several other kinds of evidence that substantiate these quantitative investigations.

35

Direct Empirical Evidence

I hate facts. I always say the chief end of man is to form general propositions—adding that no general proposition is worth a damn. Of course a general proposition is simply a string for the facts and I have little doubt that it would be good for my immortal soul to plunge into them, good also for the performance of my duties, but I shrink from the bore—or rather I hate to give up the chance to read this and that, that a gentleman should have read before he dies.
Oliver Wendell Holmes, *Letter to Frederick Pollock*

We begin with Ende and his colleagues. They presented 312 patients in a primary-care clinic of a teaching hospital with vignettes representing various levels of illness severity.[3] "On a scale where 0 indicates a very low and 100 indicates a very high preference for decision making, and 50 indicates a neutral attitude, the mean score for the study population was 33.2 ± 12.6."[4] The authors not only concluded that "patients' preferences for decision making in general were weak." Quite significantly, they found that "as patients were asked to consider increasingly severe illnesses, their desires to make decisions themselves declined."[5] Like a number of other studies, Ende's found that younger people were most likely to want to participate in decisions. More clearly than other studies, Ende's concluded that higher education, higher occupational status, and being divorced or separated were also associated with that desire. However, these factors accounted for only 19% of the variation among patients.

This study did very much resemble other studies in one consequential respect: Patients may not have been eager to make decisions, but they did want to be kept informed. Like patients in many studies, they commonly said they were anxious to be told about their medical situation. Thus, "the mean score for information seeking was [on the 0-to-100 scale] 79.5 ± 11.5."[6] This remarkable contrast between an information score of 80 and a participation score of 33 describes a pattern that is repeated in various ways in study after study.

Another striking study was conducted by Strull and his associates. They questioned 210 hypertension patients and their physicians in a community hospital clinic, a health maintenance organization, and a Veterans Administration outpatient clinic.[7] Like Ende, Strull found patients avid for information: Even though "[f]ifty-two percent of patients reported that they had received 'quite a lot' of information or 'all there is to know' about hypertension and its therapy from their current clinician,"[8] 41% "would have preferred additional information, while 58% received the 'right amount,' and only one patient preferred less information."[9]

But again, much as the patients wanted to be informed, they did not equivalently want to participate in medical decisions: "[N]early half (47%) of patients preferred that the clinician make the therapeutic decisions 'using all that is known about the medicines' but without the patient's participation . . . . One-third of the patients preferred that the clinician make the decision 'but strongly consider the patient's opinion.' Only 19% of the patients stated they wish to share equally with the clinician in making the decision, and 3% wished to make the decision themselves."[10] Intriguingly, the doctors *over*estimated their patients' desire to make medical decisions: "In contrast to the patient preferences, in the large majority of cases (78%) clinicians believed that patients wanted to help make decisions. In only 22% of cases did the clinician think the patient wanted the clinician alone to decide."[11]

The patients and their doctors also disagreed about how decisions were in fact made. "Sixty-three percent of patients reported that the 'clinician usually makes the decision, using all that's known about the medicines,' while clinicians reported such decision making in only 20% of cases . . . . Only 37% of patients, as opposed to 80% of clinicians, reported that the patient participates to any extent in decisions."[12] But whatever was happening pleased the patients. Eighty-nine percent of them "reported being 'very' or 'extremely' satisfied with their overall medical care from their current clinician, and 84% reported a 'very' or 'extremely' high degree of satisfaction with the way in which decisions about their treatment are made."[13]

Nease and Brooks asked patients (most of whom were white, male, and well educated) who faced "management decisions for symptomatic benign prostatic hyperplasia, mild hypertension . . . , or persistent low back pain" to respond to two tests.[14] The Autonomy Preference Index "frames the information questions primarily in terms of *what the patient feels the physician should do,* whereas the [Health Opinion Survey] asks *what the patient usually does* to seek information."[15] The Autonomy Preference Index "focuses on *what the patient feels he or she should do* with regard to making decisions, whereas the [Health Opinion Survey] assesses *the patient's desire to participate in self-care.*"[16] On both tests, Nease and Brooks used a scale from 0 to 1. On the Autonomy Preference Index, the mean score for information was .93, and the mean score for making decisions was .32. On the Health Opinion Survey, the mean score for information was .57 and the mean "behavioral involvement" score was .40. Nease and Brooks found that "higher desires for information and decision making are associated with younger age, more education, employment, and female gender," but that (as the studies I survey generally report) "very little of the variance we observed in the [Autonomy Preference Index] information and decision making scores is explained by the sociodemographic variables we analyzed . . . ."[17] In Nease and Brooks' study, as was commonly true, "the median decision making score decreased as the clinical condition increased in seriousness . . . ."[18]

Vertinsky and his colleagues also studied a population whose interest in being informed exceeded their interest in controlling treatment.[19] This team surveyed residents of Vancouver and asked them how they would react to a scenario in which a patient has a strep throat and the doctor does not tell the patient all the risks of either nontreatment or treatment. The factor that was least often chosen was "patient decision," which was "defined in terms of preference for retaining the final decision function in the patient's hands . . . ."[20] Indeed, "[d]irect participation ('Patient Decision') . . . was rated as unimportant by almost all subjects, although patients indicate rather strongly a desire to maintain some measure of participation ('Avoidance' receiving markedly low scores)."[21]

Another study showing that a substantial number of patients are loath to make their own medical decisions was conducted by Faden and her co-workers.[22] They asked fifty-three seizure patients to choose between having their doctor decide whether they needed medication and, if so, which medication or, on the other hand, hearing the doctor's recommendation but deciding whether to receive medication and choosing it. The former course was preferred by 44.2%, the latter by 55.8%.[23] Thus while a majority of the patients questioned preferred to make their own medical decision, a considerable minority did not. Furthermore, the patients "could be described as young, adult, married, white and fairly well educated,"[24] people probably likelier than most to want to make their own medical decisions. That they were also chronically ill patients experienced in managing their disease further increases that likelihood.

Beisecker studied 106 people "with a wide range of ailments and disabilities: recovering stroke patients, head trauma and other accident victims, patients with sports injuries, amputees, and patients with severe arthritis, chronic back pain, and muscle diseases such as muscular dystrophy" who were patients of specialists in physical medicine and rehabilitation.[25] Beisecker used a scale for measuring preferences about medical decisions in which "belief in the patient as sole locus of decision-making authority would yield a scale score of 26; belief in the doctor as the sole decision-maker would yield a score of 0, and belief that all decisions should be made jointly (or indicating that a doctor's decisions counterbalanced those which should be made by the patient) would yield a score of 13."[26] The mean score for Beisecker's medically diverse population was 8.6.

Mark and Spiro studied 102 outpatients scheduled to undergo a colonoscopy. "When asked, 'Which way would you prefer to come to a medical decision?' 57 patients wanted to share the decision with the physician, 22 wanted to make their own decision, and 23 wanted the physician to make the decision."[27] Asked about the decision to have a colonoscopy examination, "53 patients said that they shared the decision with the physician, 40 patients said that the physician was most responsible for the decision, and 9 patients said that they were most responsible." Yet despite the apparent discrepancy between how some patients said they wanted medical decisions to be made and the way the colonoscopy decision was made, "only two patients declined to say in the end that they had 'just the right amount of responsibility in making the decision . . . ."[28]

A study by Lidz and his collaborators of informed consent produced even more impressive results.[29] "[W]ith a few exceptions . . . , the patients believed that decisions about their treatment should be primarily or completely up to their physicians because of their technical expertise and commitment to the best interests of the patients."[30] Again, patients wanted information. But "only about 10% of the patients we interviewed saw themselves as having an active role in decision making."[31]

Also notable, if vaguely reported, is a study by Miller et al of 150 primary-care patients at a department of internal medicine. This study was undertaken to evaluate the way different personality types respond to threats to their health. It found that "almost no patients desired to have the final say in their medical care" and that 36.5% of one personality type and 15.9% of the other "desired to play a completely passive role in their own care."[32]

An illuminating perspective on the desire of patients to make medical decisions comes from a study by Degner and Sloan which compared the attitudes of newly diagnosed cancer patients and a random sample of Winnipeg.[33] "The majority of newly diagnosed patients (59%) preferred that physicians make treatment decisions on their behalf. The most popular first choice of patients was the statement, 'I prefer that my doctor makes the final decision about which treatment will be used, but seriously considers my opinion'. Only 12% of newly diagnosed patients preferred to play an active role in decision making."[34] The sample of Winnipeg, in contrast, seemed more interested in such participation. Sixty-four percent of them thought they would want to "play an active role in decision making if they were to develop cancer."[35]

Another Canadian study questioned fifty-two cancer patients in early stages of their disease.[36] Sixty-three percent of them "felt the physician should take the primary responsibility in decision making, 27% felt it should be an equally shared process, and 10% felt they should take a major role."[37] Again, even patients who expected their doctors to assume the primary responsibility for medical decisions were interested in receiving information.

Cassileth's team gave 256 cancer patients a choice between two statements: "I prefer to participate in decisions about my medical care and treatment" and "I prefer to leave decisions about my medical care and treatment up to my doctor." Eighty-seven percent of those aged 20–39, 62% of those aged 40–59, and 51% of those over 60 chose the former.[38] This is one of the most recruited citations for the proposition that patients *want* to make medical decisions. Yet it concludes that a substantial number of patients subscribe to quite a strongly stated desire to cede authority to their doctors. The reaction to this study typifies a common but unfortunate response to surveys—to transform a finding that a majority prefers something into the assertion that everyone wants it. As has been well said, "In health index construction, in the evaluation of the outcomes of clinical trials and in clinical decision analysis for groups of patients the use of average preference scores runs the danger of 'the tyranny of the majority': . . . [I]t essentially disregards the opinions of those whose scores are removed from the mean."[39] Majority implies minority, and minorities can be almost as large as majorities.

Furthermore, the language in which Cassileth's subjects were asked to say they wanted to participate in decisions was quite broad, while the language for declining to participate was relatively narrow. Thus even those patients who chose the former statements in the Cassileth study were only asking for *some*—unspecified—level of "participation." Some, perhaps many, of them probably wanted little more than good information and a veto power over their doctor's decisions (although presumably others actually wanted to make some decisions in some strong sense). In addition, the *relatively* strong desire for participation this study reports is in part surely an artifact of the maximally narrow range of choices—two—the respondents were given.[40]

Finally, there is the Louis Harris poll of doctors and the general public undertaken for the President's Commission.[41] Seven percent of the public wanted the doctor to present all the possible alternatives and let the patient decide. Twelve percent wanted the doctor to present a recommendation for the patient to accept or reject. Seven percent wanted the doctor to decide what should be done and do it. Seventy-two percent thought the doctor and patient should discuss alternatives and decide together what to do. Less than half a percent thought the way to proceed depends on the circumstances.[42]

This is far and away the strongest statement of a public desire to make medical decisions. However, it is not easy to interpret. Most of the respondents wanted the doctor and patient to decide together what to do, but it is unclear just how they envisioned the allocation of power between the doctor and patient. Ende and his colleagues conclude that the Harris data "seem to support the notion that patients prefer the model wherein the doctor keeps the patient informed and engages the patient in the decision making process, rather than having the patient function as the principal decision maker."[43] It is at least significant that only 7% opted for the response—having the doctor present alternatives for the patient's decision—closest to the standard formulation of the autonomy standard for patients' decisions.

What, then, can we say of the studies of patients' desires to participate in medical decisions? Like all studies, they have their limitations. Their questions can be frustratingly inexact, so that we are often left to guess precisely what allocation of authority the respondents intended. Further, I have qualms about simply asking people what role they prefer in medical decisions. These are difficult questions about which many people will not have thought much, about which they may justly be ambivalent, and about which they may change their minds with experience and on reflection. And even people who know what they want will often articulate it imprecisely. All these problems are at their most acute when, as sometimes occurs, studies ask people who are not sick to speculate about how they would feel if they were sick, or ask people who are sick about hypothetical variations on their illness. In addition, these studies neglect the daunting range of circumstances in which medical decisions are made. It matters how sick or healthy the patient is, how thoroughly the doctor and patient know each other, how trivial or consequential the decision is, and so on. It particularly matters where the decision falls on the (somewhat artificial) continuum between purely medical decisions on one hand and purely social or moral decisions on the other. Finally, it is tantalizing that none of the studies probes very far—if at all—into the *reasons* people might have for accepting or rejecting medical authority. That information might have revealed more fully and compellingly what patients want.

Nevertheless, the studies I have surveyed are not only the best systematic evidence we have about peoples' attitudes toward medical decisions, they are quite adequate to provide a basis for thinking about those attitudes. Taken as a whole, they survey a considerable variety of populations—from the perfectly well to the dangerously sick. They ask patients about their own conditions and about hypothetical illnesses. They frame their respondents' choices in various ways. Finally, they are sufficiently numerous and similar that we can make some useful generalizations about them.

Most prominently, these studies consistently conclude that, while patients largely wish to be informed about their medical circumstances, a substantial number of them do not want to make their own medical decisions, or perhaps even to participate in those decisions in any very significant way. The studies do not explain fully just which kinds of patients want to make their own decisions. They do reveal, however, two telling patterns. First, the elderly are less likely than the young to want to make medical decisions. Second, the graver the patient's illness, the less likely the patient is to want to make medical decisions.[44] This is plausible enough. The sicker the patient, the less energy and capacity the patient is likely to have, the more unfamiliar the illness is likely to be, and the worse the consequences of a mistake. But if these data are correct, those patients who are likeliest to have serious medical problems and to be making life-and-death choices are least likely to relish making their own decisions. Thus the surveys probably understate the extent to which actual patients faced with serious decisions want to exercise their autonomy.

Some Substantiating Evidence

In my belief that a large acquaintance with particulars often makes us wiser than the possession of abstract formulas, however deep, I have loaded the lectures with concrete examples . . . .   William James, *The Varieties of Religious Experience*

The quantitative studies of patients' attitudes toward medical decisions that point toward the conclusion that many patients are reluctant to make their own medical decisions find confirmation in several other kinds of evidence. First are the data suggesting that people have not swarmed to take advantage of devices designed to permit them to make medical choices. In recent years, cases like *Quinlan*[45] and *Cruzan*,[46] publicists like Jack Kevorkian, and referenda like those in Washington, California, and Oregon have brought questions about terminating life support to the fore of public discussion. Amidst this discussion, adjurations to sign advance directives have proliferated. The conventional wisdom now teaches that everybody should have one. Hospitals thrust forms on every patient they admit. Lawyers routinely offer to prepare advance directives when clients come in for estate planning. Yet despite all this, relatively few people have prepared advance directives, and many people appear reluctant to discuss such matters even with their families or doctors.[47] There are, to be sure, several reasons for this, not least that people are fearful and superstitious, that they "prefer to avoid the subject of how to manage their own dying."[48] But the point is exactly that many people have strong reasons for not wanting to grasp the nettle of autonomy.

Furthermore, many people do not believe advance directives must always be scrupulously followed. Sehgal and his colleagues asked 150 dialysis patients "[w]hom they would want to help their physician make decisions for them if they developed advanced Alzheimer's disease" and "[h]ow much leeway their physician and surrogate should have to override this advance directive if overriding were in their best interests."[49] These patients "varied greatly in how much leeway they would give their physician and surrogate to override their advance directive if overriding were in their best interests: 'no leeway' (39%), 'a little leeway' (19%), 'a lot of leeway' (11%), and 'complete leeway' (31%)."[50] In brief, if people were avid to make their own medical decisions, would they not more eagerly seize the opportunity to make advance directives, and would they not more consistently oppose meddling with those directives?

Another behavioral datum likewise implies that many patients hesitate to take control of medical decisions. If patients were ever to assert their decisional authority, it ought to be after hearing the alarming recitation of risks that characterizes the process of informed consent. That is what informed consent is for. Yet a number of studies of that process "strongly suggest that refusals attributable to disclosures are rarely, if ever, seen."[51] Similarly, a study of why patients refuse treatment found an average of only 4.6 refusals per 100 patient days.[52] The reasons for refusal were complex, and generally there was more than one "cause" per patient. But two reasons stood out: first, a failure to tell the patient about the purpose of what was proposed; second, psychological factors, prominently including "characterological factors" (e.g., refusing treatment as a way of expressing a wish to be cared for) and "other psychoses." While the first of these causes confirms the wish for information we have already encountered, neither of them is inconsistent with a reluctance to make medical decisions.[53] And the dog that didn't bark in the night is the absence of any pattern of patients who heard a doctor's recommendation and reached a different decision on the merits.[54]

Not only do patients pass up opportunities to make decisions; they also seem content with the modest extent to which they meet bioethical standards for making decisions. Two kinds of empirical data support this proposition. The first comprises studies of why patients sue their physicians. One such study found that "while the current trend in medicine stresses the importance of treating patients as active participants in the delivery of medical services, such considerations may have few consequences for disputing. At bottom, only the doctor's perceived competence and attention to the patient's health appear to influence the decision to sue."[55] The second kind of support comes from studies of patient satisfaction. They commonly conclude that patients are generally satisfied with the care they receive from their own physicians (even if they are not so content with doctors *en masse*) and with their degree of participation in medical decisions.

Further evidence of the reluctance of some patients to assume the reins of medical command comes from my own research. The doctors I have interviewed say emphatically that many patients decline to make medical decisions.[56] Doctors may have their own reasons for believing and saying patients want to cede them authority, and they are doubtless guided by their own cultural preconceptions when they interpret what patients do and say. But I am as reluctant to ignore their evidence on those grounds as I am to ignore the assertions of bioethicists and lawyers because of their considerable stakes—economic, social, and intellectual—in the issues they debate. Doctors do have notorious difficulty assessing their patients' desire to make medical decisions. But since doctors tend to *over*estimate the degree to which patients want to make their own decisions, the evidence of my interviews looks weightier.[57] Ultimately, doctors have a unique and rich perspective; they have experience too valuable to be lost and too direct to be dismissed out of hand. Thus their testimony at least seems relevant as confirmation of the other sources I have reviewed.

A final confirmation of my thesis—anecdotal, but concrete, textured, personal, vivid, and illuminating—comes from the memoirs of the sick and of family members who have cared for them. Like many of the patients questioned in the empirical studies I have described, some of these memoirists sought decisional authority. For instance, Cornelius Ryan, the author of books on D-Day and Operation Market-Garden, resolved to research his disease in the same way that he researched those battles.[58] Harold Lear, a physician who suffered from heart disease, was another patient anxious to control his own treatment.[59] Gayle Feldman, a journalist who like several of her relatives suffered from breast cancer, wrote that although she "would have to cede much of the control of my life to my doctors during the coming days and weeks, I knew that the final decisions had to rest with me . . . ."[60]

One of the closest approximations of the patient-as-decider is William Martin, a sociologist at Rice.[61] He had prostate cancer, the disease which, with breast cancer, has attained perhaps the most public attention as presenting a genuine and controversial choice of treatments. Martin approached the question with relish, as though it were a nifty problem in sociological research.[62] He set out not just to pick a doctor, but to choose among radiation, surgery, or "watchful waiting." He spoke extensively with his doctors. He read articles, popular and professional. He consulted medical friends and acquaintances. He eventually chose surgery because he discerned a medical consensus in favor of it for people at his stage of the disease. Then he got his friends to advise him who the best available surgeon was. Martin, in short, was the very model of a modern patient.

One wonders, of course, how typical Martin is even of other professorial patients. But perhaps more significant is the fact that a striking number of patients' memoirs—extensive and intensive accounts of sickness—conspicuously fail even to comment on their authors' participation in their medical decisions. Many patients do not complain about their failure to be included in those decisions, even though few if any of them achieved the level of participation in their medical decisions that contemporary bioethics would require.[63] They do not say they wanted to participate to anything like that degree, and some of them say more or less plainly that they did not. I originally began to read patients' memoirs to learn how they made medical decisions. Those works turned out to be a poor source because so many memoirists spent so little time talking about those decisions. Mary Greene, for example, wrote an account of her forty years with type I diabetes to guide other diabetics.[64] She is not uncritical of doctors, recommends firing them when they perform badly, and has fired them herself. She urges diabetics to follow her example of controlling her blood sugar meticulously. But she neither advises patients to participate in medical decisions nor describes having done so herself.

To be sure, it is hard to draw reliable conclusions from negative evidence. However, the people who write these memoirs are by and large well-to-do, well educated, well situated, self-conscious, self-assured, and articulate. They are commonly writers, journalists, celebrities, academics, and doctors—exactly the people one would think likeliest to want such authority, to feel comfortable exercising it, and to notice and criticize its absence. It seems probable, therefore, that their silence indicates that such participation was, even on a memoirist's reflection, not prominently important to them.

The memoirists' silence might be due to a reluctance to criticize the doctors and nurses who had cared for them. But memoirists are patently willing—sometimes determined—to express their unhappiness, even their bitterness, with medical deficiencies. That willingness is exemplified by the explanatory note with which Sue Baier opens her account of her travails with Guillain-Barré syndrome, her doctors, and her nurses: "The names of the hospital and all medical personnel have been changed to protect those who were less than kind."[65] These memoirists often volunteer appreciation and even enthusiasm for doctors who were conscientious, kind, and competent. The same Sue Baier whose acid note I just quoted dedicates her book "to all who cared, so they will know how much they did."[66] But these memoirs regularly relate grievances, sometimes angry and horrifying grievances. The nature of these grievances is illuminating, for they generally concern not paternalism, but medical errors, scanty information, physicians' lack of sympathy and understanding, the insolence and inefficiencies of medical bureaucracy, and doctors who were not there to attend to the case.

Furthermore, a number of memoirists expressly state their reluctance to make medical decisions. Strikingly, doctors are prominent among them. One, for example, said, "I found an excellent otologist, did what he told me to do, and am not fool enough to think that I know more about his business than he does."[67] And another one wrote, "My doctor asked me who I wished to be referred to: an orthopaedic surgeon, a neurologist, a rheumatologist, etc. I did not know. All I wanted was to be told what was wrong and what should be done about it."[68]

Even patients who seek "alternative" medical treatment do not necessarily wish to supervise their decisions in the way bioethics expects. Indeed, they often approach such treatment credulously, trustfully, and incuriously. Laura Chester, for instance, sought not just conventional treatment for her lupus, but also the "smorgasbord of therapies there were available in Berkeley,"[69] including a potpourri of dietary remedies, homeopathic medicine (particularly anthroposophical medicine), a "healer" who "didn't fit into any neat category or particular movement,"[70] a specialist in Ortho-Bionomy, one in kundalini yoga, a chiropractor who worked with a psychic, and a Psychosynthesis therapist.[71] Chester was skeptical of some of these methods and abandoned several of them. She was making her own medical decisions in the (quite nontrivial) sense of choosing her own modes of treatment. However, once she had made that choice, she seems not to have expected the briefing required by the doctrine of informed consent nor any choice about how a therapy was to be conducted.

In sum, not only does the survey literature make it plain that a significant number of people do not yearn to make their own medical decisions, but that literature is substantiated by a variety of other kinds of evidence. It is impossible to number these patients precisely: Even the survey evidence looks at patients in different ways and in different circumstances, the other kinds of evidence I have recruited are not designed to produce exact numbers, and exactitude in descriptions of complex attitudes is never possible. Nevertheless, the direction of the evidence is clear.

It is necessary, though, to resist the easy slide from "many patients decline to make their own decisions" to "no patients want to make any decisions." One of my themes is exactly that the attitude of even a single patient toward making medical decisions is likely to be ambiguous, ambivalent, and labile and that the preferences of patients as a whole stoutly resist facile generalization. While the direction of the evidence is plain, the preferences of patients are hardly straightforward. As the discussion in the next chapters will indicate, there are many complexities to be considered. For instance, patients believe they want "information."

But the evidence hardly tells us which kinds of information patients want, how much of it they want, when they want it, why they want it, or when they might not want it. I interviewed one patient who distinctly wanted to know what was going to happen next, but not until right before it was going to happen, since he did not want to dwell on unpleasant prospects. Many other patients I have talked with wanted information that would be helpful in handling day-to-day problems more than information for making medical decisions. And so on.

Or consider the evidence that many patients are reluctant to assume full decisional power. This does not mean they want none. Even patients who delegate decisions may wish to retain residual authority to countermand particularly troublesome ones: Patients may want information partly so they can monitor their treatment and intervene to prevent egregious errors. Furthermore, that patients want to cede authority does not tell us to whom they wish to cede it. For example, some patients accord authority not to their doctors but to their families. Victor Cicirelli reports, for example, that 27% of the elderly women he studied felt their adult daughters (who were providing "some degree of care" for their mothers) should make decisions about health matters for them.[72] Dallas High found that 90% of his subjects would trust family members to make decisions for them when they could not do so for themselves.[73] Not infrequently one encounters delegations from one spouse to the other. The tradition of some American subcultures (like Korean Americans and Mexican Americans) is that families and not patients should make decisions about whether to use life-sustaining technologies.[74] Nor do families and even friends exhaust the people to whom patients might defer. One doctor told me, for example, that some of his Jewish patients consult their rabbi about their medical choices and even bring him along on visits.

Further, as we will see in Chapter 4, not all medical decisions are the same. For example, that patients do not want to make "medical" decisions does not mean they are similarly reluctant to make social or moral decisions raised by their illness. Thus a patient might refuse to decide what kinds of treatment to receive but insist on retaining the power to reject a treatment as socially impractical or morally wrong.

In sum, the empirical evidence leaves questions to be answered and uncertainties to be clarified, but it compels at least one telling conclusion: A significant—and perhaps quite a substantial—number of people are not hungry to make decisions about their medical problems. What, then, should we should make of this counterintuitive proposition?

3

The Reluctant Patient
Can Abjuring Autonomy
Make Sense?

To the soul, lost, confounded in the darkness, the long night, neither charts, nor the chart-making mind, were of service. Nor, indeed, was the temper *of the charter—"strong masculine sense . . . enterprise . . . vigilance and activity" (as a contemporary wrote of Captain Cook). These active qualities might be valuable later, but at this point they had nothing to work on. For my state in the dark night was one of passivity, an intense and absolute and essential passivity, in which action—any action—would be useless and distraction. The watchword at this time was "Be patient—endure . . . . Wait, be still . . . . Do nothing, don't think!" How difficult, how paradoxical, a lesson to learn!*

Oliver Sacks
A Leg to Stand On

I have been reporting that there is in the empirical evidence on medical decisions reason to ask how far the autonomy paradigm and patients' preferences coincide. The paradigm calls for patients to make medical decisions. The evidence suggests that some significant number of patients are loath to assume that authority. What are we to make of this disjuncture?

There is, I think, a paradigmatic answer to that question—that all professions are conspiracies against the laity, and that, in particular, patients have succumbed to the demand of physicians that patients obey their professional authority.[1] Like Sacks, patients have "felt not only physically but morally prostrate—unable to stand up, stand morally before 'them,' in particular, before the surgeon."[2] The autonomist's paradigmatic answer, then, is that these patients do not want medical authority because they have never been permitted to have it and that, were they permitted it, they would learn to realize and relish its benefits.

47

This "false consciousness" answer no doubt contains a good deal of truth. There is a powerful, pervasive, and persistent tradition in medicine that doctor knows best, and many doctors insist even today on the prerogatives of their station. Physicians have weighty kinds of power over patients, armed as they are with learning and skill the patient always needs, social standing the patient usually lacks, and professional standing the patient can rarely match. But I doubt life is so simple that this standard response is anything like the whole answer. What, then, if we assume that patients are not merely cowed, but that they are making considered decisions not to assert their autonomy to the full? Could anything be said for their conclusions?

I want to suggest three justifications that even entirely competent patients might reasonably proffer for declining to make their own medical decisions. First, that patients may feel less competent than their doctors (or even than a relative or friend) to make wise medical choices. Second, that the sick may be too debilitated to deliberate actively and well. Third (and most problematically), that sometimes patients wish to cede decisional authority in order to be manipulated into courses of action they in some sense wish to pursue but find themselves resisting.

I will survey these three rationales with two aims. First, to substantiate further the evidence I adduced in the last chapter: If patients have plausible reasons for refusing to exercise medical authority, we may more confidently believe the evidence that some significant proportion of them do not wish to make their own medical decisions. Second, the nature and weight of those reasons will tell us something about how we should react to a patient's wish to confide a decision in another person and about the scope of a patient's practical incentives and moral duty to make medical decisions.

Let me explain what is to follow a little differently. Mandatory autonomy represents an extreme position. The patient who altogether rejects making medical decisions also represents an extreme position. But these two extreme positions are worth investigating because of what they can tell us about more conventional positions. Today, few doctors can get away with or even believe in a strong form of paternalism. And individual patients will vary considerably in their desire to make their own decisions. One way to put into relief the whole range of the attitudes and behavior of doctors and patients is to scrutinize the ends of the continuum. That is a crucial part of what this chapter does.

The Daunting Difficulty of Medical Decisions

[H]ow intricate a work then have they who are gone to consult which of these sicknesses mine is, and then which of these fevers, and then what it would do, and then how it may be countermined.   John Donne, *Devotions Upon Emergent Occasions*

At the heart of the autonomy argument lies an implicit syllogism. All people want to make the decisions that shape their lives. Few decisions are more consequential than the life-or-death, sickness-or-health, able-bodied-or-crippled choices medicine poses. Therefore patients must want to make their own medical decisions. *Quod erat demonstrandum.* In this section I will begin to investigate that syllogism. Particularly, I will explore the first of the three reasons people might not want to make even crucial decisions: Patients may shrink from their paradigmatic role in medical decisions because they recognize that such decisions are problematic beyond any ordinary range. They may conclude that their own frailties as decision-makers, their inexperience with medical science, the grievous dilemmas of medical decisions, and their doctor's relative dispassion, experience, and expertise argue for having their doctor—or someone else, especially a family member—decide for them.

At the core of this rationale is the uncommon difficulty of medical decisions. That difficulty is hardly unknown. But its scope and severity are easily forgotten. A survey of its causes should remind us of their number and demonstrate its extent. Such a survey may serve another purpose. The prime legal mover of bioethics' autonomy paradigm is the doctrine of informed consent. That doctrine rests on some unarticulated assumptions about what medical decisions are like and how doctors and patients make them. Our survey of what makes medical decisions hard should test those assumptions.

The Intellectual Work of Medical Decisions

Making decisions of *all* kinds can be cruelly, repellently hard, and all of us bring serious and systematic defects to that task. Irving Janis and Leon Mann—two leading students of decision—observe that someone "under pressure to make a vital decision affecting his future welfare will typically find it painful to commit himself, because there are some expected costs and risks no matter which course of action he chooses."[3] In addition, serious decisions exact uncomfortable expenditures of time, attention, thought, and anxiety. Thus Janis and Mann see *Homo sapiens* "not as a rational calculator always ready to work out the best solution but as a reluctant decision maker—beset by conflict, doubts, and worry, struggling with incongruous longings, antipathies, and loyalties, and seeking relief by procrastinating, rationalizing, or denying responsibility for his own choices."[4]

We dislike making decisions because we know we do it badly. Scholars of decision now widely believe that "people reach judgments based on simplifying heuristic rules and search until they find an acceptable solution, not necessarily the best."[5] Even this stripped-down process is beset by troubles, for "[b]iases have been observed in virtually every context that a statistician could imagine . . . ."[6] Janis, for instance, discerns "five main types of errors in estimating probabilities: (1) overestimating the likelihood of events that can be easily and vividly imagined; (2) giving too much weight to information about representativeness; (3) ignoring information about base rates; (4) relying too much on evidence from small samples; and (5) failing to discount evidence from biased samples."[7] There are yet broader and more basic "flaws and limitations in human information processing, such as the propensity of decision makers to be distracted by irrelevant aspects of the alternatives . . . ; the tendency of decision makers to be swayed by the form in which information about risks is packaged and presented . . . ; their reliance on faulty categories and stereotypes . . . ; and their illusion of control . . . ."[8] In short, during the last few decades an extensive literature has charted in convincing detail the many ways human decisions are distorted by human peculiarities. I suspect many people sense their limitations as deciders and tacitly avoid decisions. After all, "[m]ost of us feel uneasy about our decisions, primarily because we have made decisions that did not turn out well and we live with the clear understanding that we will someday regret decisions that we have not even made yet."[9]

One other general impediment to making sound decisions deserves mention. Patients represent the full range of intelligence, education, attentiveness, lucidity, and literacy, to say nothing of experience and skill in complex decisions. All these ranges are large and can affect people's ability to choose wisely and comfortably. If people at the top of these ranges often find decisions befuddling, people at the bottom will have a cruelly hard row to hoe. And which of us is at the top of all of them?

All these are challenges everyone faces in making any kind of decision. But even under the best of circumstances—even when doctors are truly trying to thoroughly inform an able and attentive patient and are truly willing to have the patient make the decision—a patient's medical decisions will often be infected with perplexities, perplexities so marked and many that they bear extended recital. Primary among them is that the information the doctor can present to the patient will frequently and unavoidably be rife with uncertainty, roiled by complexity, awkward to articulate, and hard to assimilate. This is true even under the rare best of circumstances, where the doctor has taken serious time and trouble to try to communicate with the patient and where the patient has reciprocated with thoughtful attention, clarifying questions, and intelligent reflection.[10]

The problems start with the doctor's many impediments to reaching reliable medical conclusions. Simply assembling information about the patient's disease is a process strewn with pitfalls, barriers, false turns, and dead ends. Extracting adequate information from the patient can demand all the doctor's skill and sensitivity, patience and perseverance. As one physician reflected,

> The most important part of the patient examination is the history. It sounds so simple: just ask and you'll be told. But it ain't so. You seldom get a straight answer. Taking a history is not so simple. It is an art that will take you a lifetime to learn. You think that people will tell you why they have come to see you, but they won't. They forget, they exaggerate, or they ignore what is important . . . .[11]

And yet, "[w]hen a physician sees twenty to thirty patients a day, day after day, it all becomes routine. He depends on the patient to call attention to problems . . . ."[12] Where routine dulls alertness, even the most basic information may never be collected.

Providing doctors the information they need often demands all the patient's acuity, perception, memory, and cooperation, commodities which may be in short supply.[13] With the best will in the world patients may be hard put even to describe their ailment. As Virginia Woolf ruefully remarked:

> The merest schoolgirl, when she falls in love, has Shakespeare or Keats to speak her mind for her; but let a sufferer try to describe a pain in his head to a doctor and language at once runs dry. There is nothing ready made for him. He is forced to coin words himself, and, taking his pain in one hand, and a lump of pure sound in the other (as perhaps the people of Babel did in the beginning), so to crush them together that a brand new word in the end drops out. Probably it will be something laughable.[14]

The patient strains not just to describe the indescribable, but to remember the unnoticed. Did those pains begin two weeks ago or four? Were they worse after eating? On the right side or the left? Dull or sharp? Throbbing or piercing? Continuous or intermittent? Apparently, "[a]part from the display of a more luxuriant technical vocabulary," even doctors do not provide very good histories. Perhaps this is because "the study of self is the least practiced of human virtues . . ." and because of "our resistance to the unpleasant . . . ."[15]

The doctor's task of understanding the patient is made yet harder because patients see their symptoms through their own lenses. One asthmatic's "inclination has been not to describe how severe and disabling my symptoms are, but, instead, to try to tolerate them. The truth is that I've forgotten what wellness feels like. I have become so used to living with discomfort that I realize I must learn to be more explicit about what I'm suffering."[16] Some patients repress ominous developments: "Patients, when they're describing their symptoms, often try and confuse doctors, hoping that fooling us into making a less serious diagnosis will actually change the nature of their illness, perhaps moving it from one organ to another."[17] Other patients—the hypochondriacs—stray in the opposite direction, turning every sniffle and twinge into death's overtures. Fear is, if not the patient's constant companion, always lurking around the corner, and fear distorts the patient's perception and account of illness.

Doctors know patients cannot always report symptoms accurately, and so they must interpret patients' accounts in light of their experience. But interpretation is hazardous. Done stupidly, it can be brutal. Arnold Beisser was paralyzed by polio. "Lying still with no muscles that moved made it impossible for me to generate my own heat. So, shivering, I would call the nurse and ask for another blanket to cover me." However, "[t]he room seemed comfortable to her, so she would doubt my judgment. In order to check, she would usually reach down to feel my leg. Then she would say something like 'Oh, it's all right, you're not cold.'"[18] Even when interpretation is less ham-handed, it can infuriate patients: "Since pain can neither be verified nor denied in many cases, the person in pain is doubted—are you malingering or overdramatizing?—which only then amplifies the pain. With only vivid, but subjective comparison to 'defend' ourselves with, we can hardly communicate at all."[19]

Gathering technical data presents its own problems. It can be unclear what laboratory tests and investigative procedures to perform. Some of them are not always worth their cost in money, delay, pain, and risk. Many of them yield information of dubious reliability, even relatively reliable tests frequently produce equivocal results, and interpreting test results is often challenging.

All these factors—and the inevitable defects in the physician's medical talent, training, and experience—will impede accurate diagnosis. Even if the diagnosis is accurate, there will not be consistent, complete, and trustworthy knowledge about the disease, its etiology, its prognosis, and its treatment. The teaching of formal sources may conflict with the doctor's clinical experience. In sum, the great fact about the "information" the doctor reasons from and presents to the patient is its insistent uncertainty. Uncertainty "is clinically commonplace. It is rarely the case that signs and symptoms are unambiguous markers of specific diseases. Signs and symptoms often do not appear exactly as described in textbooks, and the full constellation that describes the 'classic' presentation of a disease is often not seen."[20] Medicine "is engulfed and infiltrated by uncertainty"[21] and practiced "in a sea of doubt and uncertainty,"[22] so that "judgements must inevitably be made on the doctor's personal experience of past cases; the comparison of the present size, sound or feel of something with what is remembered; and on what a clinician believes to be the problem, based sometimes on very scanty evidence."[23] Or, yet again, "Largely because what the physician decides to do (and not to do) on behalf of a patient is generally based on less than perfect knowledge, it has been said that 'in a sense [his] every clinical act is an investigation.' . . ."[24] Indeed, this uncertainty is an old commonplace:

> "Well, you know, Standish, every dose you take is an experiment—an experiment, you know," said Mr. Brooke, nodding toward the lawyer.
> "Oh, if you talk in that sense!" said Mr. Standish with as much disgust at such non-legal quibbling as a man can well betray towards a valuable client.[25]

A jolting modern view of that uncertainty comes from a report that "[i]n less than half the cases in [a] prospective study was the clinical diagnosis of cause of death confirmed at autopsy."[26]

In short, the data a doctor receives from the patient and from medical science may be partial, tenebrous, and ambiguous. All this makes diagnosis arduous and uncertain, however skilled, practiced, and shrewd the practitioner.[27] Therefore the information the patient receives must often be frustratingly uncertain. Worse, the more serious and therefore complex the medical problem, the likelier the uncertainty and the worse its consequences. The data, the diagnosis, and the prognosis may be uncertain, and the extent of those uncertainties may itself be uncertain. So the patient struggles from the start in the disquieting position of working from possibly unreliable information. Thus one sophisticated patient concluded, "One of the barriers to informed consent is lack of information. For many treatments, particularly experimental ones, there is limited information on how the treatment is supposed to work, experience to date with the treatment, expected side effects, and potential benefits. Both the patient and the physician are working with many unknowns and uncertainties."[28] Yet how far do most patients understand the pervasiveness of uncertainty? Even when it is explained to them, do they believe it? If not, will they appreciate, for example, that diagnostic uncertainty often means that treatments must be chosen before the disease is identified and that treatment itself can be a diagnostic tool?

Even if the information presented to patients were always entirely reliable, it would still often be opaque. Information about diagnosis and prognosis must often be phrased in terms of odds, and most people find odds mystifying.[29] (Indeed, much of the population has trouble just working with fractions.) Even if you understand statistics, they can be hard to apply. One patient, himself a doctor, read that 75% of patients treated for cancer of the larynx were alive after ten years. He reflected that "the life expectancy for a man my age is nine more years. But these statistics say I have a 75 percent chance of being alive in ten years, so does that mean I will live longer because of my throat cancer?"[30] It has become common for doctors to tell patients and patients to tell themselves that "you are not a statistic," that, as Fox more accurately puts it, doctors' statements "about the problems of their particular patients are based on aggregate statistics that apply more accurately to large populations of patients than to individual cases."[31] This is true, but if patients should not consult statistics, what should they consult? In short, when diagnosis and prognosis are so routinely seen as calculations of complex odds, when screening and treatment are so commonly analyzed in cost–benefit terms, the primitive and even defective statistical sense patients bring to decisions must often be deplorably limiting.[32]

Further, each possible treatment may involve an incommensurable mix of advantages and disadvantages (medical and social), and there may be many plausible courses of action.[33] Yet another layer of uncertainty may be added if the patient seeks a second opinion, if a general practitioner and a specialist disagree, or if the patient talks to friends who have stories or convictions of their own. As one doctor with cancer comments:

> I know how some of my patients felt when I referred them to another doctor for a second opinion and the opinion was different. Now I, too, have to wrestle with several opinions. I, too, don't know which one is correct.
> Here's the score so far:
> Dermatologist 1: It's erysipelas.
> Dermatologist 2: It's a virus, maybe a lymphoma.

> Radiologist: I don't know. It's not due to X-ray therapy, and it doesn't belong in my department.
>
> My son Jim: It's shingles.
>
> Myself: I hope it's an insect bite, but it must be a lymphoma.[34]

Nor do these problems vanish when patients flee to written sources. One cancer patient discovered "reading doesn't necessarily help. Every new theory spawns disagreement, and around the corner is always someone else with an even newer idea of how to get healthy."[35]

Faced with such disagreements, many patients, like Joyce Wadler, are baffled:

> It all seems crazy to me, but there's nothing I can do. I have two doctors who have looked at the same slides and made different diagnoses. I have been thinking of medicine, I realize, as a science of absolutes. I assumed a doctor would look at a cancer cell and tell you with certainty what it was, just as one looks at the amount of liquid in a measuring cup and gives you a precise count. But breast cancer is apparently not like that; it's more like two coaches disputing a play at a basketball game.[36]

Such patients often abandon the idea of evaluating alternative treatments and instead hunt for other grounds of choice. Wadler, for instance, elected to "stay with the team with Cancer Research Center on their jerseys,"[37] since she had learned working in newspapers "how much information you pick up just being around other people. At a cancer research center, with department meetings and visiting specialists, it's bound to be the same way. If I can't have a cancer contractor, I want a place where all my records and doctors are under one roof. I have that at Sloan[-Kettering]."[38]

Furthermore, the information conveyed to the patient is often dynamic, not stable: Medical circumstances frequently change with time, as new information filters in from tests, as the patient's condition ebbs and flows, and even as science marches (or stumbles) on. Treatments themselves alter the patients' health—for better or for worse—in ways that may raise new questions. As the husband of one mortally ill patient said, "Well, options and situations change around here so fast that it's hard to keep track, and harder to know how to assess the options."

Wise medical decisions should be informed by a sense of the trajectory of illness, of what is likely to come next, of how causes, symptoms, treatments, and side effects interact. It is hard for patients to acquire such a sense and for doctors to realize patients lack it. Thus a wife making decisions for her husband after his stroke was surprised he had developed aspirative pneumonia and surprised at the gravity of that illness. "Throughout Jay's ordeal, I was reacting to one isolated situation after another. There was no time to consider the whole picture; each portion was more than enough to handle. I thought of this pneumonia as an isolated and 'chance' event."[39]

Thus far, I have spoken as though patients have only one disease at a time and make only one decision about a single treatment at a time. But many patients, especially seriously ill patients, suffer several illnesses simultaneously, each of which may be treated in multiple ways. Worse, their several diseases and various treatments will often interact elaborately, obscurely, and consequentially. Such patients will need to do onerous amounts of the forbidding work I have been describing if they are to make their own decisions.

Doctors who try to inform a patient fully must struggle not to proffer a bolus of unfamiliar, abstruse, and technical information patients cannot assimilate at the time, much less recall later on. Much information is readily and fully comprehensible only to someone with medical training. This problem has two aspects. First, the physician reads and speaks the language of medicine; the patient does not. Translations are notoriously difficult: Something really *is* lost in the translation. But more than translation is required. The language of medicine is not just foreign. It incorporates, abbreviates, and expresses a mass of arcane and elaborate learning about which most patients have hardly a clue. (Indeed, some physicians believe that medical language is so imprecise that it confounds doctors as well as patients.)[40] Doctors may try to simplify this information and explain it as clearly as they can. But the language of medicine developed partly because it efficiently communicates complex information, and many physicians (who as a class are perhaps not notoriously articulate) have trouble with the translation. The gulf between the lay and medical vocabularies is suggested by Ben Watt's confession that it was only when he became ill that he "learnt that I had two bowels—a small bowel, sometimes called the small intestine, where all the digesting is done, and a large bowel, or colon, where the waste is processed. I'd always thought 'bowel' was just a colloquial term like 'guts' and meant somewhere near your arse."[41] Even a sterlingly educated and formidably intelligent patient like Gillian Rose finally said,

> Medicine and I have dismissed each other. We do not have enough command of each other's language for the exchange to be fruitful. It is as if, exiled for ever into a foreign tongue, you learn the language by picking up words and phrases, even sentences, but never proceed to grasp the underlying principles of grammar and syntax, which would give you the freedom to use the language creatively and critically. You cannot generate the grammar of judgements in order to pursue alternative questions and conclusions.[42]

There is, in addition, the problem of euphemism. Doctors want to inform patients without upsetting them. Euphemism is the traditional solution to this problem. There is much to be said for precision, much to be said for tact, and something to be said for euphemism. Eric Hodgins, for instance, decided "cerebro-vascular accident,"

> being more specific, is an honest improvement over "stroke," although no one who has had a CVA can question how it gained its earlier and still persisting name. But medical nicety goes still further; it is good form to speak of *a* CVA, meaning a stroke which has stricken someone else, but "*your* CVA" is a little too blunt, so

when a physician must use the possessive pronoun his standard reference is to "Your, uh, Episode." *Episode* carries with it the tone of something which once was, but no longer is: "an incidental passage in a person's life." In these terms it is a total falsity, but perhaps it is also a desirable falsity, and I think I am for it.[43]

Nevertheless, euphemism is clarity's enemy.

Furthermore, there are the problems of capacity and interest. Some people have a keener aptitude and appetite for scientific learning than others. Many patients find technical medical information uninteresting, even though they realize how momentous it may be. As one man said of his multiple sclerosis, "After awhile the subject could not help but become altogether boring."[44] Tim Brookes, a journalist writing a book about the asthma which beset him, discovered that even though he "had every intention of learning about the cellular mechanisms of asthma, as soon as I started reading, my mind slid off the subject and started converting science into science fiction, like a rebellious thirteen-year-old in his first biology class."[45]

The more serious the decision, the likelier fear is to corrode concentration. A paramedic said of being told she had cancer: "I was in a bubble. I saw his mouth moving and I was aware of a flow of words, but I was unable to process most of the information. He might as well have been speaking a different language."[46] Even after her subsequent visit to her doctor she left his office with her "mind blank."[47] Another patient wrote mournfully, "When it comes to discussing cancer, especially my own, I usually hear about every tenth word. Which is why I always bring extra ears to the doctor's. On Monday, I brought Joni's, my friend Henrietta's, and my tape recorder's. And with all that listening power, I think we got about a third of the information."[48]

Even people who become interested in their medical problems and try to educate themselves may encounter difficulties talking with their physicians. Indeed, their very sophistication may beguile their doctors into overestimating their understanding. William Martin, for instance, is the sociologist whose diligence in making decisions I described in Chapter 2. Yet even he recounts an occasion when, "in my ignorance, I thought the virulence of my tumor had just been elevated from a three to a seven. Since Dr. Carlton thought I knew what I was talking about, it didn't occur to him to straighten me out."[49]

In short, patients often fail to understand what doctors tell them. It is thus not surprising to hear patients saying things like: "I'm having trouble assimilating all this, and from the look on his face, so is Herb. We're two liberal-arts guys suddenly thrown into Columbia Medical School."[50] Or to hear Tim Brookes reflecting, "The doctor's order comes out as cogent and direct as a column of smoke rising from a cigarette; but after a time that is impossible to calculate it wavers, then breaks up, eddying in all directions."[51] Or to see Agnes de Mille wanting to respond to her surgeon's assertion that a decision about an operation was " 'between you and me entirely' " by saying "something polite to the effect, 'Don't be an ass.' I did clearly say, 'How can I possibly voice an opinion? I don't know anything.' "[52]

But beyond the struggles doctors face in translating from an arcane language, there is a second aspect of the problem of communicating unfamiliar and technical information. People trained in skilled work learn to reason in ways that elide many steps and that they themselves do not fully realize or understand. As Kuhn observes (quoting Polanyi), " 'much of the scientist's success depends upon "tacit knowledge," i.e., upon knowledge that is acquired through practice and that cannot be articulated explicitly.' "[53] Experts are different from novices: they have more experience. That experience gives them a set of patterns they implicitly consult in making decisions and lets them "see a situation, even a nonroutine one, as an example of a prototype." [53a] Through experience, these prototypes become so well developed and can be consulted so readily that we can say that expert thinking is "intuitive." In other words, "it is executed under low control and conscious awareness, rapid rate of data processing, high confidence in answer and low confidence in the method that produced it . . . ."[53b] Novices lack this experience. Thus they lack those prototypes. And thus effective "intuitive" reasoning is foreclosed to them. They must work out step by step what experts see at a glance. The classic illustration of this difference in reasoning comes from chess. Chess masters look at a board and see patterns of force and possibility. Beginners see discrete pieces and ask how many spaces a pawn can move. Because experts perceive and reason about the world through prototypes and novices do not, it is fair to say that "[p]eople with greater expertise can see the world differently."[53c] This disjuncture in the way professionals and the laity perceive, analyze, and talk about problems must further inhibit and distort communication.

Not only do doctors think differently from patients; they also see their work differently. Barbara Creaturo's memoir illustrates one aspect of this problem.[54] She was anxious that her cancer be treated by "top" doctors using the latest techniques. This sent her toward researchers. She was not unsophisticated: she was a graduate of Vassar and Harvard and an editor of *Cosmopolitan*. Yet her understanding of what medical research involves differed sharply from the standard professional view. She did not see why anecdotal accounts of treatments carry little weight, why a research program using one protocol might reject an applicant who was part way through another protocol, why competition among researchers might be desirable, why researchers might not publish all their results the instant they came in, or even why researchers could legitimately disagree about how to interpret medical literature. And (one infers) Creaturo's doctors did not understand that she did not understand or what she did not understand, since to them it seemed so self-evident, so much the basis of their professional lives.

There are yet further impediments to communication. Patients commonly want to know what life will be like under the courses of treatment the doctor offers. But doctors may be hard put to say. I once asked a doctor how it felt to be in-

tubated, and she quite reasonably said she didn't know, she had never been intubated. Or, as Robert Zussman observes, "[N]either the doctors nor the nurses
. . . are at all sure of how much pain their patients are suffering. Pain is a notoriously difficult phenomenon to measure."[55] After all, "no gauge, no thermome-
ter exist[s] for pain."[56] Even if doctors comprehend how some patients experience their illness or treatments, they may not anticipate how any particular
patient will, for different patients react differently to the same symptoms and the
same treatment.[57] Even if the doctor can explain what life would be like on, say,
dialysis, the patient may flounder trying to envision it. Both too little and too
much imagination can be a curse here. As one patient remarked after reading a
protocol for treating her cancer, "My mind is reeling. I find it hard to connect all
of this to me, yet there are little flashes that it could be me, in a totally new environment. This feels a little like reading school catalogues before September, pic-
turing what it's going to be like. It was never what I had imagined. I wonder if
this will be the same."[58] These problems are intensified by the reluctance patients
commonly feel to acknowledge they are seriously ill. This makes them "a not
particularly receptive group for counseling about post-operative life, because
they [are] resistant to the very idea that there would be a post-operative state at
all. Even where people do have accurate information, some find it extremely difficult to anticipate what life is going to be like."[59]

Patients misinterpret doctors' information for yet another reason. Thoughtful
patients realize what physicians are fond of pointing out—that no doctor can
truly present information neutrally and that how information is framed shapes
how it is understood.[60] David Orentlicher, for instance, describes a study in
which "patients chose treatment 30% of the time when it was characterized in a
positive way but only 12% of the time when it was described negatively. Moreover, 17% of the patients changed their minds when given a different characteri-
zation of the treatment."[61] Anspach nicely captures the common physicians' assumption that they determine how patients make decisions by the way they
present issues. She quotes a doctor who says "the parents make their judgments
largely on the basis of the information the physician gives them. . . . So the
physician has . . . the matter completely in his hands. I think having the parents
well informed is always well informed on your grounds. . . . It's the way you
see it. So ultimately the decision is made by whoever is calling the medical
shots."[62]

But even when doctors recognize that biases must be present, they may not
know how to identify and assess them or how to express a choice "neutrally."
And even when patients recognize the doctor faces these problems, they may not
know how to discount them. Is the doctor being frank? Does the doctor believe
patients in general ought not be told much? That this patient would be upset by
hearing too much? By hearing too little? That complex or distressing information
should be doled out slowly for the patient's sake (or for the doctor's)? That it is

better to hang crepe early than to drizzle bad news down later?[63] So a woman trying to evaluate her doctor's advice to stop fertility treatments mused, "What if Dr. Kuneck was wrong? What if he was a certain type of personality, very conservative, who himself gave up too soon?"[64] And so Wilfrid Sheed

> got it into my head for God knows what reason that Doctor X. at the hospital had not been leveling with me about my condition but was sitting on worse news than he could bring himself to tell. X. seemed like a kindly sort of guy, and he might have taken one look at the pitiable wreck I imagined myself to be that day and decided "We can't tell this man the truth—now or ever. It would probably kill him," or whatever doctors say to themselves. But what could I do about it now? Call up X. and say, "Tell me the real truth, so long as it doesn't hurt too much. And try to make it *really* convincing this time"? What's the answer to a guy who won't accept good news and can't handle bad?[65]

Furthermore, since patients are increasingly treated by doctors they have not known long (if at all), they will lack a good basis for interpreting them.[66] Most crucially, patients can rarely judge how reliable, learned, or skilled their doctor is. Yet what other information would better help patients decide how to receive advice? Finally, even if the doctor is completely neutral, aggressively frank, admirably assiduous, and uncommonly competent, the patient may still fear the doctor is simply wrong.[67] One patient captures much of this confusion when she describes her reaction to hearing her doctor propose a radical treatment for her cancer:

> I look at Ken and consider him carefully; golly, he's so nice, so accessible, is he trying to snow me? I want a cure desperately—can I trust him? What does he want? He's created something that could make medical history if it works, that would be a peak experience for any scientist. Can he retain his clinical judgment? Would he risk my life foolishly? Can I trust him with my life?[68]

In all this, the addled person's usual refuge—asking questions—is often barred. Patients often know too little to assimilate what they have heard and to formulate questions. As a patient who was "a part-time college instructor said, 'I didn't know enough even to know what questions to ask. You can't ask a doctor, "Well, if A, should I B?" unless you know B exists.'"[69] All too often patients lack experience and skill in framing inquiries, analyzing answers, and articulating new questions. For many patients, their best hope is the *coup d'escalier;* their usual fate is never to see what they should have asked. Thus it is common to find reports like this: "[D]espite plain evidence of lack of understanding on the part of many, the parents of only two families asked for amplification."[70]

Another refuge for people confused by their doctors' advice is to look for information in writing. Written advice at least can be read, and reread, at leisure and one's own pace. But reliable literature that speaks at the right level directly to a particular patient's problems can be hard to find. One reporter's doctor told him that the "popular medical literature and basic textbooks have not kept up with the advances." The reporter pressed his doctor, who lent him journal articles. These the reporter found "incomprehensible—discussions on 'MOPP versus the 3 and 2 technique for total nodal irradiation.'"[71] My own experience with the pamphlets hospitals and doctors distribute illustrates the opposite problem: They are so superficial that they leave you as befogged as before.

Even if patients get reliable information in a comprehensible form, they must still process it. This is not always easy. Complicated and foreign uncertainties are hard to analyze. And the cure for ignorance can import its own frailties. The primary legal principle of medical ethics—informed consent—tries to solve the problems of patients' decisions by securing more information for them. But patients can drown in a river of information just as they can be parched in a desert of ignorance. Medical issues regularly require their solver to keep in mind a dismaying number of factors. Yet, Amitai Etzioni reports that "[p]eople are able to hold only some seven items (or perhaps as low as three) in their immediate mental grasp . . . ."[72] When those factors are so unfamiliar and complex as to be difficult to assimilate and remember individually, this problem must become even more severe.

Even patients given just the right information in just the right amounts at just the right moments can encounter another problem processing it. Patients must evaluate what they are told in light of what they believe about illness and the body. All too often, this means that patients interpret information against a background of active misinformation haphazardly collected or hazily assumed in casual inattention to the unreliable medical information that pervades our folkways and airways.[73] That information is unreliable for a number of reasons. The press, for instance, reports medical information selectively. Statistically frequent causes of death are rarely reported; statistically infrequent ones are trumpeted.[74] Single studies with dramatic results are reported with fanfare and without qualification, however shabby their method and shoddy their conclusions. Unreliable information is thus mixed with reliable information and filtered through memories that are both selective and porous.

In short, the patient's vision is often—usually?—clouded by the haze of fable, fantasy, and superstition we assimilate over a lifetime of inattentive reading, careless listening, forgotten science, and antique learning.[75] Until Joseph Heller wrote a memoir of his encounter with Guillain-Barré syndrome, he "harbored a naive conception of the mechanics of human respiration. It was my erroneous notion that breathing, particularly deep breathing, began in the nose and/or mouth with a sucking down of air that inflated the lungs and thereby expanded the chest. They tell me now it is the reverse that occurs."[76] Tim Brookes concluded, "Virtually all conversations about illness are conducted on the level of folk belief and mythology—and I'm not talking about the small percentage of poor souls who take every word of the *National Enquirer* as gospel. We simply have no idea what we're talking about most of the time."[77] Even a journalist whose mother had died of breast cancer, who had long feared contracting it herself, and who had been collecting books on it "realized [when the disease struck her] that what I knew about breast cancer was a mishmash of memories—anecdotal, uninformed, imprecise . . . ."[78]

The ill are also likely to receive medical advice of—at best—mixed soundness from their family and friends. One cancer patient not only got conflicting counsel from his doctors, but was bombarded by friends who advised "visualization[,] . . . macrobiotic diets, multivitamin/mineral supplements, acupuncture, massage, oriental herbs, and kelp."[79] He asked himself, "Are there rays I should be taking, herbs I should be digesting, regimens I should be changing? As individual tales are related around the table, icy fingers of fear and doubt tweak at my nerve strings. Am I the fool? Have I missed something?" In the end, the best he felt he could do was trust his doctors and his "instincts."[80]

Patients may even be misled by accurate information from unimpeachable sources. For example, sound information can become obsolete. One of my interviewees resisted hemodialysis well past the point of good sense (as he now sees it) partly because he retained a vivid but anachronistic impression of it from seeing a dialysis unit in his youth. Patients may not recognize misinformation for what it is and thus may analyze accurate new information in a distorted way.[81] Furthermore, correct information may be applied to the wrong problem. Most of us, for example, have learned something about an illness from the experiences of our families and friends. But this information is rarely conveyed in its full and exact context, and applying it can thus be risky. Aunt Betsy had pneumonia, she was given antibiotics, and she promptly recovered. We infer that antibiotics reliably treat pneumonia. What we haven't grasped is that Aunt Betsy did not have viral pneumonia and that it is not treatable with antibiotics. If we have pneumonia, our physician might set us straight. But suppose we have been told pneumonia is a risk of a proposed treatment (or of refusing a treatment). We may underestimate the consequences of getting pneumonia because we mistakenly believe it can be easily cured.

One way people improve their decisions is by asking how well previous ones worked. But it is hard to tell whether your condition improved because of the decision you made and whether a better decision would have produced a better result. This is common enough. As Gary Klein writes, "We often cannot see a clear link between cause and effect. Too many variables intervene, and time delays create their own complications."[82] As one physician noted, patients "are more likely to classify a previous decision as a mistake if an adverse effect occurred and the final result was not optimal. Yet the same adverse effect may be viewed more favorably if the outcome was successful."[83] Patients may also "use their previous perceived state of good health as the reference point and not appreciate that cancer, AIDS, or other chronic diseases are associated with an inevitable and progressive loss of functioning. So, when therapy fails to maintain or reestablish the perceived reference performance level, the decision to be treated is judged to be a mistake."[84] All this is problematic because, as Klein observes, "In domains that are not marked by opportunities for effective feedback . . . , mere accumulation of experience does not appear to result in growth of decision expertise."[84a]

Tim Brookes engagingly sums up patients' problems acquiring and analyzing information:

> Our consciousness experiences illness like George III experiencing the American War of Independence: as a series of messages of wildly varying reliability bringing mostly disturbing news from a country he has never seen. And all this while he is receiving hourly reports from every corner of the realm on countless subjects, any of which—fluctuations in the cost of tobacco or tea, an insufficiently deep bow from a foreign ambassador—may be affected by the war, or by a different war, or by something else entirely. And in hearing advice from friends, family, and physicians we are just like poor George, surrounded by courtiers of dubious integrity and advisers of doubtful perspicacity. Who can blame us for going off our rocker, issuing contradictory instructions to the body politic, ordering quick fixes to only the immediate problems, or wanting to let the war wage itself and let us get on with easier problems of government, such as chewing the carpet?[85]

I have been talking about medical decisions made under good conditions, but they often must be faced in bad and even terrible circumstances. Sometimes patients are flatly unable to make any kind of decision (and the graver the decision, the likelier the patient is to be incapacitated). Patients may be mentally enfeebled by decay, disease, and distress; their minds will frequently be clouded by drugs and other treatments. Patients with kidney disease often comment that when they have been uremic for a long time, they lose any sense of what it feels like to be healthy or of how sick they are. In the hospital battling a rebellious immune system, Ben Watt found he "couldn't care. I couldn't care at all much of the time. About anything." He "regularly seemed to leave myself, and became ego-less, free-floating, non-doing, motionless but for my eyes flickering and blinking, like a lizard on a rock, basking in the alcohol-like fug of Voltarol or the pleasure of being temporarily released from the effects of drugs or pain . . . ."[86] Even decisions that should have been small and pleasant distressed May Sarton after her stroke:

> For anyone who is for any reason feeling weak in the head it is not advisable to suggest solving a problem that requires *choices*. Yesterday I spent an hour choosing finally a flowering plum tree, from Wayside Gardens, a birthday gift for Mary Tozer and two white azaleas for Anne Woodson. It sounds pleasurable but was actually the hardest hour I have spent for a long time and I cried at the end.[87]

Simply being in the hospital can be intellectually disorienting and psychologically debilitating, for you are deprived of much that is familiar and that makes you what you are, and you are isolated from the world, the seasons, and even the time of day. As Max Lerner writes, for example, "Sleep in hospitals is at best intermittent, broken by 'procedures,' tests, and schedules, and dreams are often transformed by pain and drugs into hypnogogic states, between sleep and waking. The result for me was that the dividing line between reality and imagining got blurred, and I spent much of my time in a haze."[88] This problem can become so severe in ICUs that it has acquired a diagnosis—ICU psychosis.[89] The very experience of prolonged illness is itself disorienting. As a patient with chronic fatigue syndrome said,

> it is very confusing to be chronically ill. The machine of my body is broken; a delicate poise between body and spirit is disturbed. I have been cut off from my past as an athlete, as a member of the work force, as a vital human being. Family relationships and friendships have altered. Whether I have sinned or lived wrong, expended too much or held too much in, deserved my virus or was stricken arbitrarily, my life has been changed utterly. This is difficult to grasp, even now.[90]

Even if the patient is competent, decisions may be warped by fear, by panic, by a passing preference for short-term comfort, by pain, by bitterness, by guilt, by depression, by despair. Patients' decisions may be distorted even by hope: As her doctor described retinal surgery to her, one patient, with her "usual aptitude for selective listening, . . . didn't pay much attention to his professional assessment: a 50–50 chance of success. What I forgot is that often means a 50–50 chance of failure, too."[91] But fear, especially, torments patients. "Fear," Tim Brookes writes, "is the counselor to whom we listen, whose terminology we use, and whose advice we take, no matter how irrational."[92] Fear shatters the mind's clarity. A patient facing breast cancer "reported severe impairment of critical thinking and concentration, together with elevated anxiety rates."[93] Another such woman came to "see clearly how one set of fears led to the next poor judgment, which in turn led to the next wrong choices."[94] Philip Roth saw his father (whose enduring strength he admired) collapse in the face of his medical choices:

> [M]y father was hardly equipped to make the decision to go ahead on his own. He'd conducted himself gallantly with the two brain surgeons, but now, caught in the vise of their differing proposals, he succumbed to a wild helplessness. He began to say things to me that didn't make much sense, and then for longer periods said nothing or suddenly, unprovoked, lashed out at Lil so uncontrollably that even he was startled afterward by his vehemence and meekly apologized.[95]

One more quotation is necessary to convey the mind-distorting terror that can wrack patients.

> For the next few days I sense I've changed. My hands shake, my concentration is nonexistent, a pile of magazines sits neat and dusty on the nightstand as I lie wakeful and alert through a wilderness of sights and sounds. There is sensory stimuli and a network of raw nerves at the mercy of a chaotic universe with no order, no security. Questions arise, both medical and ontological, having to do with my sanity and the nature of this terrible new awareness. . . . At times I become strangely de-

tached from the environment, particularly in the midst of loud noises or multiple conversations. I am accosted by the everyday, overwhelmed by the mundane. And the symptoms are terrifying; I break out in a hot sweat, become dizzy with the secret but powerful secretion of adrenaline, my mind boils with disparate thoughts as the world transforms itself into an elaborate disaster. All I know is that I am naked and alive. During the brief stretches of calm I attempt to ponder my condition, and slowly it occurs to me that these symptoms could represent some subtle brain damage incurred during the surgery. But mere explanations of course provide no relief, because all I now know is that I am deeply and irrevocably out of my mind.[96]

It is, then, easy to see how even patients committed to the principle of making their own decisions can become ambivalent in the face of fear. One patient's "wish all along" had been to

be included in all aspects of my medical care. To be included, so that, if I had to go through all this, it would at least be my journey and not just some ride that I was taken on, blindfolded, like a hostage. Now that the opportunity was being offered, I found myself paralyzed with fear. For the first time, I had an inkling of why so many people don't want the doctor to share too much with them.[97]

As the paramedic-become-patient commented, "At one of the most frightening moments of my life, I suddenly had to become a researcher and make cool decisions in a field I knew nothing about. It was not a likely time to be a smart consumer."[98]

Finally, whatever the patient's condition, medical decisions are harder under time and economic pressures. Most illnesses are best treated promptly, and most patients want to ease their symptoms quickly. Furthermore, the machinery of medical care rolls along, doctors become impatient, procedures must be scheduled, and so decisions must be made. Thus one cancer patient would "question the almost universal recommendation to take the decision-making process into your own hands," since "you cannot find out enough to save your own life in two or three frantic weeks of searching."[99] Inadequately uninsured patients also face intensified perplexities. Troyen Brennan describes a not-uncommon patient. She has hypertension, high cholesterol, diabetes, and a family history of heart disease. Finding the right combination of medicines would be tricky under the best of circumstances, but this woman has no health insurance, so at each meeting with Brennan "she takes out her medicines and we go over the cost of each. We try to decide what to add, and then figure out what to subtract in order to bring the total cost down."[100]

The Structural Context of Medical Decisions

I have argued that medical decisions are daunting because they overwhelm patients with baffling questions they are ill-equipped to grapple with. Those decisions are further complicated by the structural context in which they arise. Perhaps in the traditional medical setting this was less true, for the patient modally dealt with a single doctor who was responsible for handling most of a patient's medical problems, so decisions could be made in a few face-to-face discussions. However, the developing structure of modern medicine is changing—and complicating—the context of medical decisions. Increasingly, that context is what we may loosely call bureaucratic. Medical knowledge has burgeoned; medical technology has proliferated. Doctors have become more specialized, and they are increasingly assisted by specialized technicians. More and more services can only be delivered in institutions large enough to afford expensive equipment and staffs.

A bureaucratized and technologized medicine costs so much that those who write the checks for it—private employers and public agencies—are pressing doctors and hospitals to save money. Among the classic solutions to such pressure is one medicine has adopted—economies of scale. Hospitals have consolidated, not just locally but nationally. Physicians increasingly practice in groups, in preferred-provider organizations, in HMOs, and as employees of hospitals. For example, as Bradford Gray wrote several years ago, the "employment of physicians (in hospitals and elsewhere) is growing and now involves more than one in four physicians. The trend seems likely to continue, since the percentage of employed physicians is highest among the younger doctors."[101] In short, as the medical–industrial complex[102] swells and burgeons, medical services are more and more delivered by large and elaborate—and thus bureaucratically organized—structures.[103]

The forces that drive the bureaucratization of medicine can only intensify. Indeed, the trend is part of a larger social development, for "over the past decade, in all the human services but most strikingly in the health services, there has been a distinct increase in pressure toward strengthening administrative powers and, in fact, an effort to encourage by legislation the consolidation and formal organization of everyday medical practices that in the past have been typically organized on an individual and informal basis."[104] This change is a momentous one which is already transforming the practice of medicine and the course of medical decisions. In two respects it makes decisions more difficult for patients. First, by complicating the way doctors arrive at proposed treatments. Second, by making it harder for patients to get information and influence treatment.

Put differently, the bureaucratization of medicine pushes the process of decision toward complexity and confusion. First, bureaucracy exacerbates the problems I described earlier by complicating the way doctors acquire information. Doctors in a bureaucratic setting find some information easier to obtain, since bureaucratization makes possible more sophisticated and thorough testing. In many ways, however, it attenuates the reliability of information. It can make so much testing possible that the resulting mountains of data become hard to keep track of and interpret. Furthermore, information in large hospitals must be passed from person to person, so that residents tell attendings what the nurse told them about the family's report about the patient's first symptoms. As Anspach notes, "[P]hysicians are often forced to rely on information that has been preinterpreted by nurses and social workers, sometimes entered as cryptic notes in a patient's chart, devoid of behavioral referents . . . . [I]nformation about the family can be transformed and even distorted as it filters up the nursery's occupational hierarchy and even further transformed as it is entered in the patient's case record."[105] This problem of communication among medical personnel may be aggravated by the depersonalization of relations among them.[106] In addition, in a modern bureaucracy gathering and analyzing information is impeded because "the accumulation of medical knowledge and its resultant splintering can make a particular physician a 'lay person' *vis-à-vis* the physician (or technician) who is an expert in another specialization."[107]

Once doctors have gathered information, bureaucracy can complicate reaching a decision. As Bosk observes, decisions in hospitals are frequently made by "a network of consultants, house staff, and attending physicians. . . . [U]ncertainty in diagnosis leads to seeking multiple opinions, multiple opinions produce a fragile consensus about what is really the problem, and the fragile consensus exacerbates the problem of making decisions." When the consensus is fragile, doctors may hope "that the next laboratory value or the next drug combination will resolve or reduce the remaining uncertainty." And that "uncertainty combined with group pressures introduces the temptation, opportunity, and, many times, the obligation to reopen debate."[108]

Bureaucracy complicates not just the way doctors acquire information and make decisions, but also the way patients do. It does so primarily by diffusing information, expertise, and responsibility among the people who care for the patient. A bewildering array of people may contribute (more or less officially) to a medical decision because a proliferating variety of people have information or skill that is relevant to the decision or have an interest in its resolution. Patients, family members, friends, co-workers, employers, fellow patients, teachers, clergy, paramedics, nurses, physician's assistants, medical students, interns, residents, fellows, attending physicians, private physicians, consulting physicians, surgeons, anesthetists, psychiatrists, psychologists, pathologists, radiologists, pharmacists, respiratory therapists, physical therapists, occupational therapists, speech therapists, dieticians, technicians of many sorts, drug-company representatives, social workers, discharge planners, hospice personnel, nursing-home personnel, peer-counselors, support-group members, hospital administrators, lawyers, risk-management staff, ethics committees, utilization-management personnel, insurance-company representatives, governmental bureaucrats, "patient advocates," and so on and on may have something to say—directly or indirectly—about a given medical choice. All these people bring to bear their own professional and personal experiences, perspectives, and interests.[109] The patient will never even hear about, much less meet or consult with, some of them, even though they may crucially affect the decision. Utilization-management programs, for example, may effectively preempt a physician's recommendations without the patient even realizing that such programs exist.[110]

Contributions from the many players may be made in a welter of times and places, as interested people happen to be present, as fresh information presents itself, and as the patient's condition ebbs and flows.[111] The players may change regularly, as the patient moves in and out of the hospital and specialized units, as specialists are consulted, as shifts change, and as doctors rotate in and out of units.[112] It is commonly said nurses provide some stability, but "with rotating nursing schedules, shifting assignments, the short turnaround time of many nursing tasks, and the constant turnover of nursing personnel, it is not clear that nurses provide continuity at all."[113]

In this disorienting world, patients first need to discover who has the information or advice they need. Then they must work out who can and will release it. Carol Heimer's study of neonatal intensive care units shows how demanding these tasks can be: "Part of the problem is that there is a division of labor between medical (i.e., physicians) and other personnel, and 'non-medical' personnel are not supposed to give medical information. . . . But parents have more contact with non-medical people, especially with nurses, and in some cases with social workers or therapists."[114] Yet parents cannot learn all they need to know even from nurses, who may not provide some kinds of information, do not have other kinds, and are constrained by fears of conveying false information. Nurses "*are* supposed to give reports to parents about how well the child is eating, whether he or she has had any apneic spells, what the ventilator settings are, and the like, but the nurse need not give anything but the 'objective' information, and can even shade toward misreporting by interpreting questions about the baby's status to be questions about whether there is any immediate crisis."[115] Doctors are responsible for relating the information nurses may not provide. But though they

> consult extensively, they may not give entirely consistent stories, and parents with precarious understandings of what is happening in the rollercoaster of their child's hospitalization are surely sensitive to small changes in the message and unsure whether these variations mean that the baby's situation has changed, that individual physicians have slightly different perspectives, that some physician has misread a chart, or that the same message is being given in slightly different words.[116]

These problems sharpen where there is bad news to tell. Fred Davis learned in his study of families of children with polio that in

> the bureaucratized hospital setting, the resident staff doctor is prone to take a narrowly circumscribed view of his professional responsibilities to the family of the patient. Were he to break the bad news of the child's handicapped outcome to the family, he would, as likely as not, have a "weeping and emotional" parent on his hands, a situation that many staff doctors eschew because it is time consuming, difficult to handle, and disruptive of their tightly scheduled routines.[117]

In short, bureaucratization means that acquiring information for, making, and carrying out a decision may demand contributions from many people with different training and experience from several units of the hospital. This not only diffuses responsibility for decisions but diffuses it in ways that the participants may not understand or agree about and that vary from case to case. The observer in a hospital sees, for example, both efforts to "turn out" patients to other units and efforts to prevent consultants from hijacking a decision about "our" patient. As Chambliss observes, "[I]n multiple ways the organization presents opportunities for the setting aside of individual responsibility. It provides a setting for individual action . . . that is largely technological, dense with expertise, hierarchical, and roughly fragmented."[118] Being effective in such an environment requires medical sophistication, knowledge of how the institution works, and acquaintance with the players. Patients are outsiders in the bureaucracy, and they often lack all these assets. This leads to situations like the one in which the adult child of a nursing-home patient met its director and was soon "embroiled in deadly verbiage, and quickly outwitted by her facility with administrative loops and tangents. . . . I wonder what the rules are in such situations. Is this the only way to learn them?"[119]

Patients repeatedly discover they cannot tell who is responsible for what. A cancer patient worried: "I had the problem most patients face in this age of specialization: too many doctors involved. I had the chemotherapist, the radiotherapist, the internist, even the surgeon. Who was 'in charge' of my case?"[120] A woman with Guillain-Barré syndrome "tried to understand how [one doctor] was connected to my case, especially when he began giving orders to the staff concerning my care. . . . No one ever explained how he got authority over my care—specifically, over the setting of my respirator. But even Bill [her husband] was recognizing him as one of my doctors."[121] Sometimes the patient must not just find out who is in charge, but must persuade those in charge to cooperate:

> Dr Lord left the room. In a few minutes she returned with Mr Wong. Then bedlam broke loose: "I will not talk to my colleague. I will not change my position. This is my cancer." In the ensuing ten minutes I summoned all the resources at my panicked disposal. I pleaded, cajoled, begged, flattered, inveigled Mr Wong to talk to his colleague, Mr Bates. I argued that my respect for my consultants was such that I could not proceed unless I understood the relation between their different views of my condition.[122]

In short, as a man learned when he complained his wife's care was not coordinated, "'Medical care *is never coordinated!*'"[123] That is the lesson taught by a patient who needed cardiac surgery and who "wanted to call a board meeting! Not of his firm—but of all the doctors. He said, 'Let's get all the M.D.'s. Get them all here—cardiology and the surgery people—and we'll run a board meeting. We'll have an agenda: *Will's Health.* We'll hear all the opinions, hear all the options, go through a stepwise, logical process, hear the motions, take a vote if needed.'" But Will's doctor "was laughing, listening to this. In an institution the size of Duke University Medical Center—a medical-industrial complex—it would be a logistical feat to get *everyone* involved into the same room for a 'board meeting.' "[124]

Medical decisions, then, are often not made—and often cannot be made—in the neat way informed-consent doctrine visualizes. Decisions are often not presented to a single identifiable decision-maker at a single moment when all the relevant information and all the relevant people have been assembled and when everyone realizes a decision has to be made and what is at stake. Rather, a decision is often a prolonged and jumbled process of small steps falteringly made.[125] Patients may not even realize a decision is being made, even if they are kept thoroughly informed. The Simmons study, for instance, reports that in some of their cases "the donor *never* felt he had decided to donate a kidney, or he felt that he had made a series of small exploratory steps and then found himself locked into donation."[126] Even where patients grasp that a decision is being reached, they may be so uncertain whom to talk to, so frustrated by delay, so confused by conflicting data and opinions, so unclear about the roles of the people they are dealing with, that the already onerous task of decision becomes even more daunting.

To some extent, the complexity of bureaucratic decisions protects patients because it means many people are thinking in different ways about their problems. It can mean that decisions are made incrementally, cautiously, experimentally, and (relatively and within important limits) reversibly.[127] It can mean that patients have multiple points of information and influence. But it can also lead to complication, confusion, and chaos.

The Nonmedical Aspects of Medical Decisions

I have been saying medical decisions are and must be uncommonly perplexing because medical information is uncommonly hard to acquire, assimilate, and analyze. But what of the nonmedical side of the equation? The patient is supposed to "provide the values—his or her own conception of the good—with which to evaluate these alternatives, and to select the one that is best for himself or herself."[128] This task is hardly as simple as this schematic formulation makes it sound.[129] Those "values" raise the most imponderable questions human beings ask. Because they are so hard to face, to formulate, and to employ, those values are usually unexplored and undeveloped. Particularly if they are unexamined, but even if they are well considered, people's beliefs are complex, contradictory, and confusing. In short, patients will often lack what autonomists too readily assume—"a set of preferences which are clearly-defined, well-understood, and rank-ordered so that people can make logical tradeoffs among them."[130] Max Lerner, for example, was a thoughtful and reflective man who had spent a long lifetime "explor[ing] the sovereign mind and its capacity to create its environ-

ment by choices."[131] One of his sons was a doctor and one of his daughters had
died of cancer. Nevertheless, he found he

> was—as so many cancer patients are today—in a crisis of belief. I had strong
> doubts about the bruising effects of medical technology in these extreme illnesses,
> yet I could not get myself to embrace the still dubious alternative treatment whole-
> heartedly. So there I was, a self-tormented creature, doubting while I strained to be-
> lieve, caught between a medical world that was suffering sharp challenge and one
> that had not yet come to birth.[132]

Further, people's values and their resulting medical preferences will often—
understandably and even admirably—change with time, as they confront new
and revealing problems and answer in grim reality questions they had only considered in abstract theory.[133] As Etzioni comments, "Often, goals are in continual
flux, as means are chosen, and decision-makers do not set out with clear goals
(let alone clearly ranked goals), but discover what they are after as they proceed."[134] Orasanu and Connolly write that it seems "rare for a decision to be
dominated by a single, well-understood goal or value. We expect the decision
maker to be driven by multiple purposes, not all of them clear, some of which
will be opposed to others. . . . These conflicts and tradeoffs . . . are often
novel and must be resolved swiftly, and . . . the situation may change quickly,
bringing new values to the fore."[134a] Howard Becker explains that commitments
"are not necessarily made consciously and deliberately. Some commitments . . .
arise crescively; the person becomes aware that he is committed only at some
point of change and seems to have made the commitment without realizing
it."[135] Yet more emphatically, Lee Clarke suggests preferences may "follow
rather than precede behavior"[136] and may thus be "little more than devices that
tell people what they have done rather than what they desire."[137]

These observations apply with special force to medical decisions. Illness is
disturbing at the deepest level. It is psychologically and morally disorienting. It
makes people strangers to themselves: "The sick person who says he doesn't feel
quite himself today has it exactly right. Sickness is like a hostile takeover in
which the part of your mind which hurts manages completely to dominate and silence the rest of you."[138] Not just one's self, but one's moral situation is confused
by illness. Arthur Frank, a sociologist who had cancer, found serious illness a
loss of the "destination and map" that had guided his life.[139] "However cancer
may be anticipated in fantasy, the reality is different. When I was told about the
lymph nodes on my chest X-ray, I was amazed at what a narrative wreck I was: I
who spend my life telling stories about illness, my own as well as others. Somehow the stories we have in place never fit the reality, and sometimes this disjunction can be worse than having no story at all."[140]

The literature on the stability of patient preferences is preliminary and equivocal, but it seems to confirm what one would suppose—that people learn from and
change with experience and that uncertainty and ambivalence lead people to

waver and equivocate. Thus even patients who seem ideally situated to make a stable decision—pregnant women deciding in advance whether to have an epidural during delivery—change their minds in nontrivial numbers during childbirth.[141] Experience with cardiopulmonary resuscitation apparently decreases the wish for it.[141a] A study of twenty male ICU patients over the age of fifty who were interviewed upon transfer out of the ICU and one month later found that "approximately 10–15 percent of patients who had desired a particular life-sustaining treatment while in the ICU expressed their wish to forego this treatment at the follow-up interview. Similar numbers changed their mind in the opposite direction."[142] A larger and longer study asked patients to write advance directives and requestioned them after six and twelve months. It found 72% agreement over time.[142a] A yet larger and longer study questioned people over two years about whether they would want various life-sustaining treatments if they were terminally ill. "Instability was substantial during the 2-year period in patients' preferences for a given treatment."[142b] More specifically: "Of the patients who answered 'yes' to any of the questions at baseline, only 18% to 43% answered 'yes' to the same question at follow-up. Patients responding 'no' to baseline questions were more consistent, with 66% to 75% still answering 'no' at follow-up."[143] As still another study explained, "Patients may change their wishes for life-sustaining therapy because of their experience with their illness, changes in their subjective appreciation of their 'quality of life,' or changes in their evaluation of the benefits and burdens of life-sustaining measures as they realize the imminence of death."[144]

Patients' memoirs confirm what these studies attest—that experience changes opinion. One doctor-turned-patient wrote frankly, "While I had expressed a strong rejection of amputation prior to the biopsy, like most people who do not have to face the problem squarely, I promptly abandoned this point of view."[145] Ernest Hirsch had originally regarded multiple sclerosis as a "strange, somewhat bizarre, frightening illness," but he found that as it developed it lost those qualities.[146] He was relieved to observe that things he could no longer do "lost much of their importance. Such things as driving, running, walking and standing are no longer within the sphere of possibility and are therefore not missed as though they were possible."[147] He discovered that "[g]radual changes have taken place in my outlooks, in my likes and dislikes, in what I feel to be a natural part of my life and in what I had always regarded as a necessity for happiness."[148] He concluded, "Probably had I known in 1956 what would be the symptoms that have appeared by now, I would have been anxious about and discouraged by the prospect of the future. Now that I actually find myself here, however, it seems that things are not nearly so bad as I would have thought then."[149]

These examples of the way experience changes preferences are primarily instances of people who learned that staying alive was more important and disabilities were less intolerable than they had thought. An oncologist tells the story of a patient whose beliefs moved in the opposite direction. Jerome Groopman's patient was an aggressive short-term investor with badly metastized kidney cancer. Initially, Groopman told his patient what every other doctor had—that nothing could be done. The patient insisted on treatment: " 'If you will help me, I'll undergo anything. The worst side effects. They can't be worse to me than'—he paused—'being dead.' "[150] Groopman's treatment was astonishingly successful. But when the cancer recurred, the patient was apathetic. He had found during his remission that " 'my deals and trades seemed pointless, because I was a short-term investor. . . . I had no interest in creating something.' " He concluded that his wife and children would be " 'fine without me' " and that he was " 'a self-absorbed, uncaring shit.' "[151] In short, attitudes that had seemed an inextricable part of his personality—" 'I'm not ready to just pack it up and die. I'm a fighter.' "[152]—were displaced by their diametric opposite under the pressure of recovery.

Developing experience can change preferences. And so can fluctuating emotions. A patient awaiting a heart transplant underwent "pendulous mood swings, which, in turn, are dictated by my current state of health."[153] Wilfrid Sheed found that "the imagining self can give you a bad day at any point and, either way, always seem to be either far ahead or behind the rest of you at accepting the new regime, bouncing in with impossibly good news one day and inconceivably bad the next, as optimism and regret war for your attention."[154] Such unstable emotions can alter one's very perception of reality. For example, Etzioni describes a "typical study" which found that when subjects are "sad, negative events are viewed as more likely and good outcomes as less likely than when subjects are in a neutral mood. . . . In short, mood biases cognition."[155] How much more, then, must mood bias preference?

Even a patient whose beliefs are well considered and well established may be hard put to deduce what conclusions about medical care should follow from them, for it is perilous to infer courses of action from statements of principle. As lawyers have special cause to know, general principles do not settle particular cases. They do not settle cases because often several conclusions can be reached from one principle. One of the most common principles is "I am a fighter." But does that mean that you want to try every treatment unto the bitter end or that you don't want to wage a war you can't win? General principles do not settle cases because no one can anticipate all the circumstances in which they might apply. "I do not want to be intubated" is a principle many patients adopt because they associate intubation with the pointless prolongation of life; they have not anticipated a brief intubation leading to recovery. General principles do not settle cases because they usually contain terms whose definition is uncertain. "I don't want to endure hopeless treatments" is another common principle, but "hopeless" both demands and resists definition. General principles do not settle cases because one principle usually conflicts with others: "I want to live" often fights with "I want to avoid pain."

Finally, principles do not settle cases because they often require comparing incommensurables. For example, the Simmons study tells of a donor "who attempted to follow the classical deliberation model and found himself frustrated by having to weigh normative obligations against a risk to the self and by his lack of expert knowledge in evaluating the risk."[156] Today's cliché says "quality, not quantity." But quantity matters, and what scale tells you how much gain in quality is worth how much loss in quantity? As a thoughtful cancer patient said: "There is less than twenty-percent chance that chemo could extend my life six months at the end. Traditional chemotherapy has no curative and limited palliative value for my thyroid cancer. While still squirming over the very nature of such a choice, I decline the offer (not recommendation) of chemo. Thirty-percent? Forty? What odds warrant what gambles? I don't know. Six healthy rather than sick months? Probably."[157] Or consider the statement of values Betty Rollin gave her doctor: "I looked at him and decided to say what I had been thinking. . . . 'Do what you think is best. But I want to be sure you understand what is important to me. I do not want to die. That's number one. And number two is—I am vain. OK? I am vain. I—would like not to be very hideous, if—if that's possible.' "[158] How much guidance could her doctor—or Rollin herself—derive from these two principles? How much extra risk to life is to be tolerated for how much gain in appearance?

For all these reasons, general principles do not settle cases. For all these reasons, we do not know in advance what general principles actually mean or what we actually believe. Each new case puts a principle to a new test, a test that may reveal that we did not understand or did not really accept the principle. Each new case may thus lead us to reexamine and reformulate the principle. Ultimately, we learn what our principles mean and refine them only by repeatedly applying them to concrete cases.

The opacity of principles is illustrated when we draw inferences about what incompetent patients would have wanted from our knowledge of their beliefs. Several studies find family members (and even more physicians) are often hard put—despite their long and intimate knowledge of the patient—to predict what patients would want in even relatively simple circumstances. As one review of the literature concluded, "studies addressing the utility of the substituted judgment standard have documented substantial lack of accuracy in proxy determinations of patient preferences for care at the end of life under diverse clinical circumstances."[159] This might be because people do not develop clear enough principles while they are competent, but that ought to be less true where patients have written advance directives. Yet despite the clarity for which these documents strive, they often turn out, when applied, to be remarkably ambiguous.[160]

Data take patients only so far. Often "values" take them little farther. An AIDS patient commented, "It was time to make a choice. All of the questions in the world, answered and unanswered, couldn't help me."[161] Another patient wrote that when her doctor "had mentioned Clomid, she had talked as if it were no big deal. But I thought taking something like that into one's body, messing with one's hormones, was serious business. To me it meant another decision, and as usual I didn't know everything I'd like to know—such as, *Is this a good idea or not?*"[162]

Under the autonomy paradigm, patients may rely on doctors for help in amassing, assimilating, and analyzing medical data. But patients are supposed to be unique authorities on their "values," on the principles which guide their medical choices. In this section, I have suggested those principles are often obscure. Many patients lack considered religious or philosophical convictions. Even if they have such convictions, they may be puzzled about how to deduce principles of medical care from them. Even if those principles can be securely deduced, they may change with the experience of illness and treatment. Even if those principles remain stable, patients may find it hard to deduce decisions from them. In short, even someone who has built a careful structure of beliefs and analyzed them well may struggle to supply the "values" needed in making medical decisions, for human goods conflict and tragic choices are inevitable: "We ask, 'What course without evils?' but we know that no true answer will give us comfort."[163]

Conclusion

We launched this investigation into the difficulty of medical decisions to learn why patients might not crave the decisional authority the autonomy paradigm envisions for them. I have argued that those decisions are so complex, so foreign, so tumultuous, so recalcitrant, so confounding, so demanding that patients might reasonably hope to escape them. They might, like Eileen Radziunas, believe they are not "qualified, able, or willing to continue to coordinate my complicated health care."[164] They might, that is, reasonably conclude that someone else— their doctors, their families, their friends—would make their decisions better than they. They might decide that referring their decisions to someone else was the course of prudence. They might agree with one patient I interviewed, a person of the most exceptional education and intelligence, who was intellectually aggressive and strong-minded, who was socially forthright and even fierce, who had exerted himself to find good doctors, and who had worked assiduously to be well informed:

> I think I have a tendency with all experts with whom I deal to believe that you get the information from the reputation of who is the best person you can get and then you rely on that person. That basically, that even if I read all this text [i.e., medical literature], I will never in a short time absorb what they have had over a period of time to be able to make that kind of judgment. I want to know a lot about the person that I am dealing with and, once I have done that, as I have said, I feel that then I am paying him for his best judgment. My best chance is to use his best judgment, not mine, at that point.

Delegating medical decisions is not the only reasonable strategy for patients, nor always the wisest. Patients who want to make their own decisions—and there appear to be many—should be helped to do so. But the survey we have just completed suggests one plausible reason for the disjunction between what the autonomy paradigm calls for and what the empirical evidence suggests some substantial body of patients seems to want: Many patients delegate medical decisions because they believe someone else will make them better than they can.

The Life of the Sick

It takes time for an ill person to understand her needs. The caregiver cannot simply ask "What do you need?" and expect a coherent reply. A recently diagnosed person's life has already changed in more ways than she can grasp, and changes continue throughout critical illness. Part of what is "critical" is the persistence of change. Being critically ill means never being able to keep up with your own needs. Except for the need to hear that it is all a mistake—the lab results had the wrong name on them; I'm fine, really—the ill person does not know what she needs, though the needs are very real.   Arthur W. Frank, *At the Will of the Body*

To appreciate the force of the second reason patients might reject the leading role in their medical decisions, we should recall the syllogism that lies silent at the heart of the autonomist paradigm: People want to make all decisions that shape their lives. Few decisions matter more than medicine's life-or-death, sickness-or-health, fit-or-frail choices. Therefore patients want to make their own medical decisions. I argued in the previous section that this syllogism is flawed because some patients conclude they will reach wiser decisions by deferring to the expertise and judgment of someone else. But the syllogism errs in other ways, ways suggested by what Talcott Parsons called the "sick role, with how people feel when they are ill."[165] The autonomy paradigm rests on assumptions about the natural desire of all people to control themselves and their surroundings. As I will contend in Chapter 4, these assumptions are overstated even for the population at large. But sick people differ from healthy people, for they often feel frightened, discouraged, dull-witted, abstracted, uninterested, and weary. These feelings, I will now suggest, may inhibit them from making medical decisions.

The Work of the Sick

We have just seen how arduous and distressing medical decisions can be. Even healthy people sometimes (indeed, regularly) cede control over decisions in the face of untoward demands on their energy, intelligence, interest, time, and attention. How much more, then, might sick people—even sick people who felt intellectually prepared—wish to escape so onerous and unpromising a burden? Oliver Sacks, surrounded by fellow patients, realized that "[w]e had all, in our ways, been undermined by sickness, had lost the careless boldness, the freedom, of the well."[166] Thus some patients will accept that they lack—if only temporarily—the vigor, the persistence, the dispassion, the alertness, the concentration, the courage, the will—to resolve the riddles and face the bafflements of their medical distress. Such sick people may avoid all kinds of work, especially the fierce, foreign, and forbidding work of medical decisions. As one doctor-turned-patient observed,

> Too sick at first to respond in any other than an automatic "reflex" way, it was only now that I could bring out any new response which took into account the new facts. It was as though all before had been on a low level and only along lines ingrained from previous beliefs and behavior patterns. While words made sense, evaluations and thoughts did not. Nature seemed to reserve all energy for combating the disease. The transition of response was gradual and the evolution of critical appraisal and facing facts cannot be labeled as having occurred on any one day or in any one week.[167]

And Reynolds Price

> was plunged into degrees of pain and realistic depression that produced a dangerously passive state. In that psychic bog of helplessness, like most trapped sufferers, I was transfixed by the main sight in view—my undiminished physical pain. And in such a trance state, for that's what a heavily drugged life is, any personal crusade for sane alternative therapies was literally unthinkable to me. It was all I could do to focus my scarce strength and clarity on one main aim beyond plain endurance.[168]

Exhaustion dogs patients' lives. Their reserves of energy depleted, the severely ill barely stumble through the day. They lose the physical strength and emotional fortitude to keep their houses clean, their families cared for, and their friendships alive, much less to earn a living. They can hardly rise out of bed, brush their teeth, or make breakfast.[169] One cancer patient was so weary he could not "read a newspaper for more than 15 minutes."[170] Another said: "Weakness was the central experience—a bankruptcy of strength and energy. A few hours in the morning used it all up, and there was no reserve account on which to draw. I was overdrawn at the energy bank."[171] In these straits, the labor of living preempts the work of medical decisions.

All these are calls on patients' reserves that are a normal part of life. But those reserves are also sapped by the special demands of illness. Patients must devote resources to recovering from their disease and coping with it physically, mentally, and spiritually. Some of this effort is tiring because it is hard physical work, like rehabilitation after a stroke. Some of it is psychologically wearing. As Herzlich and Pierret write,

> Mentally, some persons find it very difficult to be responsible for their own treatment. . . . The young secretary acknowledged: "Always, *always having to pay attention,* that . . . is something that people have trouble accepting. *This is the thing that's hard to learn,* because the shots . . . . I am always worried, but I do it. The analyses are not hard to do, but what is so constraining is that one has to pay attention at all times." The older diabetic also said, "That is why we who are sick are so tired, because we always have to gather up our will power to do the things that have to be done, and that one couldn't deal with if one let oneself go."[172]

Many patients also must strive to manage their emotions, to sustain their spirits, to stop the slide into soul-sickening anger, frustration, and depression. As a doctor with cancer wrote, "I only know that during this time I felt blighted physically and overrun psychologically. I am sure that deep within me I was furious at the fates which had brought me to my knees in youth. Had I had the energy and a target, or even a surrogate target, I imagine I would have broken out in rage. But I was past being angry. What I do remember feeling was despair."[173] In addition, patients must work to adjust to the fact of their illness and their damaged future. Thus Michael Kelly says the decision to have surgery for colitis "is not about the absence or presence of particular information nor about its distortion, it is about the individuals changing their view of themselves so that they define themselves as sick. . . . The process is one of aligning the self with the public identity of prospective and actual surgical case."[174]

These kinds of work can mount up to become all-demanding, so that medical decisions seem too expensive a distraction which can better be shuffled off onto intimates or experts. James Johnson, for example, had to decide about a skin graft after a long hospitalization for dire heart problems. He could hardly face even this relatively trivial decision, for he "suffered from battle fatigue. I'd had my fill of doctors and hospitals." So "[a]t this point, I knew I could not go on trying to figure it out."[175] When considering whether she should make her own medical decisions, Joie McGrail concluded "it would be wasteful to use energy that would be desperately needed to fight my disease in simply asserting my personality, so I allowed myself to be trundled about, poked, prodded, kept waiting and rushed."[176] Eileen Radziunas wrote sorrowfully that she "carried the burden of being the one to suggest ideas, ask about tests, and question possible diagnoses. I felt overwhelmed with all this responsibility, and I needed the *doctors* to take control so that I could use all my energy for recovering."[177] Thus Kenneth Cohn found it "comforting to be treated by competent dedicated professionals. Their skill allowed me to eschew the medical literature on lymphoma and to focus on being a patient."[178]

Agnes de Mille captures so many of the reactions of so many sick people to making medical decisions that she must be quoted at length. When she had a stroke, she was not young, but as a dancer, she had lived vigorously. As a choreographer she had bustled with energy until she was, literally and figuratively, stricken:

> I was taken up with the minutiae of living. Everything was so extraordinarily difficult and so new to perform. Every single act became a contest of skill; and games can be tiring. I did not concern myself with the medical details. There are patients who do, and presume, after a short while, to advise the doctors and to interfere in their conferences. I wanted none of that. . . . I watched them at it and I was glad for their expertise, but I did not seek in any way to share it, and even when they tried to explain it to me I resisted. I was reluctant to learn because I didn't think the horrid details would help me to keep my energies where they belonged—on survival. The dreadful possibilities were entirely the doctor's business.[179]

In sum, illness lays strength and stamina to waste. Thus the sick may decline to make their own medical decisions because they have too little vitality and too much to spend it on.

The Burdens of the Sick

Recall what it is like to be sick: "[A] little cooling down of animal excitability and instinct, a little loss of animal toughness, a little irritable weakness and descent of the pain-threshold, will bring the worm at the core of all our usual springs of delight into full view, and turn us into melancholy metaphysicians."[180] The only benefit, the only comfort, you may find in being sick is that other people will care for you, and you can let them, let them fix your meals, bring your pills, rub your back. May Sarton captures both these aspects of the sick person's life: "How I have enjoyed complete passivity! Being 'looked after' like a Paddington bear—listening to the bustle in the corridor as though from very far away so even the noisy voices didn't trouble my floating. But I still feel frightfully tired and so I dread going home."[181] Even patients who always resented dependence may savor it when they are ill. Agnes de Mille reflects, "Up to May 15, as far as it was possible for a woman to be independent, I had been independent. Now, not so. I cared nothing. Let me lie still. Let me be. As far as I was concerned, people could wait on me, serve me, help me in every way."[182] And a doctor fallen ill found that

> [f]or one of the few times in my adult life, I felt that I was being taken care of completely. Everything was being provided for my care. I did not have to make any decisions or take any responsibility for my thoughts or actions. It was an especially good feeling to be cared for, and secretly I still cherish those days that I spent in the hospital although not the reason why I had to be there.[183]

As that doctor gratefully recognized, people may particularly spare you the travail of decision. As another patient put it, "I allowed myself the forgotten luxury of childhood: other people were in charge."[184] Jay Katz remorselessly disparages "the regression to more childlike functioning that can result from illness [and that] becomes augmented by a patient's wish for caretaking by a patient-physician who, as memory informs, will immediately alleviate all suffering."[185] But I believe Sacks speaks with wiser tongue when he observes more sympathetically that, "though as a sick patient, in hospital, one was reduced to moral infancy, this was not a malicious degradation, but a biological and spiritual need of the hurt creature. One *had* to go back, one *had* to regress, for one might indeed be as helpless as a child, whether one liked it, or willed it, or not. In hospital, one became again a child with parents (parents who might be good or bad) and this might be felt as 'infantilizing' and degrading or as a sweet and sorely-needed nourishing."[186] Such patients may accept the comfort of relief from the burdens of decision.

In addition, even more than most of us, the sick may wish to escape not just the wearisome labor of medical decisions, but also the responsibility for such savagely difficult choices, choices on which their own happiness and that of their friends and families may so much depend but which are so bewildering. When decisions go wrong, many patients blame themselves and feel blamed. Thus one study of kidney donors concludes, "[W]here the costs of failure on both sides are so great, our impression is that individuals frequently wish to absolve themselves of the responsibility of the decision. Deliberation and a conscious decision emphasize the freedom of one's choice and one's responsibility for the choice. To hold oneself responsible for a potentially disastrous outcome is painful, however."[187]

Robert Murphy, an anthropologist dying of a spinal tumor, put this observation into more personal form. He acknowledged that "the patient is responsible for his own recovery, and this has many positive aspects." However, he learned it has its drawbacks too:

> [If] his efforts can yield improvement, then any failure to improve can be an indication that he isn't trying hard enough, that he is to blame for his own condition. This load of culpability is often added to a lingering suspicion among family and friends that the patient was responsible, somehow or other, for what happened to him. And the patient, too, is often beset with guilt over his plight—a seemingly illogical, but very common, by-product of disability.[188]

The authors of a study comparing the desires of cancer patients and the general public for participation in medical decisions generalize this point: "The strong effect [on the desire to make decisions] of the presence or absence of cancer suggested that decision making preferences might be influenced by diagnosis of a life-threatening illness. In that context, being freed of responsibility for making treatment decisions can produce an immense sense of relief, with treatment failures becoming the responsibility of the practitioner rather than the patient."[189]

The problem is not just that a baneful sense of responsibility may impede decisions in the first place and make living with them tormenting. It is also that that sense warps decisions. Thus the study of kidney donation I quoted a moment ago found that people burdened with this sense "are motivated to regard the decision [to donate] as inevitable—as the only possible alternative, given the enormous moral obligation, or the social pressure, or the fact that another family member volunteered first, or the perception that this issue is not one's moral responsibility. Thus, while the outsider sees the potential donor as making a choice, the potential donor himself is likely to describe it as 'no decision at all.'"[190]

Medical decisions may repel patients for yet another reason. Such decisions cannot ordinarily be made well without acquiring thorough information about one's illness and analyzing it carefully. But not everyone finds that learning and thinking interesting, or pleasant, or even tolerable, particularly at the level of intensity and persistence needed to make complex and unfamiliar decisions. Some patients—like William Martin, the sociologist with prostate cancer—may "want to keep on looking stuff up and trying to make sense of it for as long as I can," and they may become "totally engrossed in trying to unravel the riddles of prostate cancer, sometimes almost to the point of forgetting just why I had developed such a keen interest in the subject."[191] But other patients will not have made research their life's work, will not know how to do it, will not enjoy it, will not like learning a new vocabulary and thinking in foreign ways, and will find better things to do with their time. Indeed, some people find medicine, and even their own ailments and treatments, boring. Few subjects are universally fascinating, and medicine is not one of them. As Wilfrid Sheed writes,

> I've never been the least interested in the nuts and bolts of sickness and health. In fact, even when I've been so ill myself that there's been no avoiding them, my position has always been "Just tell me what I'm supposed to do, and who do you like in the World Series?" or the Oscars, or any damn thing that doesn't require thermometers and blood tests every half hour.[192]

Even people who once were fascinated by medical questions may see them pall after months of the tedium of patienthood. One couple put the point bluntly: "*We are both so weary of this medical junk.*"[193]

Furthermore, many patients—especially the gravely ill—will not relish having to think about the terrible and terrifying things that are happening to them, the cruel uncertainties they must endure,[194] the wretched alternatives they confront, or the bitter prospects they face. For just such reasons many people resist buying life insurance, writing wills, preparing advance directives, signing organ-donor cards, seeing the doctor,[195] and even visiting sick friends.[196] In short, some patients will be disqualified from making decisions by their reluctance to learn enough about their illness.[197] For Lance Morrow, "Having a heart attack and waiting for another at any moment results in an especially wearing and unlikeable introspection. It is a physical introspection entirely, an in-peering anxiety, my focused self standing like a peasant outside the castle walls, awaiting the caprice of a lord who is given to drunken rages."[198] Joseph Heller says wryly: "My attending doctors . . . had adopted the sensible approach of not giving me any distressing information about my illness unless they had to; and I had adopted the sensible defense of not seeking any."[199] The mother of a child with cancer wrote that "the few articles and newspaper paragraphs I have read are certainly inadequate; yet I do not intend to become an authority on Carol's leukemia. Intuitively, I desire to keep all bitter informants at bay, to study no discouraging life expectancy charts or bleak percentages."[200] Ernest Hirsch, a psychologist and a thoughtful man with multiple sclerosis, shunned the literature on his disease, since in it "the illness tends to be described in its most acute, extreme and often final form. Such an account naturally makes reading about the illness depressing, particularly to a patient who is afflicted with it."[201] Reynolds Price, a writer with cancer of the spinal cord, reports,

From the start of the trouble, I made a conscious choice not to open my file and confront what doctors believed was the worst—I saw in their eyes that they had slim hope, and I knew I must defy them. On balance I think the choice of a high degree of ignorance proved good for me. All my life I've tended to try to meet people's hopes. Predict my death and I'm liable to oblige; keep me ignorant and I stand a chance of lasting.[202]

Finally, Molly Haskell reports that when a doctor told the mother of her desperately sick husband that he (the doctor) "couldn't promise he wouldn't have brain damage," Haskell was "stunned, outraged, first, that he should say such a thing to her, and second, because it was a possibility I hadn't allowed myself to even think about. How dare he answer a question that nobody had asked! I told him from now on not to volunteer grim information unless we asked for it."[203]

Such patients do not warmly welcome the practice of informed consent: "I signed everything without reading any of it, and tried not to listen while he told me in great detail what would happen later that morning. All I wanted to know was, would it hurt?"[204] And: "I signed it quickly, not noticing too much of any of it. If it were going to happen, it would happen. But it was a bit frightening as I thought of that long list."[205] Even less formal communications can be disturbing: "Another sort of drowning is inflicted on us patients by doctors who think out loud while they examine you. These physicians not only expose you to their full conclusions, they expose you to the full process by which they reach these conclusions. As your examination proceeds you hear all the malfunctions you might have, as well as those you do have, and you have twice as much to worry about."[206] Thus one ill doctor "learned how simple words from a physician can strike absolute terror into the hearts of patients. A well-meaning internal medicine resident remarked offhand, as he pushed on my belly, that my liver seemed 'a little enlarged.' The fear of metastatic malignancy nearly turned me to jelly."[207]

As this last example suggests, even patients who are professionally equipped to understand their illness may not wish to know too much. One doctor afflicted with cancer wrote,

I am terrified at the thought of examining my own chart for fear that someone has recorded in it a poor prognosis. I know that's illogical and that I should look to see if there's an error that could be corrected. But I am no longer able to function as my own doctor. My confidence has been worn down—by my fears about my illness, of course, but also by something more subtle, something that's happened psychologically over these past months.[208]

Another doctor with cancer observed, "I knew as much as anyone about X-rays and easily could have examined my own on the way back to the clinic. I never did. The possibility that I would again discover trouble in my chest was so horrifying to me that it quenched my curiosity."[209] Yet another doctor acquired an aversion "to learning anything new or even remotely pessimistic about my dis-

ease and its complications." He reasoned, "It is a doctor's job to search diligently
for the worst. The *patient* hopes eternally for the best. When they are the same
person, the conflict becomes extremely difficult (perhaps impossible) to recon-
cile."[210]

But even if patients' curiosity is not quenched, even if they want information,
the same fear that deters them from asking for it may keep them from assimilating
it. When some of the colitis patients Michael Kelly studied were told they needed
surgery, they "expressed great surprise when the operation was first mentioned to
them, this in spite of the fact that several had been attending surgical out-patient
clinics over many months."[211] One such patient "tried not to think about it. 'I just
blocked it out. I just didn't want to know. I just couldn't picture it at all. All I knew
was that you would have a bag. I just didn't want to know.'"[212] Another patient
"refused to acknowledge that she was a prospective surgical case, even after she
had been admitted to hospital for the operation . . . . She claimed that she
thought she was going into hospital for tests."[213] And Gerda Lerner believed her
husband "undoubtedly 'knew' before I told him" of his brain tumor,

> and certainly many times refused to "know" after I told him. He was already deeply
> caught up in the process of dying and conscious knowledge was only a minor as-
> pect of it. Just so it is with me now: the fact of his death, his absence, is incontro-
> vertible. I "know" it in many different ways and with many different modes of per-
> ception. Yet, to this day, I still do not "know" it the way I know other facts. It shifts;
> it wavers—sometimes it is as true as a rock; sometimes it is as true as a bad dream.
> I imagine it must be that way for the dying until that final stage when they really
> "know"—then they let go.[214]

To put the point somewhat differently, patients may prefer to "deny" their illness, avoid information about it, suppress thoughts of it, and try to go about their
business as though they were well. Popular psychology has cursed "denial" with
a bad name, perhaps with some cause.[215] But denial has its uses, for happiness
"has blindness and insensibility to opposing facts given it as its instinctive
weapon for self-protection against disturbance."[216] Paul Monette observes, "This
force of life continuing is what they mean by 'positive denial.'"[217] Robert Murphy said he "once asked the neurologist how bad it could get, and, with a pained
expression, he answered, 'Do you really want to know?' I didn't."[218] Murphy
commended the "well-tuned repression mechanism, the ability to become detached from one's emotions, to benumb the inroads of fear."[219] He acknowledged
that "[t]his kind of repression is bought at considerable emotional cost, but it has
its positive uses. Some fears and sentiments are better left unstated, and those
that I harbored as I entered the hospital in 1976 were among them. What I refused
to contemplate was the progressive and total destruction of my body, the reduc-
tion of all volition to quietude, the entombment of my mind in inert proto-
plasm."[220] And a seriously ill doctor thought "psychiatrists only preach nonsense
when they say: 'Adjust to reality.' We can only really endure life if we cherish

healthy illusions, if we have faith no matter how fantastic, or the kind of healthy-mindedness that shakes off, as a dog shakes off water, the disagreeables of now and the future."[221]

These opinions have even found scholarly defenders. Arthur Kleinman, for instance, writes, "[D]enial and illusion are ready at hand to assure that life events are not so threatening and supports seem more durable. . . . In short, self-deception makes chronic illness tolerable. Who can say that illusion and myth are not useful to maintain optimism, which itself may improve physiological performance . . . ?"[222] And Kelly argues, "Rather then perceiving denial in these circumstances as evidence of a malformed psyche incapable of dealing with reality or as an automatic psychological defence, it is better to regard it as a *realistic* response in the absence of the necessary skills to deal with the illness."[223] Evidence that "denial" can sometimes be sensible also comes from empirical studies showing, for instance, that "[a]lthough some patients seek out information prior to surgery, such information does not always reduce their arousal levels or promote recuperation from surgery . . . . Indeed, information may actually increase arousal and retard recovery . . . ."[224] Thus, Miller and Mangan note that while laboratory studies show that most people want information about an aversive event, "in less artificial studies that mirror real life . . . , the preference reverses: The majority of individuals then prefer to distract themselves from threat-relevant information . . . ."[225]

Many memoirists put these opinions in terms of hope, "the only fuel that keeps them going."[226] Natalie Spingarn writes: "I have found no skill more important (no matter how it is gained) than the ability to believe in my survival, for at least a bit longer. For this, I am dependent on how my fellow human beings—doctors and nurses, family and friends— . . . reinforce the hope that sustains my life."[227] She tried "to avoid the medical mighties who with their harsh 'honest' words—and I cannot say it often enough—deprive me of the hope that I can fend off my enemy, death."[228] Their "blunt, tell-it-like-it-is" way of speaking may reflect "the common wisdom that *knowing all the news, whatever it may be, is 'good' for you,* conversely, [that] it is *'weak' to try to avoid even a single cancer statistic inferring bad news, even if it helps deprive you of hope."* But Spingarn disapproved: "Hope, I repeat once again, is the essential ingredient. Without it, we patients can find no reason for struggling to survive; without it, we find it easy to give up and stay in bed."[229] Thus she remained "peeved at the physician who told me over the telephone when my second breast cancer was diagnosed, 'We have to stop talking in terms of cure and begin talking in terms of control—one year, maybe two.' "[230] In sum, while some patients may cope with disease by visiting a medical library and tackling the relevant literature, others will be anxious to avoid learning about their illness, contemplating their perilous condition, acknowledging their grim choices, imagining their possible fates, or making medical decisions.

Many of my points about how being sick disinclines one to seize control of one's medical decisions are captured in a provocative article by Franz Ingelfinger, an editor of the *New England Journal of Medicine* stricken with the very illness he had specialized in as a physician. He

> received from physician friends throughout the country a barrage of well-intentioned but contradictory advice. . . . As a result, not only I but my wife, my son and daughter-in-law (both doctors), and other family members became increasingly confused and emotionally distraught. Finally, when the pangs of indecision had become nearly intolerable, one wise physician friend said, "What you need is a doctor." He was telling me to forget the information I already had and the information I was receiving from many quarters, and to seek instead a person who would dominate, who would tell me what to do, who would in a paternalistic manner assume responsibility for my care. When that excellent advice was followed, my family and I sensed immediate and immense relief. The incapacity of enervating worry was dispelled, and I could return to my usual anxieties . . . .[231]

Ingelfinger is not alone. The editors of an anthology of doctors' accounts of illness report,

> Autonomy may be lauded for modern patients, but it is not something sick physicians usually choose for themselves once they have found a doctor. Sick doctors want to be taken care of, even if they try to remain in control; we find the most relief when someone else takes over. Here we are, a group with special knowledge, and often trying to exert control beyond the bounds of reason, and yet almost to a man or woman sick doctors who express an opinion suggest that they want to be taken care of so that they can give up their lonely vigil. Most of them want to be cared for, have decisions made for them.[232]

Perhaps doctors' testimony on this score should be doubted (although they seem especially suited to make their own medical decisions). But a similar reaction appears in the memoirs of lay patients. One wrote, "I think my husband helped me to transfer worry and responsibility to the doctors' shoulders instead of carrying the burdens myself. That was very important. It gave all of us something to lean on."[233] A patient with infertility found "something reassuring in the order that [her doctor] imposed on the situation, the idea that there was a definite path to tread, and she'd take me by the hand. When I left the office, I was excited and relieved."[234] Another kind of evidence comes from Ellen Annandale's study of a birth clinic which appealed to women who wished to be unchained from the bonds of medical authority. Even there, studying clients who were presumably vigorous, independent-minded, and healthy, Annandale witnessed the relief of abdicated autonomy: " 'I didn't need to worry about making decisions and could leave it all to [the midwives] . . . . I felt utterly relaxed being at home and having complete faith in those around me.' "[235]

I have been suggesting reasons the sick may be in no mood to plunge into medical decisions. Let me close with one other. The standard argument is that patients should make their own decisions because those decisions so much affect them. By the same token, becoming immersed in your medical decisions means thinking intensively about yourself. Even in our psychologized, therapeutic society, not everyone believes this is a good idea. Some see a moral duty to temper their interest in themselves and invest it in their neighbors. Others are skeptical on prudential grounds. Sheed, for example, counsels against self-absorption. He admonishes advice columnists: "So tell your readers to go dancing, overeat at least once, or buy a book about Napoleon (*not* about self-help, or self-anything. Tell them to forget themselves for five minutes. The air outside is wonderful)."[236] Sheed's attitude is so resonant that we have a word—valetudinarian—for people too fascinated by their illness and themselves.

Conclusion

The points I have made in this section may helpfully be seen in light of patient's memoirs. As I suggested earlier, often they are not primarily about making medical decisions, or even about patients' relationships with doctors. Rather, they are about what it means to be a person who is sick. They are about how illness ravages the body, staggers the rhythms of daily life, distorts personal relationships, and destroys the familiar. They are about how illness savages the mind and leaves it brooding and afraid. They are about how people struggle with pain and uncertainty. They are about how people labor to make sense of their pasts and their futures, their lives and their deaths. These memoirs suggest, then, that while medical decisions may have crucial consequences for patients, they will not always be most central, most pressing, or even most interesting to patients. To people "wrestling with the crises of their fate,"[237] medical decisions may seem a distraction, not a duty.

For many patients, medical decisions are both above and beneath their attention. Above, because patients are concentrated on day-to-day coping. They try to perdure with their lives despite their disease, to make it to work, to get a full night's sleep, to see their families, to get the laundry done and the lawn mowed, to pay the bills and call the plumber. They do not ignore their illness. But their attention is concerned with adapting to it, not treating it. They ask how they can learn to walk after a stroke, find a ride to dialysis sessions, avoid insulin shock, cope with incontinence, follow their diet, or manage their drugs and lives to reduce the risk of seizures.

On the other hand, medical decisions fall beneath patients' attention because illness urgently presents the largest kind of questions to them, questions about their religious faith, about whether their lives have been well led, about what a good life is. Patients ask why they became sick, whether they managed their careers well, whether they loved and were loved, whether they enjoyed their lives, whether their lives were spiritually fulfilling, and, as to all these questions, how to do better in whatever future might remain. This leads some patients to become preoccupied with their emotional and spiritual development. For patients who have sought "alternative" therapies, the psychological, the spiritual, and the medical can become as one and become everything in their lives. Thus David Tate's experience with Hodgkin's disease (and later a heart attack) helped take him from Roman Catholicism and a career in the law and real estate to life as a psychotherapist and a New Age stand-up comic who found meaning in, among other things, Silva Mind Control, Edgar Cayce readings, acupuncture, psychic healing, Carlos Castaneda, Jonathan Livingston Seagull, Paramahansa Yogananda, spiritualism, Esalen, and transpersonal psychology, particularly psychosynthesis.[238]

Even if patients are not preoccupied with their spiritual situation, they may be absorbed by moral crisis.[239] As Sheed writes, "The details of any illness are too tedious and repetitive to occupy you for more than part of the time and what you do with the rest is critically important in this case, as you bet your whole self against death."[240] Thus "[t]he interesting part is all provided by you, an average citizen and image of God, finding out for probably the first time what's been in you all along."[241] Here Sheed is reflecting on his three illnesses—the polio he endured as an adolescent, the depression and addiction he fought in middle age, and the cancer he suffered as he emerged from the depression and addiction. To Sheed, illness is crucially a battle of character and courage. The news he brings from the front is hopeful. He writes, for instance, "Numerous people who have had to care for critically injured patients have testified, as polio nurses once did, to how amazingly quickly the patient's spirit seems to take over and begin to pull *them* through, as if it were a new presence in the room, preternaturally strong and self-assured."[242] Nevertheless, much of what absorbed his attention and energy in his illnesses was the moral problem of managing his response to the depredations of disease and the menace of death.

Now in principle, none of these concerns—whether quotidian or cosmic—has to preclude a patient from making medical decisions. But in practice, such concerns often divert patients' interest, attention, and energy away from the process of informed consent and the tasks of medical choice. The concerns I have been describing not only consume patients' time but are emotionally and intellectually draining. The sick will often prefer to treat their medical decisions as fixed points about which they need not worry and around which they can work.

Patients who cede authority to make medical decisions for the reasons I have examined in this section obviously run risks—the risks classically associated with paternalism. But the reason they run those risks differs from the usual justification for paternalism. These patients do not necessarily say someone else knows their situation and interests better than they. Rather, they say that, whoever might make the best choice, they do not wish to bear the weight of formulating a decision. Nor are these patients necessarily delegating decisions to the ordinary paternalists—their doctors. In my research, I have often encountered people who instead (or as well) ceded authority to their families, in whose concern, vigor, wisdom, and faithfulness they reposed their trust.

We may admire people who take on the burdens of illness, chart their own course, and, resolute, remain captains of their fates and masters of their souls. But surely we can understand sick people who shudder at the labors of analyzing their own medical problems, who ask to forget the terrors that assail them, who yearn to share the responsibilities that crowd upon them, who hope to husband their resources for other conflicts, who long for comfort and for care. For such patients, shrugging off the mantle of decision can be appealing, appropriate, and liberating.

The Divided Self

Zwei Seelen wohnen, ach! in meiner Brust.   Johann von Goethe, *Faust*

The free doctor . . . doesn't give orders until he has in some sense persuaded; when he has on each occasion tamed the sick person with persuasion, he attempts to succeed in leading him back to health.   Plato, *The Laws*

In this chapter, we are exploring three flaws in the autonomist syllogism. That syllogism holds that people want to make every decision that shapes their lives. Few decisions matter more than medical ones. Therefore patients must want to make medical decisions. The third flaw in this syllogism is related to the first and second. Patients sometimes want their doctors not to accede, or at least not to accede too readily, to their decisions. They occasionally want doctors to persuade them to some course of action, perhaps by logic, perhaps by cajolery, perhaps by persistence, perhaps even by manipulation. Autonomists believe people should be given thorough, dispassionate, and objective information so they can make informed and free decisions. But most of us wage what Thomas Schelling calls the intimate contest for self-command.[243] We try to maneuver and trick ourselves into doing what we espouse in principle but have trouble managing in practice. Many of us recruit allies in this conflict: we often enlist doctors to help us get ourselves to do what we should. As Schelling writes, "Doctors report that when patients are flatly told that their condition makes it imperative they cease smoking at once, the patients quit not only more reliably than when they are left any choice, but far more comfortably."[244]

Apostles of autonomy see this differently:

Have the familiar symptoms recurred because the patient has failed to take the medication as prescribed? If so, chances are we'll label him as noncompliant, a word that quickly shifts any blame from care givers to patient. Moreover, using "noncompliant" rather than "uncooperative" tells us that a good patient doesn't cooperate, he obeys. This inadequate, complaining wretch is back again because he hasn't followed doctor's orders. Orders? Where are we? On a battlefield? Perhaps. I think we know who the generals are. But who is the enemy?[245]

However, from the perspective of patients who want help persuading themselves, terms like "doctor's orders" and attempts to induce "compliance" are, so to speak, just what the doctor ordered and just what the patient wants. The problem lies not in maneuvering patients; it lies in telling which patients "want" to be maneuvered and in recognizing the borderlines of the "desired" manipulation. Not all patients put their request as clearly as the woman who begged her doctors to let her leave the hospital: "They were close to relenting, but were reluctant. Finally I said, 'I will say anything to get out of here. I'll shamelessly bribe you and play on any emotion. I'll even lie. So it's probably better if you don't listen to me and do what you feel is best."[246] Not all patients recognize their ambivalence as quickly and clearly as Joseph Heller. He told his doctor, "tearfully and heroically, that I would rather be dead than remain [in the ICU]. I told him frankly that I would have to go mad if I stayed. I could not bear being there." But when his doctor refused to move him, Heller "felt better already. I know ambivalence when I can no longer shut my eyes to it and I can recognize repression when it smacks me in the face."[247]

The story of a gastroenterologist with Crohn's disease (a disorder, potentially grave, of the stomach and bowel) illustrates the problem of the divided self and medical decisions. David Hein's illness worsened savagely, but he did nothing because (he later thought) he was afraid that admitting he was ill would jeopardize his practice and because he "feared what I might learn about my physical state."[248] Finally, Hein went to his internist, who recommended that he see a gastroenterologist. Hein selected his "closest medical associate." Hein greatly respected his colleague's skill, but his "[a]dvice was given in a nonauthoritarian manner—from colleague to colleague or friend to friend—and there was little actual follow-up regarding results of the recommendations." Hein later perceived "that subconsciously I was protecting myself from the reality of my situation."[249]

Hein eventually became so debilitated that another gastroenterologist told him he looked dangerously ill. This time, Hein went to an out-of-town hospital and began to make progress with his disease. He concluded, "Positive influences on my recovery were (1) a physician who served as an authority figure for me, (2) an excellent communication channel through my local physician and concerned partner who could work with me in carrying out my doctor's specific recommendations . . . . I needed strict and positive guidance from afar plus ongoing and enthusiastic contact locally."[250] In short, Hein's is a story of a patient who despite his expert understanding of his disease aggressively avoided treating it. He needed to enlist a doctor in his cause who would help him persuade himself to find and follow an effective course of treatment.

Distinguishing between patients who are ambivalent and those who are not is difficult and even dangerous. But I suspect most patients regard their physicians as advocates for life and health.[251] They expect their doctors to try to persuade them along the path toward those goals, and even to do so with some passion and persistence. Particularly when they are sick and sorrowful, they hope their doctors will buck them up and pull them through. Thus Gretel Ehrlich writes warmly of her cardiologist, "One of Blaine's gifts is a belief in the resilience of the human. His ardor is contagious: it's made of his cockeyed optimism and our own vital force. However weakened by illness, a thread of vitality pulls through: his vitality becomes ours and we revel in its presence, no matter how long it lasts: an hour or fifty years."[252] Patients may feel puzzled and even abandoned when their physicians defer too abruptly to their initial decisions. They may wonder how much their doctors care about them, or whether their doctors are too ready to follow the course of least resistance in acceding to whatever a patient seems to say. One study, for instance, tells of a "patient whose doctor agreed, acceding to *her* protest, to perform minor surgery in his office rather than in the hospital. This patient told us, 'He's the doctor. Why was he so quick to change his mind?'"[253]

To put the point differently, in important respects many of us have divided selves. One self may yearn to give up the struggle for health and even life. But another self wants to be encouraged to persist. The former self may eclipse the latter. But often the eclipsed self reemerges and prevails. I am not arguing that that latter self is the "true" self, since I am supposing there are multiple selves, each "true" in some genuine sense. But I think the great preponderance of patients would regard that self as their "better" self, the self of "my reason and my more composed judgment,"[254] the self they expect their doctor to help them contend for: "It was myself indeed in both the wills, yet more myself in that which I approved in myself than in that which I disapproved in myself."[255]

Two kinds of patients may be specially prone to the problem of the divided self. The first includes those who have grown discouraged in a long course of treatment, who vacillate between a desire to persevere and a longing to succumb. The second includes patients who run medical risks that are not easily perceived, who find it all too beguiling to neglect even simple measures that will prolong their health and lives.[256] As chronic illnesses become an increasingly large proportion of medical problems,[257] the former category will presumably grow. As medicine shifts its emphasis from curing to preventing disease[258] and as more medical interventions grow out of screenings of asymptomatic patients for such factors as high blood pressure,[259] the latter category may similarly burgeon.

Arthur Kleinman recounts one example of a patient who might well have fallen into the former category.[260] "Alice Alcott" was a diabetic who had fought for years against the debilitations of her disease. However, she became embittered, depressed, and discouraged, although "her state did not warrant the clinical diagnosis of major depressive disorder or any other serious psychiatric syndrome. Her problem was not a mental disease but a reaction, in large part . . . justified by her suffering and disablement."[261] As she began to resist further treatment, her family, doctors, and psychiatrists responded with efforts at encouragement. Eventually—although not permanently, one assumes—she decided to "do my best again to fight back."[262]

But let me offer a radically provocative and disquieting case from my own research. I interviewed a husband and wife who both had serious chronic diseases and were both told they needed transplants. These operations might kill them and were likely to leave them with onerous medical troubles and tasks. They were told they would certainly die without the operations. They talked with physicians, hospital employees, survivors of similar operations, and their family. They both reported that while they were told a good deal, no one made the kind of full disclosure of risks the law of informed consent and the autonomy paradigm require. One spouse's operation and recovery went brilliantly, the other's disastrously.

Had they been fully warned of the risks and consequences of the operations? Certainly not, they said. Given their perturbation at the time, they would surely have refused the operations had they been well informed. Would they have been wrong? They certainly would. Because then they would be dead and could not enjoy the pleasure they would feel that very afternoon when their grandson walked through their front door. And did they now fully disclose all the drawbacks of these operations to people who came to them to ask whether to undergo them? Of course not. Because then those people would refuse an operation they would ultimately be grateful for.[263]

There is some sketchy but plausible evidence that my interviewees are not unusual. One patient tells of a nurse who was worried about his failure to gain weight and who put him on a scale. "Unknown to me, she had hiked the lever up five pounds. When she told me I weighed 155, I hugged her. She did it to give me a life, even if she had to 'manipulate' a little. Even later when I found out that she had tricked me, I was grateful."[264] Another couple I interviewed had to decide what kind of dialysis to use. They rejected home hemodialysis, since they doubted they could handle it well. The clinic disagreed, and, as the wife said, "they kind of pushed us into it." The husband (the patient) agreed: "We didn't have time to think about it or decide." Nevertheless, they thought the clinic had been right about their capacity and right to insist, and the husband eventually concluded "it was the best decision they [the clinic] made." Similarly, Michael Kelly quotes a colitis patient who reports, "'I had been in hospital four days and they said I needed an operation. I felt they could do anything to me, but I didn't want a bag [a colostomy]. Then the doctor said, "It'll be fine when you get your bag." Maybe it was a good thing in a way, because if I'd had time to think about it, it might have been a different reaction, but I just felt numb to it.'"[265]

A key reason for such success stories is that patients are often less well situated than doctors to understand what life will be like under a treatment regime. As one man observed,

> When I was young and physically strong, to live life from a wheelchair was unthinkable. When I became disabled it was unacceptable, but gradually, over the

years, not only did it become acceptable, but I found it satisfying as well. Now, at those times when even the freedom I have in my wheelchair is threatened, I wonder if there is anything that is really unacceptable from the subjective standpoint. Or if, on the other hand, I will not be willing to accept most things.[266]

Likewise, Wilfrid Sheed reflects: "What distinguishes the only three illnesses I've ever had . . . is that all three are generally deemed incurable, and that each has caused me to lose something quite irreplaceable, something I would have sworn I couldn't live without."[267] He "quickly learned" that "cancer, even more than polio, has a disarming way of bargaining downward, beginning with your whole estate and then letting you keep the game warden's cottage or the badminton court; and by the time it has tried to frighten you to death and threatened to take away your very existence, you'd be amazed at how little you're willing to settle for."[268] Sheed came to believe that there must be a point at which life is worse than death, but reports that, so far, "[a]fter each of my 'unbearable, insupportable' losses, I have felt not only undiminished and unready to die, but quite goofily elated . . . ."[269]

In an important sense, patients may not even know what the life they are leading is like. Patients with poor kidney function, for example, often lose track of how it feels to be normal and only recover that sense after initiating dialysis. Patients on dialysis similarly forget what it is like to have a working kidney, and only recover that sense after having a transplant. Yet patients resist both dialysis and transplants because they think they already feel "normal." And it can be frustratingly hard for doctors to make this emotionally as well as intellectually clear to the patient.

Similar hints come from a less anecdotal source. Commenting on evidence that patients with colostomies are less willing than patients without them to trade a risk of death for a chance of avoiding a colostomy, one study suggests "patients may regard a particular outcome of treatment as highly undesirable but then become accustomed to it when it is directly experienced, and learn to tolerate it well."[270] As Gillian Rose wrote of her colostomy, "It makes all the difference: it makes no difference at all. It becomes routine; my routine is unselfconscious about the rituals and private character of your routines. Thus, I handle my shit."[271] Interestingly, "[t]he utilities obtained from physicians actively involved in the treatment of rectal cancer were in general similar to those of patients with a colostomy."[272] But how far should a doctor go in persuading, or even maneuvering, a patient who resists a colostomy because of an aversion the physician believes from experience will soon diminish?

In one sense, in one important sense, all this is paternalism with a vengeance. For patients who would not "truly want" my interviewees' operations, this approach could be calamitous. For patients who might want the operation but who would genuinely want to make their own informed decision, this approach is an affront. For my interviewees, it was just right. The question is how to structure medical services, to develop a medical ethos, to train doctors, and to acquire the insight as a doctor to serve all these kinds of patients well—if that is possible.

How Do Patients Make Medical Decisions?

O reason—ambidexter implement for effecting the irrational!   Gillian Rose, *Love's Work*

I have argued that patients have good reasons not to enter as fully into medical decisions as their bioethical and legal counselors would have them do. I now want to look briefly at how patients actually make medical decisions. I do so for two reasons. The first is to provide yet more evidence that not all patients want to make all their own medical decisions. The second is to confirm and amplify the arguments I have adduced to suggest that patients have their reasons for that reluctance.

We can say sadly little about how patients make medical decisions. Those decisions have inexplicably been studied only rarely. And, of course, we have few good ways of measuring their quality. The autonomy paradigm posits that there are no universal standards for gauging the success of a treatment. And even if we could somehow be sure a patient had accurately established some "true" standard of success, we would still grope to determine what effect the decision had on the patient's progress to that goal and whether some other path would have reached it better. If we want to evaluate patients' decisions, then, we find ourselves relegated to asking whether patients follow sensible procedures in making them. Here we are helped by the fact that bioethicists and the law of informed consent have some ideas about what "sensible" might mean: surveying all the available choices; assembling all the relevant information; identifying all one's interests, beliefs, preferences, and goals; and analyzing all these factors carefully, systematically, and rationally.

As I said, the evidence about how patients make decisions is partial and primitive. But it is quite suggestive. It suggests that the way patients make decisions is far less rationalistic and rational than the law and much bioethical writing assume or than patients themselves might want. This is hardly surprising. It is what one would expect from the arguments I have developed so far in this chapter. Most people find decisions difficult. Medical decisions are especially hard decisions made under especially onerous circumstances. Thus Janis says of patients that "the stresses of making major decisions and the various ways people deal with those stresses . . . frequently result in defective forms of problem solving that fail to meet the standards of rational decision making."[273]

Most prominently, patients often decide with a rapidity which forecloses the systematic deliberation students of decisions prescribe and the doctrine of informed consent presupposes. A study of kidney donors, for example, reports that despite elaborate attempts to have donors give truly informed consent, "[n]ot one of the donors weighed alternatives and rationally decided. Fourteen of the donors and nine of the ten donors waiting for surgery stated that they had made their decision immediately when the subject of the kidney transplant was first mentioned over the telephone, 'in a split-second,' 'instantaneously,' and 'right away.'"[274] In short, "all the donors and potential donors interviewed . . . reported a decision-making process that was immediate and 'irrational' and could not meet the requirements adopted by the American Medical Association to be accepted as an 'informed consent.'"[275]

A much more extensive study of kidney donors and recipients likewise describes radically abbreviated decisions. Simmons, Marine, and Simmons interviewed 178 recipients, 130 related donors, and numerous family members.[276] They too found that donors tended to make decisions that were procedurally short-circuited, for at least "62% of the donors would be classified as making an immediate choice." Thus "the majority of donors *volunteer immediately upon hearing of the need* without any time delay or any period of deliberation, and they themselves regard their choice as no decision at all."[277] Only "25% of the donors . . . seem to have approximated a classical decision-making pattern," since they "had done some *deliberating* and weighing of costs and gains."[278] For most donors, then, "the term *decision* appears to be a misnomer. Insofar as decision-making implies a period of deliberation and a conscious choice of one alternative, most individuals do not feel as if they made a decision."[279]

These figures are striking enough. Also striking is how truncated the decisions even of the "deliberators" were. Although a "sizeable percentage" of them sought out information, a "large proportion" did not. "In fact a predilection to donate and key initial acts were taken based on very little new information other than that provided by the family. Only two or three deliberators in the blood-tested relative group had done any reading about donation between the time they found out about the need for a donor and the time of the blood test, and only two out of twelve had consulted a physician."[280]

The Simmons study identified yet another defect in the way patients approach decisions. It discovered that a few prospective donors simply delayed making a decision "so long that they feel they have never reached a moment of conscious self-directed choice. The decision is made *for* them not *by* them."[281] For such people "the process is a *drift*-process rather than a deliberative decision-process."[282] This decisional approach led either to making or not making a donation without the prospective donor having decided anything. Some of these postponers would agree to take initial tests, accede to the next and more extensive tests, and discover that with each step "more and more of the relevant actors—the patient, the other relatives, the physicians and nurses—assumed he had already made the decision to donate,"[283] so that withdrawal became ever more awkward. Other prospective donors never brought themselves to volunteer, and "before they felt they had to make a decision, someone else volunteered or a cadaver was found, or they discovered they were the wrong blood type or a less good match than someone else."[284] This looks like a tacit decision not to donate, but the authors of the study say that that is not how the prospective donors saw it and that many of them "appeared willing to donate if necessary."[285] Postponement, in this view, is "a pattern of avoiding choice as long as possible. Each step is taken with the purpose of seeing whether one will or will not be compelled to make a decision, because the outcome of the stepwise action . . . may allow one totally to avoid the problem."[286] This urge to postpone rather than make decisions is common. Thus the Simmons study points to evidence that people often choose careers by small steps taken without considering where each step is leading and that people generally drift into crime rather than choose it as a career.[287]

I have been describing studies of kidney donation because that is one of the best-examined patients' decisions. It might be said that that decision is not really "medical" because the decision whether to donate a kidney ordinarily rests partly and even largely on "nonmedical" grounds. I am skeptical of that argument. Donating an organ involves an undoubtedly medical procedure (surgery) and undoubted medical risks. And many medical decisions are made on nonmedical grounds.

In any event, the processes the Simmons study describes seem to characterize other kinds of medical decisions. Penny Pierce, for instance, investigated a classical medical dilemma—the choice of procedure for treating breast cancer. She found "perceived salience" the leading "influence on decision-making behavior."[288] She explains, "Subjects who responded to the salience of one option over another did not report conflict about what course to take or the need for further information or deliberation."[289] And however far this way of deciding may seem from the bioethical model, it corresponds to the reality students of decision describe. Nisbett and Ross, for example, observe that

> once subjects have made a first pass at a problem, the initial judgment may prove remarkably resistant to further information, alternative modes of reasoning, and even logical or evidential challenges. Attempts to integrate new information may find the individual surprisingly "conservative," that is, willing to yield ground only grudgingly and primed to challenge the relevance, reliability, or authority of subsequent information or logical consideration. As a result, the method of first choice— and we believe heuristics and schemas to be such methods of first choice—may have disproportionate impact, while other methods (notably, methods considering pallid base lines, mitigating situational factors, possible sources of unreliability in the data, and the like) have relatively little impact.[290]

In my own research among renal patients I have found similarly truncated courses of decision. The patients I have observed and interviewed rarely gather all the relevant information and then deliberate about it. Rather, they often seem to listen until they hear some arresting fact and then make it the basis of their decision. For instance, as soon as some patients hear that hemodialysis requires someone to insert two large needles into their arm three times a week, they opt for whatever the alternative is.[291] When some other patients hear peritoneal dialysis means having a tube protruding from their abdomen, they choose "the other kind of dialysis." Many patients rest a quick decision on a single practical consideration. I recall with special affection one patient whose only interest was finding the method that would least interfere with his bowling. When he was told he could bowl while using either method, he announced he did not care which method the clinic wanted to use. Some patients did conduct more extensive inquiries. However, none of the patients I observed and only one of the patients I interviewed asked the question the law of consent assumes is central to a properly made discussion—which method will keep you healthy the best and alive the longest.[292]

Many patients' memoirs report similarly abrupt decisions. One breast cancer patient "knew right away what my decision would be; I had known it fifteen minutes after my diagnosis, although it had been only the fear talking then."[293] When her doctor surprised Betty Johnson by telling her she needed a heart transplant and suggested she take twenty-four hours to think about it, she "didn't think about it for any twenty-four hours. I figured I didn't have to think about it."[294] When Carobeth Laird's doctor "said that I had to have immediate gallbladder surgery, but at my age and in my physical condition, the chances of coming through it were not good," she replied "'OK, go ahead.'"[295] Reynolds Price "instantly declined" his doctor's recommendation that he needed surgery, since Price feared (without evidence) that his employer, Duke University, would want him to retire if he did not finish teaching for the semester.[296] For Mary Alice Geier, "[n]ot even a split second was needed to opt for chemotherapy despite all I had heard about it."[297] And often memoirists felt their medical decision presented them with "no choice."[298]

Not only do patients often make decisions quickly and consult only a few criteria—or even a single criterion—but even patients sufficiently well educated and reflective to write memoirs frequently describe no decisional process at all. Instead, they invoke intuition, instinct, and impulse. An AIDS patient, for example, started off making decisions on what seemed to be a rational basis: "I was frightened of the side effects of radiation and chemotherapy. Interferon produced less severe, flu-like symptoms. I chose interferon because it was the least toxic. I had no idea what I was getting myself into."[299] Eventually he came to make decisions in a frankly nonrational (although in his view successful) way: "I've learned to listen to my inner voice for guidance when choosing treatments. If I get what Louise refers to as a 'ding' (a strong instinct) about a vitamin, herb, drug, or other treatment, I try it."[300] A patient with metastatic melanoma reported "making the decisions and going on my own best instincts."[301] A heart-transplant patient and her husband "sensed there was something right about Stanford. We cannot explain why."[302] Anatole Broyard defended this approach expressly, even if wryly: "I think that if a man should ever give in to his prejudices, it's when he's ill. . . . I mean all prejudices, instinctive likes and dislikes. I'm convinced that my prejudice in the matter of medicine reflects the intelligence of my unconscious, and so I go with it. I need my prejudices. They're going to save me."[303]

Some patients defend decision by intuition less irreverently. A multiple sclerosis patient "got a flash,"[304] found that a "little light flashed inside my head,"[305] came to "trust my instincts and intuition,"[306] and asked why she should not "play my hunches."[307] She believed that "[i]ntuitive knowing is a higher form of knowing than rational knowing."[308] She may have meant what a woman with kidney cancer said more directly, that decision by intuition is therapeutically sound because of the influence the mind has over the body and its illnesses. She reasoned, "I know my healing has to come from within. I know I need to get out of my own way and let the healing in. . . . That means deciding on my own program, sorting out the myriad alternatives, choosing those that intuitively speak to me . . . ." She thus sought to "sort out all the available alternatives, and decide on the ones I instinctively feel will work out for me." This was "one of the most important steps I take on my path to healing, for it is necessary to both believe in, and be comfortable with the choices I make."[309] It was also necessary for her to "'connect more deeply to [her] source of inner intuitive knowing, which is essential to the process of personal empowerment and healing.'"[310]

Even people committed to making rational decisions often fall surprisingly short. Michael Korda's effort to choose a treatment and doctor for his prostate cancer is instructive. He is the editor in chief of Simon & Schuster and the author of books with titles like *Success!* and *Power!* He believed in understanding his prostate cancer and making his own decisions. He consulted a well-known surgeon to get a second opinion about a recommendation that he have an operation and asked some practical questions about the procedure and the recovery. But then he found that his "mind had gone blank" and that he was "feeling the inevitability of the thing." When the surgeon left, Korda realized that he had made his decision. He "felt a curious sense of relief. The decision had been made at last—had simply fallen into place, without any real debate on my part. I had put my fate in Dr. Walsh's hands, and he seemed to have no doubts at all about his ability to deal with it."[311] An actor named Evan Handler was also committed to seizing control of his own medical decisions. He describes the ultimate basis for one choice: "In the end, quite simply, I went with my heart. . . . I reminded myself that I had been in the top 5 or 10 percent of almost everything I had done in my life, and so, in forgoing any more treatment, I still had a 10 or 15 percentage-point cushion to feel comforted by."[312] Even that model patient, the Rice sociologist William Martin, sometimes worked in an uncannily similar way: "Without knowing precisely why or being able to provide a clear rationale, I decided I would ask Peter Scardino to perform my surgery."[313]

An illuminating example of how patients approach medical choices may be found in the one decision patients must make without professional guidance—the decision to seek that guidance. Fear, among other factors, terribly often causes people to put off seeking help no matter how evident the problem and exigent the need: If it be possible, let this cup pass from me. "Over 30 percent of cancer patients have been found to postpone seeking a diagnosis for three or more months after they first notice growths or other symptoms that they know could be danger signs."[314] Many people having heart attacks delay calling a doctor for four or five hours because "the decision making process gets jammed by the patient's inability to admit that he is mortally sick."[315] As one writer comments ruefully, "In full health, I imagine minor ailments to be dangerous symptoms, or else, from fear, ignore them away. I do not submit routinely to preventive medicine. What may it not show up?"[316]

Sometimes patients may delay getting medical attention because they fear its expense. But patients' memoirs are full of stories of well-to-do people who put off getting help for even serious symptoms. More systematically, Janis and Mann note that even where medical care was free, "a study of a representative sample of families in the London area showed that over one-third of the families had a member who was suffering from pain or discomfort but was not receiving medical treatment."[317]

Delays might also be due to medical ignorance, but again the evidence suggests otherwise. People who know cancer's danger signs are *likelier* to postpone seeing a physician than people who do not.[318] And a collection of doctors' accounts of their illnesses is a veritable cavalcade of lessons in how trained people can ignore horrible diseases.[319] Even people who have known for years they are chronically ill may feel as Brookes does: "[H]oping against reason, we prefer to believe that our illness will simply go away by itself. To seek medical treatment is to admit the disease . . . [and to] have our chronic fallibility, our mortality, exposed."[320] As one physician who postponed investigating his cancer symptoms said, "I wondered why I had been so foolish. Why had I waited so long to see Du-Vall? In spite of all the excuses I had made to myself, I knew the reason. I had acted like many of my patients had, accepting the [less worrisome] diagnosis to avoid facing something else."[321] Reynolds Price puts it vividly: "Inquisitive to a fault though I'd been all my life, some deep-down voice was running me now. Its primal aim was self-preservation. *Don't make them tell you, and it may not happen. Whatever they tell you may be wrong anyhow. Stay quiet. Stay dark.*"[322]

In sum, patients often do not make decisions the way students of decisions, or even most people, would advise, and certainly not the way the law of informed consent contemplates or autonomists expect when they speak of "substantial *understanding*" and "substantial *absence of control* by others,"[323] of "the informed exercise of a choice" with the "opportunity to evaluate knowledgeably the options available."[324] But these expectations of patients should be evaluated against the background of the way people ordinarily make even momentous decisions.

How often does anyone reach those standards of knowledge, or reflection, or freedom? Consider, for instance, how people choose careers. People have a rousing interest in thinking about that choice and plenty of time—years—to make it. Yet when I ask my law students—who have extraordinary leisure and resources for choosing careers—why they want to be lawyers, the modal answer, at heart, is that they do not know. They say they want to serve mankind, but they rarely take jobs that (in their view) let them do so. Before they come to law school few of them know much about the practice of law generally, and I rarely meet an entering student who realizes what kind of practice our school's graduates routinely join. They generally know even less about the alternatives to a legal career they might pursue. When they choose among the firms that court them, they are swayed by little blandishments and by the place on the status hierarchy their fellow students have—for the nonce—assigned each firm. One is reminded of how Hans Castorp found a career:

> He looked about for a profession suitable in his own eyes and those of his fellow citizens. And when he had once chosen—it came about at the instance of old Wilms, of the firm of Tunder and Wilms, who said to Consul Tienappel at the Saturday whist-table that young Castorp ought to study ship-building; it would be a good idea, he could come into his office and he would keep an eye on him—when he had once chosen, he thought very highly of his calling. It was, to be sure, confoundedly complicated and fatiguing, but all the same it was very first-rate, very solid, very important.[325]

I say all this not to criticize my students. On the contrary, my point is that even people as bright, engaged, and fortunate as they make even this consequential choice just the way people regularly make all kinds of critical decisions—with little information, after modest reflection, buffeted by social pressures, scrabbling to postpone decisions, scratching to "keep their options open," yearning to avoid commitment, leaving much to chance. And I suspect that career decisions are everything an autonomist could want compared to, say, selecting a spouse. If this is how people ordinarily make life's pivotal decisions, will medical decisions be any different?[326]

That patients make decisions rapidly and on sketchy data need not mean their decisions are bad. If doctors propose only good alternatives, any decision may be reasonable. I believe many patients rely exactly on the assumption (which may flout the principles of informed consent) that any alternatives presented to them will be sound. In addition, the crucial fact patients seize on may be precisely the fact they care about most. Many kidney donors can decide instantly to donate because they overwhelmingly want to help someone they love and because they axiomatically believe they have a duty unto death to help their brothers and sisters, their parents and children. (On the other hand, this is harder to credit about some reasons for choosing dialysis modalities.) Nor does the fact that patients make decisions on eccentric grounds prove they are being improvident. The prospective dialysis patient whose sole criterion was the effect each method would have on his bowling may truly have valued bowling above all else. Further, people can sometimes make rapid but reasonable calculations about their choices. Finally, perhaps exceptionally difficult decisions are also decisions that will be right (or wrong) whatever one does and that no amount of cogitation will improve.

Nevertheless, patients clearly make medical decisions in ways that are less than optimal and quite different from the ways lawyers and bioethicists assume. Rapid decisions cannot account well for the many factors medical decisions raise, and decisions made on the basis of only one or a few factors usually scant others. The prominence of "practical" factors at the expense of "medical" factors is often sensible, but it can also mean patients simply avoided the harder questions. And decisions patients cannot explain will frequently be decisions they do not understand. In the end, as Flannery O'Connor says, illness is a foreign land.[327] The patient enters as a stranger, disoriented. His guides are vague about the terrain, and their directions are therefore suspect, as well as prey to all the unreliability of human communication. Confused, frightened, pressed, the patient hastily picks out the few familiar objects in the landscape and scrambles toward them, hoping, at best, to muddle through, relieved to have made *some* decision. Often he wanders on, uncertain of the goal, uncertain of the path chosen, uncertain of the distance yet to cover.

This is not how good decisions are made. But most of us make decisions rather badly. And illness poses especially problematic choices under particularly trying circumstances. Patients generally realize this and are delicately sensitive to the likelihood that they will err. For all these reasons, then, patients may feel confirmed in their choice to delegate medical decisions.

How Can Doctors Make Medical Decisions?

If the clinician seems knowledgeable and authoritative, and if his reputation and results seem good, he can be condoned the most flagrant imprecisions, vagueness, and inconsistency in his conduct of therapy. The clinician does not even use a scientific name for his method of designing, executing and appraising [treatments]. He calls it clinical judgment.

Alvan R. Feinstein, *Clinical Judgment*

How might sophisticated autonomists answer the argument that many patients are reluctant, hasty, clumsy deciders who wish to delegate medical choices? One such reply suggests that people

who doubt the ability of patients to make fully rational medical judgments implicitly assume that the judgment of physicians is significantly more reliable. Many studies have suggested, however, that physicians' decisions are influenced by a wide variety of factors that are unrelated to a patient's specific medical problem. These factors include practice setting, degree of specialization, and physician age.

Other studies have shown that physicians may misunderstand quantitative medical information and that they may manifest some of the same "irrational" biases in decision making to which patients are claimed to be susceptible.[328]

If doctors make decisions improvidently, is not the case for mandatory autonomy strengthened? Should not patients make decisions to counteract the unwisdom of the doctor?

There is evidence that, although "[p]hysicians are obviously much more educated than the average citizen, yet their judgments—in their area of specialized training—are subject 'to all the flaws of human reasoning . . . .'"[329] For example, one study asked if it mattered whether radiation were presented as a treatment for lung cancer in terms of the chances of living or the chances of dying to patients, doctors, and business-school students who had completed courses in statistics and decision theory. Not only was the mode of presentation's effect "large (25 per cent vs. 42 per cent) and consistent," but "the effect was not generally smaller for the physicians (who had considerable experience in evaluating medical data) or for the graduate students (who had received statistical training) than for the patients (who had neither)."[330] Other research suggests that many doctors misunderstand statistical analysis[331] and that training in statistics, while beneficial,[332] improves their decisions less than one might hope.[333]

Doubts about the quality of doctors' decisions have been enlivened by the "many studies [that] have suggested . . . that physicians' decisions are influenced by a wide variety of factors that are unrelated to a patient's specific medical problem. These factors include practice setting, degree of specialization, and physician age."[334] Furthermore, "[w]ide variations in the incidence of medical and surgical services are the *norm,* not the exception,"[335] although much of this variation is concentrated in areas where there is professional disagreement about the best treatment. Also, there is evidence "that as much as 25 percent or more of expenditures for medical care is for unnecessary or inappropriate services."[336]

In addition, doctors may have interests of their own. This is no disgrace. Some of those interests are thoroughly admirable, as when physicians treating patients are simultaneously conducting medical research. Nevertheless, bioethics was born partly in response to the failure of researchers to treat their subjects properly.[337] There are now procedures intended to minimize such abuses, but researchers who are also treating patients may willy-nilly face conflicts of interest.[338] To some extent, these conflicts are built into the structure of research. For example, patients in the control group might be better off receiving treatment, while patients receiving treatment bear the risks of experimentation, risks that include the failure of the treatment and the danger of side effects.

These conflicts in the doctor–researcher's role are largely unavoidable. Others are not. Pearl Katz, for instance, describes a case in which surgeons were signed on to a research project by their chief of surgery with, Katz suggests, little chance to reflect or refuse. A surgeon then recruited a patient into the project without providing adequate information. The surgeon did not know how to do the procedure, and the resident who had seen it done elsewhere had trouble with it. The procedure caused more injury to tissues than had been anticipated, the surgeon commented he "'wouldn't want my mother to go through this,'" and the chief of surgery said, "'We're going to have an increase in post-operative infections with these patients.'" But the chief's only suggestion seems to have been, "'If we get too many [infections], we'll have to look into it.'"[339]

Some of the ways doctors' and patients' interests conflict are less admirable than those in medical research, but hardly blameworthy and perhaps inevitable. The fee-for-service system, for example, notoriously invites doctors to perform services however faint the need. More broadly, Pearl Katz suggests "variables such as colleagueship, hospital organizational structure, departmental hierarchy, the influence of the Chief [of Surgery], competition (such as that between medical oncology and surgical departments), increased referrals, and conceptions of appropriate income play[ ] significant roles in the medical decision-making."[340] Katz provides the example of a general surgeon, Jeff Schneider, who had consulted a thoracic surgeon about whether Schneider ought to perform a hiatus hernia repair which he could only do abdominally, not thoracically. The thoracic surgeon told Katz,

> This hernia will probably not hold if Jeff (Schneider) does it. If he's lucky, it may hold until the patient goes home. It should be done thoracically. But Jeff is terribly worried about his income. That summer house means a lot to him, but it's above his head. He needs money now. He is my friend. It's a tough decision. But if I take it from him (i.e., decide that it be done thoracically), he'll think twice about consulting me again, knowing I'll take his patients. And he's a friend who's in financial trouble. . . . I'll let him do it.[341]

Other conflicts arise out of the entrepreneurial behavior of doctors. For instance, "[s]everal studies of laboratory and X-ray use show a direct relationship between physician ownership and rates of testing."[342] A study of hypertension patients found "there were 50 percent more electrocardiograms and 40 percent more chest radiographs among the patients in fee-for-service group practices than among the patients in prepaid group practices."[343] Even where doctors do not own businesses they may be swayed by people who do, "as was demonstrated in congressional hearings in the early 1980s into the apparently widespread use of kickbacks by manufacturers of intraocular lenses (IOL) as a way to encourage ophthalmologists and surgeons to use their products."[344]

Alternatives to fee-for-service present their own conflicts. Those arising out of attempts to control medical costs have recently attracted concern, for those attempts often give doctors direct financial incentives not to provide treatment. Even doctors whose salaries do not depend on keeping expenditures low may feel administrative pressures to do so.[345] Of course doctors with financial conflicts do not always or even often succumb to them. Yet decisions are harder when doctors must not only resist financial and social pressures but must also avoid being overscrupulous.

Even if the doctor's economic interests coincide exactly with the patient's, the doctor still faces some disadvantages making decisions for the patient. As I said earlier, physicians may be poorly situated to apprehend and appreciate the way patients see, feel, and think. One doctor with AIDS commented, "[M]any doctors aren't really aware of the side effects, dehumanization, and outright discomfort their patients experience when they follow their physician's orders."[346] One doctor I interviewed said he had advantages as a decision-maker, "[b]ut I am very cognizant, or very aware, of the fact that it is not the needle going into me. I am not the one who is going through the pain and suffering or [who will] suffer the risks. And the patient is the person who is going to suffer that." Furthermore, doctors tend to lead lives that are socially insulated from the lives of most of their patients and that are economically insulated from many common worries. Some hint of the difficulties these factors create for doctors seeking to understand patients lies in studies finding that doctors have trouble anticipating patients' preferences about medical care.[347] In short, many disabilities hamper doctors trying to make decisions that suit patients' tastes and temperaments.

I have been speaking primarily of medical decisions in a fairly narrow sense, of relatively technical decisions. Doubts about doctors' decisions apply all the more forcefully to the broader kinds of medical issues, particularly those presenting moral problems. Here doctors often seem particularly handicapped. Little in the process of selecting people to be doctors leads one to expect acute moral insight from them. Their training remains overwhelmingly technical, and there is little prospect of real change. One may even doubt that "humanistic" education or ethics courses much alter the way doctors behave when they graduate. Nor is the attitude of many doctors toward moral decisions reassuring. A disturbing number of them seem not to recognize many of the moral issues they encounter, regard them as not repaying thought and discussion, or even scorn the enterprise of moral thought, whose softness they contrast with the diamond clarity of scientific analysis.[348] For example, an internist Robert Hahn studied was animated by what Hahn calls "moral Certainty"—a belief that "some events and acts are clearly right, others clearly wrong."[349] The internist, Hahn reports, "mocks what he calls philosophical issues, quoting the medieval question, 'How many angels are there on the head of a pin?' as an example of irrelevance and insolubility."[350]

Finally, if patients are delegating decisions to doctors, or indeed anyone, in the hope of securing a truly "rational" decision, they are doomed to disappointment. Such a decision is impossible in any important area of life: Our information will always be too opaque, our preferences too disorderly, our goals too conflicting, our fears too distorting, our passions too imperative, our intelligence too limited for reason truly to govern our decisions. There is, in other words, a degree of irrationality no human—dispassionate doctor or devoted friend—can transcend.

In sum, doctors can fall into the traps that plague most human reasoning. They are influenced by the extraneous. Their interests diverge from their patients'. They cannot easily put themselves in their patients' shoes. They can claim no special gift for moral reasoning. And the goal of a truly rational decision is chimerical. All this being so, should patients ever refer decisions to doctors?

The defects in doctors' decisions are serious enough to explain why patients might want to make their own medical decisions, or at least to monitor their doctor's decisions vigilantly. But they are hardly so overwhelming or universal that all patients ought to make all their own decisions. Physicians' decisions are not always impaired in the ways I have described: Some doctors do not do research, some do not work on a fee-for-services basis, some are not unreasonably pressured to reduce medical costs, some do not own the laboratories to which they refer patients, and some rise smoothly above the temptations they encounter. Some doctors think rigorously, some empathically.

In addition, the question is not whether doctors will make optimal decisions, but whether they will make better decisions than patients. The many reasons I have already given for patients' reluctance to make their own decisions must be weighed against the defects in doctors' decisions. In such a weighing the physician's judgment often is preferable (particularly since the patients who defer to their doctors may often be the patients worst equipped to make their own decisions). Doctors have several kinds of advantages over patients. Since these parallel the reasons patients hesitate to make their own decisions I will not survey them at length. But a few of them should be noted. First, doctors' emotions are less deeply and painfully engaged than patients'. This matters because emotions distort decisions. For example, where patients feel their choices pose frightening risks, they may respond through "defensive avoidance," which is "manifested by lack of vigilant search, selective inattention, selective forgetting, distortion of the meaning of warning messages, and construction of wishful rationalizations that minimize negative consequences."[351] Because doctors' emotions are generally less violently roiled than patients', doctors should be less susceptible to such mental disruptions.[352]

But there is a more basic reason patients might, *ceteris paribus*, think doctors better equipped than they to make medical decisions. Doctors may be susceptible to the biases in reasoning that plague us all. Nevertheless, they have two crucial advantages. First, they have more experience and knowledge; second, they work in a setting which disciplines the way they make decisions.

Gary Klein argues that the "heuristics and biases" studies which reveal such extensive defects in human reasoning apply badly to experts working in their fields because experience and the expertise it brings change the way people make decisions. Experts can make decisions better than novices because they make more of them. Inexperienced people are at best relegated to making decisions in the perilous way the informed-consent model supposes—by gathering all the data, identifying all the alternatives, articulating all the goals, developing criteria for evaluating the alternatives in terms of the goals, and finding the alternative that best fits those criteria. This is commonly an arduous process that demands complex and reliable reasoning. Experts, however, often can shortcut this process. They ordinarily do not reason their way through a problem step by step. Rather, Klein argues, they use "*experience to recognize key patterns that indicate the dynamics of the situation.*"[353] Experts

> recognize [a] situation as typical and familiar . . . . They understand what types of *goals* make sense (so the priorities are set), which *cues* are important (so there is not an overload of information), what to *expect* next (so they can prepare themselves and notice surprises), and the *typical ways of responding* in a given situation. By recognizing a situation as typical, they also recognize a *course of action* likely to succeed.[354]

Experts can make decisions efficiently without working through all the steps because they have seen so many cases. Indeed, "the familiarity of the situation (or the expertise of the decision maker) is one of the most important factors in how decisions are actually made."[355] Competence even among experts seems to depend more on their experience than their powers of reasoning. Thus one study of doctors "found that problem-solving expertise varied greatly across cases and was highly dependent on the clinician's mastery of the particular domain."[356]

Klein believes that "recognitional strategies that take advantage of experience are generally successful, not as a substitute for the analytical methods, but as an improvement on them. The analytical methods are not the ideal; they are the fallback for those without enough experience to know what to do."[357] This is partly because "[i]t is usually difficult to make the estimates called for by calculational methods."[358] It is also because for experts sophisticated "decision-making knowledge is embodied in special-purpose packages, such as schemas, frames, or scripts . . . ."[359] These schemas perform more accurately the demanding calculations experts would otherwise have to attempt for themselves for each new problem.

More specifically, doctors bring to the encounter with patients a well-stocked file of patterns that describe the way bodies, diseases, and diagnostic equipment typically work. When doctors receive data, they evaluate them against those patterns. The data will generally be incomplete and ambiguous, but doctors use their patterns to check the reliability of the data, to fill in missing pieces, and to decide what further information to seek. The file of patterns then is consulted to determine which features of the data are significant or anomalous and thus to reach a diagnosis. Patterns are again consulted to establish which goals might be realistic and what treatments might promote them. Patients, on the other hand, ordinarily lack the patterns on which each of these steps depends. This is why "[p]roblem-solving studies show fundamental differences between novices and experts in how problems are interpreted, what strategies are devised, what information is used, memory for critical information, and speed and accuracy of problem solving."[360]

The preceding paragraph significantly understates the advantage experts have over novices. Even the process it sketches requires a number of steps, each hazardous. Experts' patterns can shortcut the work of each step and sometimes of entire steps in ways that make more complex and accurate thought practical. We are hobbled in analyzing problems by what Klein calls our "limited working memory," which cannot keep many parts of the puzzle and steps in the reasoning in mind simultaneously. However, "[i]f we have a lot of familiarity in the area, we can chunk several transitions into one unit. In addition, we can save memory space by treating a sequence of steps as one unit rather than representing all the steps."[361] Furthermore, "[w]hereas novices may be confused by all the data elements, experts see the big picture, and they appear to be less likely to fall victim to information overload."[362]

In sum, "[e]xperts in a field can look at a situation and quickly interpret it using their highly organized base of relevant knowledge."[363] They can do so because "[t]hey have a larger storehouse of procedures to apply. They notice problems more quickly. They have richer mental simulations to use in diagnosing problems and in evaluating courses of action. They have more analogies to draw upon."[364] And the point is not just that doctors have a good file of patterns. It is that patients often have bad ones. When people of all kinds make decisions, they "create causal models of the situation. They try to understand the significance of events and information by inferring causal relations . . . ."[365] As I said earlier in this chapter, however, patients bring misinformation of many kinds to the task of creating those causal models. The unreliability of their causal models in turn can lead them to misperceive and misinterpret even clearly stated medical information and advice.

No one reasons flawlessly, and medical school does not change that fact. Doctors' reasoning can be distorted by the "heuristics and biases" to which we are all susceptible. However, there is evidence "that decision biases are reduced if the study includes contextual factors and that the heuristics and biases do not occur in experienced decision makers working in natural settings."[366] What is more, doctors' experience endows them with the equipment to reason more acutely about medical problems than patients generally can.

Doctors not only have the advantage of expertise. They also belong to a discipline which can bring group rationality to bear. Even if doctors individually reason poorly, they have a large and sophisticated literature which subjects standard medical reasoning to statistical and logical scrutiny.[367] Further, because medical decisions are increasingly reached collectively, "[t]wo useful defenses" against error are becoming more available—"to consider the data from multiple perspectives and to discuss the issue with a person whose opinion on the same problem is different."[368] There are even medical practices—like morbidity and mortality conferences[369]—that encourage or even compel doctors to scrutinize and criticize their own and each other's work. Eric Cassell writes, "I know of no other structured area of human activity in which open self-criticism is so much a part."[370] Indeed, much of the attack on doctors' reasoning comes from medicine itself.

Finally, because patients rely on doctors for information and advice, many of their doctors' irrationalities will remain even if patients make their own decisions. Few patients can regularly detect those irrationalities and offset them. Patients thus may fear that, by making decisions, they are merely compounding their doctors' irrationalities with their own.

Notice, too, how far the discussion of doctors' role in medical decisions has come. Much of the impetus for the law of informed consent was the argument that doctors could not make decisions for patients because they did not know patients' beliefs. The solution was to require doctors to lay out the medical choices so patients could apply their beliefs to the data. As the attack on medical paternalism has mounted, it is increasingly said doctors reason imperfectly about medical questions. This certainly should invite doctors to modesty and caution. But what should patients make of the evidence about doctors' reasoning? If medical decisions are so challenging that doctors botch them, if the human mind is too muddled for anyone to make good decisions, what should you do? Follow your own prejudices, however unsound and unexamined? Try to make yourself an expert? The criticism of physicians is that they are insufficiently rigorous, systematic, and scientific. Who thinks patients can do better on these scores? The solution for physicians is sharper science and better training. Who thinks this a solution for patients? But if it is not, what is?

In this section, we have been investigating the argument that patients should make medical decisions because doctors make them badly. I have argued that for most patients most of the time, the issue is not whether the doctor reasons badly, but whether the patient reasons worse. I have suggested that expertise and context matter and that experts have significant advantages over novices in specialized reasoning. This takes us back to the original justification for patients' authority—that their preferences should prevail. This justification essentially contemplates that doctors will do the medical reasoning and that patients will decide which medical alternative best fits their preferences. Under this model, patients may seem to be relieved of medical reasoning and need only think about their preferences. However, my discussion of how experts and novices make decisions raises questions about even this more modest position.

The questions are of two kinds. First, can this procedure in fact serve its goal of making patients' preferences dispositive? What we know of decisions suggests that they are rarely made in the linear way the standard bioethics formulation I quoted in Chapter 1 posits:

Instead of analyzing all facets of a situation, making a decision, and then acting, it appears that in complex realistic situations people think a little, act a little, and then evaluate the outcomes and think and act some more . . . . Decision event models assume all options, outcomes, and preferences are known in advance and thus are amenable to evaluation. The decision cycle approach treats the development of this knowledge as an integral part of decision making.[371]

But if this is true, if "the decision process consists more of generating and clarifying actions and goals than of choosing among prespecified alternative actions . . . ,"[372] the danger (though not the certainty) is that doctors will already have done much of the work of integrating preferences into the decision by the time they present choices to their patients. For

goals affect the way we evaluate courses of action, and the evaluation can help us learn to set better goals. The goals determine how we assess the situation, and the things we learn about the situation change the nature of the goals. Goals define the barriers and leverage points we search for, and the discovery of barriers and leverage points alters the goals themselves. The way we diagnose the causes leading to the situation also affects the types of goals adopted.[373]

In short, while doctors work their way through a medical problem they are likely to be making choices that shape and reshape the goals of treatment. Thus the more of the medical reasoning the doctor does alone, the more decisions about goals are likely to slip away from the patient's grasp.

Second, the autonomous patient is supposed to select the alternative "that is best for himself or herself." The patient's special expertise is the patient's own preferences, preferences, for example, about what kinds of risks are worth running, about what kinds of side effects are intolerable, about the relative value of quantity and quality of life, and so on. However, patients ultimately are selecting a medical treatment, and an effective treatment will often be the strongest of the patient's preferences. We can say patients should simply accept the doctor's assessment of medical efficacy. But once patients take on a decision, they will often try to make sense of the alternatives, to put them in some frame of reference, in short, to evaluate them. That evaluation is likely to affect the patient's decision. In other words, even if we say we want patients to make decisions because they know their own preferences best, we must recognize that they will also implicitly be undertaking more technical judgments.

Both these criticisms seem to me correct. Unless you make a decision yourself you are likely to lose some control over the ends the decision serves. If you make a decision yourself, it is hard to avoid evaluating *all* its components. But neither criticism seems to me to dictate any standard role for patients. Patients may prefer to lose some control over goals in the interest of better-founded technical decisions. To put the point differently, attempts to give patients maximal control over goals have costs because they increase the burden on patients to make technical judgments they are likely to make less ably than a doctor. Ultimately, as Dr. Johnson is supposed to have said, when we walk toward one blessing we walk away from another. The more patients try to retain their autonomy, the more deeply they must involve themselves in unfamiliar kinds of reasoning. The more patients rely on experts, the harder they must find it to effectuate their preferences and to detect problems in experts' decisions. The challenge, as always, is to find the right balance in each case, for much will depend on the circumstances and nature of the decision and the participants in it.

In short, no one supposes doctors are infallible. They reach bad decisions for all the reasons I have described in this section. They are human, "born but to die and reasoning but to err." Their work is exceptionally difficult. They are betrayed by vanity, cupidity, incompetence, carelessness, and sloth. But patients may nevertheless conclude that they too are human, that they too are prone to err, that they too are betrayed by their own flaws, and that their doctors have crucial advantages in medical reasoning. Often their doctors will be right. All too seldom will patients be able to tell when they are wrong. Yet less often will they be able to turn a sow's ear of bad advice into the silk purse of a good decision.

This chapter began with a puzzle: that many patients seem to have declined to seize the power of decision bioethics has proffered. In this chapter, I have argued that those patients may have legitimate reasons to shun the burdens of medical decisions: Patients may believe themselves poorly situated to understand and analyze medical problems, they may feel too ill to face serious decisions, and they may wish to be helped to overcome themselves. Furthermore, patients often seem to make decisions badly, which gives them all the more incentive to find people likelier to make them well. The obvious candidates—doctors—labor under disabilities of their own, but they will nevertheless often do better than the patient. This does not mean it is irrational or even unwise for patients to make their own decisions. But it may be rational and perhaps necessary for some of them sometimes to confide those decisions to their families, their friends, and even their doctors.

4

How Can They Think That?
Of Information, Control, and Complexity

[T]hroughout my stay in the Convalescent Home, I saw that one must oneself be a patient, and a patient among patients, that one must enter both the solitude and the community of patienthood, to have any real idea of what "being a patient" means, to understand the immense complexity and depth of feelings, the resonances of the soul in every key—anguish, rage, courage, whatever—and the thoughts evoked even in the simplest practical minds . . . .

Oliver Sacks
A Leg to Stand On

On hearing the evidence and arguments you have just read, some of my colleagues have been disbelieving. They assure me that this is not how they react to illness and that they know no one who does (except their parents and, perhaps, a few friends, and, as they think about it, maybe even some colleagues).[1] I am not surprised. This is not how I would expect lengthily educated, endlessly analytical, and professionally aggressive academics to respond to illness (although many of them do). But most people lack these characteristics, and for them other approaches to illness—and life—make sense. In this chapter, I will sketch how this might be possible. I will thus be continuing the work I began in Chapter 2—showing there are patients who would rather not make medical decisions. As in Chapter 3, my technique is partly to substantiate Chapter 2's empirical data by showing how declining to exercise autonomy to the full can make practical and psychological sense. This enquiry also advances another of Chapter 3's projects—better understanding the patient's view of bioethical problems generally and of the relations between doctors, patients, and decisions specifically.

In this chapter I want to address explicitly a question Chapter 3 addressed implicitly: the role of control in people's lives. As before, I emphasize that people's situations and preferences are more varied than the autonomy paradigm, with its universalistic aspirations, allows. I consider that complexity in three respects. First, I examine the apparent tension between patients' strong desire for information and their relatively weak desire to make medical decisions. Second, I investigate the contemporary certitude that people's lives are at heart a struggle to assert control over their environment. I ask how far this is true and what "control" might mean for the ill. Third, I show that the category "medical decision" is deceptively capacious and that different kinds of medical decisions may evoke different levels of desire to exercise control by making medical choices.

Knowledge

Asking questions, you feel less powerless, yet you end up not much wiser or even better informed.   Paul West, *A Stroke of Genius*

If people do not wish to make their own medical decisions, why do they want to know about their medical condition? Why would they want information about something they cannot—or will not—control? The first answer is that, while studies suggest the desire for information is stronger than the desire to make decisions, they also suggest that not everyone wants information. Here again we see the truth of the proposition that for every majority there is a minority. Furthermore, not everyone who wants information wants it all the time, or wants all kinds of information. And they may be right not to want it. For example, a review of attempts to provide information about "aversive events" concluded that "no straightforward relation has been found between the receipt of information about an event and reactions to that event."[1a] And we have already seen that some patients fear learning about their illness. As Stewart Alsop wrote, "A patient should be told the truth, and nothing but the truth—but not the whole truth. I find scribbled in my notebook . . . : 'A man who must die will die more easily if he is left a little spark of hope that he may not die after all.' "[2]

Second, many patients want not so much information as good news, as reassurance. They want to hear that their illness is not serious, or if it is, that it can be cured. Alsop admits when discussing how fully patients should be informed, "For myself, I'm ambivalent. I like to know where I stand, but I don't at all like being scared."[3] A cancer patient acknowledged she "only wanted confirmation of what I had already heard, to know from some other authority that what the doctors I'd already seen had recommended was the right thing to do."[4] Thus we find a number of patients who regret their snacks from the Tree of Knowledge, even patients as aggressive as Cornelius Ryan:

I have been reading a book called *End Results in Cancer*. Could any title be more oppressive? It is a little tome filled with records and statistics about the kinds of cancers there are and how long it takes particular age groups to die from each one. . . . The median survival time for my age group with cancer of the prostate is 5.5 years. That means I have a 50/50 chance of living that long after diagnosis.

    I wish I had never acquired this book.[5]

Similarly, a doctor with cancer remarked, "Now for the first time since my illness, I have the courage to read some texts on laryngeal cancer. One author recommends that cancer of the vocal cords be treated by surgery, not by X-ray. I wish now that I hadn't read it."[6]

Third, information about your health is interesting. It absorbs you; it is a currency of conversation that attracts astounding virtuosi. As Broyard remarks, "When people heard that I was ill, they inundated me with stories of their own illnesses, as well as the cases of friends. Storytelling seems to be a natural reaction to illness. People bleed stories, and I've become a bloodbank of them."[7] Furthermore, people are expected to answer friends' questions about their illness and are embarrassed when they cannot. Thus the mother of one kidney patient thought placing pamphlets in waiting rooms would not only allow family members "to be clear in their own minds as to what certain procedures are but also help answer the thousands of questions they are asked by friends and relatives."[8]

A weightier reason patients want information is that they care about their own welfare and their prospects for health and happiness. They wonder whether they will be able to work or will be disabled, whether they will live in pain or comfort, whether their lives will change or continue in their course, whether they will live or die. Wilfrid Sheed, for instance, "would have sold my soul cheerfully (if I could have done anything cheerfully) just to hear from someone else who had passed this way and could tell me what was actually happening to me and what to expect next."[9] Quite as urgently, people fear pain, disability, and death, and they crave information that can alleviate their fears. As one epileptic patient said, "'I wanted them to tell me [the] kinds of things I've seen in the literature. What a seizure is and basically, more important, what a seizure is not. I think that's the biggest fear I have. Can I die? Can I choke? Can I . . . ? Oh, big fears. I wanted my bigger fears allayed . . . ."[10]

While patients prefer good news to bad, they may prefer bad news to silence, for uncertainty can be as agonizing as physical pain. Molly Haskell writes: "As the puzzle continued, my spirits sank to a kind of subsistence level dread. I no longer had any idea what to feel or expect, and I got no help from the doctors. We were equally baffled in the presence of a mystery that broke all the rules of suspense, spraying clues widely in all directions, no solutions in sight."[11] For the misery of uncertainty, information is the only balm.[12]

In addition, learning about your disease can help you manage the strains and stresses of illness. As Fox comments of the men in the ward she studied, "'getting a liberal medical education' provided most F-Seconders with an accessible, appropriate, and effective way of coming to terms."[13] That knowledge "gave patients a sense of achievement and unity that made it easier for them to cope with incapacity and isolation."[14] In short, as Schneider and Conrad say, "Information about the disorder can help locate the person's experience in the medical and social world. It can alleviate fears, dispel misconceptions, and give people greater understanding of their troubles."[15]

People also seek information to help them handle their practical day-to-day problems. Illness, particularly chronic illness, confronts patients with novel challenges in the management of the quotidian, with new sensations and perceptions, new defects and limitations, new tasks and trials. Sick people want to know how they must adjust their lives or prepare for their deaths, what kinds of work they can do, which side effects of a drug to watch for, what symptoms and reactions justify calling 911,[16] how they should comply with a treatment and what will happen if they do not, and so on and on. As Schneider and Conrad write of the epileptic's need for information, "Knowledge then is a resource for developing ways to manage one's life. It includes acknowledging and validating one's feelings about epilepsy, learning how to minimize the interference of seizures and stigma in one's life, managing medications and other regimens, and dealing with other people and their reactions."[17]

Finally, people want information from their doctors as a matter of courtesy and an expression of kindness and concern. They think it rude and callous of doctors to leave them wretched in uncertainty. They welcome information that diminishes the social and personal distance between doctor and patient. What they want from their doctors as much as anything—except health—is sympathy and encouragement, and information can be an expression of both. Thus an English cancer patient wrote, "What gave me such a boost was that the second doctor treated me as a reasonably intelligent human being. After taking my history he began by saying, 'Let me explain what I think is happening to you.'" This helped convince her that he was "genuinely interested in how his patients were coping with their disease."[18] A novelist mired in illness said, "To quell terror and humiliation, I asked lots of questions. I didn't always understand the answers, nor did they always answer me, but I needed to let them know I had a mind as well as a body."[19] Finally, another patient was pleased his doctors "interacted with me as a person, not just an object of his or her practice. Dr. Blum frequently took time to explain what was going on." His doctors' concern to explain things gratified him not just because it increased his confidence in their decisions, but because it showed he was "a person about whom they cared."[20]

Some confirmation that information plays this role lies in the fact that, when Schneider and Conrad describe the information patients desire, they say patients "want to be listened to, supported through their fears, and helped to make better adaptations. They want doctors to *share* more with them. For some this is very general: 'If someone had just sat down and said *anything* [about epilepsy and what was happening] to me, I would have been so grateful at that point.'"[21] Similarly, Haskell says, "I was ravenous for information, and although most of what I was being given was baffling, I was so flattered at being treated like an intelligent human being that I never asked for amplification or explanation, and simply jotted down words and phrases with the intention of looking them up later."[22]

More systematic, although oblique, confirmation of this reason patients may want information without control comes from evidence that patients are specially likely to be noncompliant when their doctors obtain information from them but give none in return.[23] Less obliquely, a literature survey reported patient satisfaction "was best predicted by the amount of information given by providers during the medical encounter."[24] This survey also noted the existence of "a growing literature demonstrating the efficacy of information-giving for a variety of therapeutic effects, including shortened hospital stays, decreased use of analgesics, and reduced patient anxiety." The survey concluded that "the mechanism by which information achieves its therapeutic effects is through both the informative content per se and through the interpreted message of interest and caring."[25]

Finally, even if patients do not want to make their own medical decisions, they may want to refuse proposed treatments that seem patently unsatisfactory. Being told about treatments in advance permits them to retain such residual authority.[26] In other words, receiving information can make a delegation of authority safer.[27] It permits, to put it in legal terms, a kind of legislative veto, the principle of which was that an administrative agency could make decisions but had to report them to Congress, which could countermand egregious actions.

In short, patients can want a good deal besides the power to make medical decisions, and information is a crucial means to many of those ends. Patients can desire information from doctors for many purposes and without wanting to make their own decisions.[28] We have surveyed some of those reasons in this section. But to understand all of them we need to turn to the question of control.

Control

"Control" in this context has two distinct meanings, both equally crucial. In the first place, "control," as you would expect, means priority and ability to manage, not to force, the compliance of others, to determine what others think or do. In the second, more elusive sense—a sense which, nevertheless, saves my life and which, once achieved, may induce the relinquishing of "control" in the first sense—"control" means that when something untoward happens, some trauma or damage, whether inflicted by the commissions or omissions of others, or some cosmic force, one makes the initially unwelcome event one's own inner occupation. You work to adopt the most loveless, forlorn, aggressive child as your own, and do not leave her to develop into an even more vengeful monster, who constantly wishes you ill. In ill-health as in unhappy love, this is the hardest work: it requires taking in before letting be.

Gillian Rose, *Love's Work*

A second question I am often asked is how people can give up control over their own lives, as patients who delegate their medical decisions are taken to do.

This question reflects the contemporary assumption that human nature dictates and the psychological literature confirms that everyone craves plenary control and struggles unyieldingly for it. And it is true that "[i]n general, the pattern of these research findings suggests that the perception of personal control results in positive reactions, whereas the perception of a loss of control results in negative effects."[29]

It is another commonplace that the sick particularly long for control: "If I had to pick the aspect of illness that is most destructive to the sick, I would choose the loss of control. Maintaining control over oneself is so vital to all of us that one might see all the other phenomena of illness as doing harm not only in their own right but doubly so as they reinforce the sick person's perception that he is no longer in control."[30] Yet more categorically, but still conventionally: "[I]llness may cause patients to lose some control over their bodies. The traditional process of medical care then robs them of more control . . . . The loss of self reliance inevitably leads to the loss of self-esteem and the inculcation of dependency . . . ."[31] This view pervades the ideology of many support groups and some patients. Thus Korda was rebuked when he told his support group he was a victim of cancer: "'A cancer survivor,' Dennis said, facing me. 'Never forget that. *You are NOT a victim!* You're a *survivor.* A victim is somebody who's helpless, who has no control over his own fate. You're not helpless. Your fate is in your hands. Got it?'"[32] Another patient writes, "It was all about control. Take away a patient's sense of control over his life, and you have hurt him more than any injury or disease. Give him back that sense of control—and you have helped him more than any drug or therapy. He can make miracles happen."[32a] John Hockenberry comments sardonically on this attitude when he writes, "People who lose control are deviants or failures. People who have control are heroes, role models, victors over adversity, people 'with their shit together.'"[33]

Conventional wisdom further holds that patients best cope with the loss of control illness brings by making their own medical decisions. As one woman said: "I did everything I could think of to try to make sure the surgery would go smoothly and successfully. This time I was not in shock; I tried to prepare, educate myself, and make my own decisions. I wanted to feel some control this time."[34]

It is one of my continuing minor themes that, even if studies find that a majority of people feel one way about something, a minority—often a substantial minority—feel otherwise and that even the majority are often ambivalent or change their minds as circumstances vary. So it is with studies of the desire for control. They regularly report that some subjects do not crave control even where its attractions look obvious. And "researchers have now uncovered many exceptions to the rule [that people seek out control]. Many studies have reported situations in which people willingly relinquish control or respond in a negative manner to the perception that their personal control has been increased."[35] Furthermore, "there is more variability in perception of and desire for control with advancing age . . . ,"[36] so that those likeliest to be sick are also likeliest to vary in their wish for control. Not only are there people for whom control is not vital, there are weighty reasons people might not want—or might even want to cede—control. In addition, even people who want control as a general matter might seek it in ways other than making medical decisions.

Many people do want control in plentiful quantities, relish it, and flourish with it. Many patients expressly say they desire control and mourn its loss. Gilda Radner wrote, "The hard part about illness and cancer is that it feels so out of control."[37] Another cancer patient wanted "to be in control of as many things that affect myself and my family for as long as I can."[38] In a number of circumstances, people and patients who have "control" seem to be happier and healthier than those who do not. However, this view is so widely regarded as self-evident that it needs no reiteration from me. Rather, my task is to explain how people might *not* feel that way. Thus I will primarily ask why patients might cede control or might seek other forms of control than making medical decisions. I will begin by reviewing research that suggests why patients might forgo—or at least seem to forgo—control over their own circumstances by rejecting the power to make medical decisions. Then I will discuss ways patients seek control without making medical decisions.

First, some personality types want control and others do not. Burger and Cooper, for example, argue that "a desire for control over events is an important psychological dimension" of human characters which varies and can be systematically measured.[39] There is evidence, to take another example, that "people who have an external locus of control and those who handle stress through repression are less likely to prefer control or to find it beneficial."[40] Such people will "be more stressed by situations in which control is available. Several studies have found that sensitizers benefitted from information about self-control options following stressful medical procedures but that the same information was counterproductive for repressors to deniers . . . ."[41] Sensibly enough, people "seem to prefer and seek out situations that match their desired level of control. For example, compared to externals on health locus of control, internals prefer control in health-related areas . . . , are more involved in their post-operative care . . . , and are more likely to practice preventive dental care . . . ."[42]

The authors of the report I have been quoting conclude that "control options that are incongruent with an individual's desired or expected level of control will not be preferred and, in some cases, may actually be maladaptive."[43] Control might be undesired or "maladaptive" in a number of ways. These ways will be familiar, for they parallel tellingly the reasons patients might decline to make their own medical decisions I explored in Chapter 3. First, control is bad for you if you are likely to use it imprudently. I argued in Chapter 3 that patients might think they are less likely to make good choices than their doctors or families.

Given the high risk and cost of error, they prefer to relinquish some control to increase the odds of retrieving their health. Such people are, in brief, behaving in accord with the "research showing that humans will refrain from exercising control in situations in which the probability of success is not high."[44]

Not only might patients believe they lack the knowledge,[45] experience, or skill to make a decision, they may be reluctant—as I suggested in Chapter 3— to take responsibility, and thus blame, for decisions that seem fated to fail: "[P]eople will often refrain from exercising control in a situation that has likelihood of failure, presumably to avoid internal attributions for the failure."[46] Thus, speaking of situations in which "the possibility of failure is high and the price for failure is significant," Jerry Burger observes that "[u]nless the increase in control brings with it some strong advantages, people in this situation are likely to opt to relinquish control, to experience negative affect (such as anxiety), and not to perform as well on the task over which they have control."[47] Irving Janis puts the point yet more dramatically: "Although the relationships between reactions of postdecisional regret and the onset of psychosomatic disorders have not yet been adequately investigated, it seems quite possible that when ill people make unsound decisions, they not only reduce their chances of rapid, uncomplicated, and full recovery, but also increase their chances of developing new illnesses."[48]

Perhaps people *should* take this responsibility whether they welcome it or not. But the problem is complex partly because people sometimes feel responsibility when they should not. Annandale writes of patients in an "alternative" obstetrics clinic, "The consequences of this ethic of individual responsibility were quite problematic; women felt that they were responsible for an outcome that was, in reality, structurally induced and beyond their control. For example, women often felt that they had 'failed when they had difficult births.'"[49] Another part of this complexity is the "possibility that believing in and attempting to exercise control leaves one cognitively unprepared for failure, and that an unambiguous disconfirmation of expected control is more maladaptive than an initial perception of no control."[50] Here we return to a key problem: For too many patients, true control is an illusion, because their disease is so unruly. Such patients reasonably ask themselves not how to maximize control, but how to cope with its irretrievable loss.

The literature on control also substantiates the suggestion I made in Chapter 3 that sick patients can find the work of making medical decisions burdensome: "There is some evidence that control options that require effort and attention to execute are no more effective than not having control, or can actually increase arousal [i.e., distress] in comparison to situations in which no control is available to influence a stressful event. . . . It appears that control options that require attention and effort may at times increase rather than reduce stress."[51] As one study found, "the stress, effort, and hassle involved in using control were frequently mentioned by respondents . . . as reasons to prefer not having control."[52] Thus before we urge patients to seek control because of its psychological and moral benefits, we need to consider that, at least for some patients and in some circumstances, control may have the opposite effect.

Control can be "maladaptive" in yet another familiar way. As I noted in Chapter 3, acquiring and processing the facts needed to make decisions means facing up to that information. Burger concludes that at least some kinds of people (particularly the "blunters" described above) may not want or may suffer from control "when the increased controllability leads to an increase in attention to the now-predictable [unpleasant] events."[53] Thus, as I argued earlier, some patients may characteristically and comprehensibly trade control and authority for (relative) peace of mind.

In sum, patients might not welcome the control popular psychology assumes they crave. They may not want it because they fear using it badly, because they want to avoid the blame for failure, because control can be burdensome, and because control means confronting disturbing realities. But not only might patients not want control, they might want control without wishing to make medical decisions. This is a centrally important idea. Control means many things to many people. Students of the subject distinguish "three types of control: behavioral, encompassing direct action on the environment; cognitive, the interpretation of events, including information; and decisional, having a choice among alternative courses of action."[54] We have discussed the last of these at some length. But there are two other forms of control, and patients may prefer to substitute one form for another.

In considering what kinds of control might satisfy patients, we may begin by asking why people might want control. The primary answer is that control allows them to alter their environment so they can get what they want from life. Patients want control over their illness so they can end or at least moderate it. But complete control of one's environment, of every aspect of one's life, is not a realistic goal for anyone, and control over illness can be particularly elusive. Where patients cannot control their disease, they may look for other forms of "control." To put the point a bit differently, people might want control not to direct their medical treatment but to relieve two miseries of illness—the senses of uncertainty and helplessness. These two feelings can often be reduced without actually mastering one's illness or dictating one's medical care. Even patients who cannot subdue their disease may be able to influence other parts of their lives. And they may be able to tame their thoughts. In particular, both uncertainty and helplessness can often be vanquished by explaining the world to oneself to make it comprehensible, predictable, and benign.

Patients may achieve many benefits of control without making medical decisions because much of the argument for control is not about control itself, but about the psychological and even moral benefits of a *sense* of control. Fortunately, you can have a sense of control without the reality. People generally and patients particularly regularly persuade themselves they have control where they do not.[55] One Swedish study hinted at this when it reported that surgical patients "tended to retrospectively perceive their influence on the decision [to have an operation] as being more significant than they did at the time when the decision was taken."[56] Ellen Langer believes patients in hospitals and residents in nursing homes acquire a sense of control if they make a few decisions, even if not crucial ones.[57] In the dialysis unit I studied patients often felt they had taken control of their medical care when they decided what kind of dialysis to have, even if they rarely made other choices.

A sense of control may even be achieved by referring decisions to someone who will do it better than you: "Control may also not be preferred in situations in which another agent is seen as possessing greater skills or knowledge than oneself. Transferring control to that person is likely to be seen as a more effective way of getting desired outcomes than is exercising the control oneself."[58] Thus, in one study of why people chose not to assert control over health issues, one of the two "most common reasons given [was] identifying a more effective agent (e.g., 'My trainer knows better than I when I'm healthy and can play, so I let him decide.') . . ."[59] This is presumably the strategy of many of the patients I discussed in Chapter 3 who delegated medical decisions because they expected their surrogates to make decisions which better heightened their chance of regaining the control sickness had taken away.

In addition, as I wrote earlier, some patients gain a sense of control by learning how their disease works. This sense of control is of two kinds. First, knowledgeable patients discover how to soften the harshness and lighten the burdens of their illness.[60] Thus ulcerative-colitis patients Michael Kelly interviewed explained their disease in terms of diet or activities, explanations which helped them reduce the frequency or intensity of attacks of illness.[61] This tactic can verge on making one's own medical decisions, but for many people it means the reverse—being especially compliant with their doctors' instructions.[62]

Second, knowledge of one's disease may impart a sense of control even where the disease's effects go unabated. One doctor with ulcerative colitis knew she was "at risk for development of malignancy" and might therefore need surgery some day. Although that was "unpleasant to consider," it was "part of the larger and welcome realization that I am likely to know what can happen to me. Knowledge is control; the comfort of reasonable prediction outweighs the sadness of what may transpire."[63] A heart patient who aspired to be a doctor was "supremely triumphant" because he could "explain why I feel worse after a large meal." His "discovery was evidence that I can master this disease, come to know it so intimately that I will be able to survive with it. I am a spy in the house of my heart."[64] In addition, the sense of accomplishment won from learning to treat oneself can stimulate a sense of control. A multiple-sclerosis patient "marked a major turning point in my life" when she learned to catheterize herself: "For the first time ever, I'd taken control and stolen something back from the disease." This victory taught her "I truly was capable of doing *anything*."[65]

Not only do patients assert control over their disease without making medical decisions. They also compensate for disease's power by controlling other aspects of their lives. Many patients strive to live their daily lives normally, productively, and happily. In my research and my reading of patients' memoirs I am repeatedly impressed with the centrality of quotidian coping, of arranging the small and mundane affairs of daily life.[66] Tocqueville was right—"It . . . is especially dangerous to enslave men in the minor details of life. For my own part, I should be inclined to think freedom less necessary in great things than in little ones, if it were possible to be secure of the one without possessing the other."[67] We live lives compounded of chores and errands, customs and routines, minor problems and modest pleasures. These foolish things interest and concern us. We do them well and enjoy them. We do not wholly regret measuring out our lives with coffee spoons. Coffee spoons matter.

Many memoirists explicitly see this as a prudent and practical way of asserting control. One cancer patient remarked that, because he "already depended heavily upon the medical profession, I needed to be in charge of some of my own battles." He thus "continued the ritualization in my suite at Apley by gathering up my electric blanket, my radio, and a trashy magazine that predicted the astrological fortunes of aging Hollywood stars. Such personal property permitted the illusion that I was controlling my hospital environment."[68] Another cancer patient said, "We take control by choosing to take action in our daily life with the sickness and the horrendous side effects of chemotherapy."[69] And Michael Korda spent the night before deciding how to treat his prostate cancer by arranging his

> travel plans for my return from the hospital. This kind of thing is a common reaction to cancer. Trivial problems take on undue importance. There is a natural human tendency to turn molehills into mountains in the face of disaster, if only because thinking about relatively unimportant or pedestrian details gives people the illusion of being in control of their fate. *You* can make decisions, after all, about travel arrangements, or hotel reservations, or which dressing gown you're going to bring with you to the hospital, or whether or not you should go for a TV in your hospital room.[70]

Control for these patients comes from maintaining the familiar basics of their lives: They affirm their ties with those they love, they get to work on time, they go bowling Thursday night.

Sometimes patients assert control over debility in more striking and even reckless ways. Gretel Ehrlich's encounter with lightning left her blood pressure so unreliable she was constantly in danger of passing out. But though she had learned "how easy it was to die," she resolved "by God, I was going to pack a few more things in before Death took me away."[71] So, not long after her injury, she journeyed from California to London to see a ballet she had collaborated on.

The trip's rigors, and thus her determination to assert herself, are betokened by her having to lie down in the taxi to avoid fainting.

Control may be attained in less admirable ways. The sick may wield "the tyranny of the helpless"[72] by using illness to quell friends, family, physicians, colleagues, or employers. Mrs. Bennet, for example, memorably berates her husband,

> "Mr. Bennet, how can you abuse your own children in such a way? You take delight in vexing me. You have no compassion on my poor nerves."
> "You mistake me, my dear. I have a high respect for your nerves. They are my old friends. I have heard you mention them with consideration these twenty years at least."

Literature's manipulative valetudinarians are hardly confined to *Pride and Prejudice;* they are as plentiful in life as in fiction. Marvin Barrett asked himself how he would use his cancer. "Am I already using it? To feel more, less guilty? To get sympathy? To make others feel guilty? To get out of things I would otherwise have felt obliged to do?"[73] Ben Watt

> watched friends stumbling over their self-consciousness and battling with over- or under-reaction. If I held out a hand I'd see them choking back a tear. If I were quiet for a few minutes they would feel they had overstayed their welcome. If I smiled weakly I'd feel I had inadvertently created a moment of unbearable poignancy. And curiously, because of this, I felt a huge amount of power over them. I realized I could manipulate their emotions, and I was fascinated at their impressionability. It seemed easy to exploit their good intentions and, if I chose, to turn a cough into a dying breath, a goodbye into a last farewell.[74]

Howard Brody reasons that if "the sick affect the healthy in deep and powerful ways, and if, as the sociologists argue, to be sick is to occupy a well-defined social role that creates reciprocal role responsibilities in others, then the sick person is ironically also in a position of great power."[75] That power sometimes gives patients control over their environment as great as, even if less admirable than, the control found in medical decisions.

Where patients cannot control their illness or their surroundings, they may wrest a sense of control by reinterpreting their lives. Some people, for example, master disease by adjusting their view of it. William James called this the "religion of healthy-mindedness":

> Much of what we call evil is due entirely to the way men take the phenomenon. It can so often be converted into a bracing and tonic good by a simple change of the sufferer's inner attitude from one of fear to one of fight; its sting so often departs and turns into a relish when, after vainly seeking to shun it, we agree to face about and bear it cheerfully, that a man is simply bound in honor, with reference to many of the facts that seem at first to disconcert his peace, to adopt this way of escape.[76]

As the paralyzed Arnold Beisser reflected:

> What became new and exciting was this idea: that perhaps the power to determine how I looked upon life was within me. Whether I considered my disability a great tragedy and a loss or whether I saw it in some more positive light might just possi-

bly be a matter of my discretion. If this was true, and it seemed increasingly likely that it was, new worlds of belief and perception were open to me, and new hope for what my life could be was waiting.[77]

And as an AIDS patient put it,

> He was changing the way he was feeling about life. It was happening not through denying his feelings however. Feelings always need to be expressed. No, he was actually changing his feelings by looking behind them toward the thoughts in his mind from which they emerged. He was now choosing to think differently. This was the one thing he could always have control of. He could choose what to think about the events unfolding in his life. He was beginning to exercise his free will.[78]

In one sect of the religion of healthy-mindedness—what James called the "Mind-cure movement"—this attitude is even thought therapeutic. "The leaders in this faith have had an intuitive belief in the all-saving power of healthy-minded attitudes as such, in the conquering efficacy of courage, hope, and trust, and a correlative contempt for doubt, fear, worry, and all nervously precautionary states of mind."[79] Under this movement's sway, "[t]he blind have been made to see, the halt to walk; life-long invalids have had their health restored."[80]

The Mind-cure movement has hardly faded in the century since James wrote. If anything, it has blossomed. Norman Cousins, the St. Paul of this creed, was told his illness was progressive and incurable. But "[s]ince I didn't accept the verdict, I wasn't trapped in the cycle of fear, depression, and panic that frequently accompanies a supposedly incurable illness."[81] He could thus deploy his will to live, "a physiologic reality with therapeutic characteristics," and "mobilize all the natural resources of body and mind to combat disease."[82] Similarly, Joie McGrail thought eliminating fear was her "best hope for prolonging my life."[83] The attraction of control through Mind-cure is put explicitly by a leukemia patient converted by two of its apostles: "What Drs. Simonton and Siegel were offering was a sense of power and control. A sense of simple cause and effect. While all the doctors were emphasizing the randomness of my history, and, more important, of my hope for recovery, here was a way of thinking that offered me some influence over the course of events."[84] Another cancer patient so believed in the power of mind over body that she came to "avoid phrases like 'to die for,' 'it's killing me,' or 'it's driving me crazy.' These thoughts, once verbalized, get internalized as fact. Often the body can't detect what is just a saying and what is actually happening."[85]

The religion of healthy-mindedness can induce patients to change from being "more or less disposed to let the doctors worry about my condition" to feeling "a compulsion to get into the act."[86] But it can also direct concern away from medical decisions and toward emotional or spiritual well-being. Thus one of James' friends came "to disregard the meaning of this attitude for bodily health *as such,* because that comes of itself, as an incidental result, and cannot be found by any special mental act or desire to have it, beyond that general attitude of mind I have referred to above."[87]

But even when the religion of healthy-mindedness inspires patients to get into the act, it does not necessarily lead them to participate in medical decisions as commonly understood. Many Mind-cure treatments require no mediating expert; they offer do-it-yourself remedies. For example, it is the rare disease someone does not try to cure through diet, and legions of patients experiment heroically with diets while undergoing conventional medical treatment.[88] Even alternative remedies that rely on experts often supplement, and do not replace, conventional therapies. Thus many Mind-curers simultaneously consult conventional and unconventional therapies. Some adherents are aggressive about choosing alternative therapies but unaggressive about participating in conventional medical decisions.[89]

Jill Ireland, for example, had breast cancer. As a movie actor in her own right, and as the wife of the star Charles Bronson, she had easy access to her doctors. However, she did little to join in their decisions. In fact, when her husband told her after her biopsy he had asked her doctors to perform a mastectomy but they had insisted on consulting her, she protested: "'Why didn't they operate while I was out? Why didn't they? No. I won't. I can't go through that again. . . . I can't face the anesthetic. I can't go through the post-operating room again. Oh, why didn't they do it while I was out. Why?' "[90] However, Ireland's ready acquiescence in the "AMA" portion of her care coexisted with her repeatedly professed desire to participate actively in treating her disease. Thus she sought out Dr. O. Carl Simonton, who gave her meditation assignments, including visualizing her white blood cells destroying her cancer cells; consulted a homeopathic doctor (as, she says, the English royal family has long done) who had her drink electrically treated water and undergo sessions on an electromagnetic wave table; saw a therapist who gave her crystals ("for focusing and energizing my mind and body"[91] and "to help change my cancer personality"[92]) and led her to begin "the hard work of self-discovery";[93] and in all these ways started "to wage war on cancer."[94] She knew that if "I allowed myself to believe I would have a cancer recurrence within the next year or two, then I probably would. But if I deeply believed I would not . . . then I knew I wouldn't suffer a recurrence."[95] In short, Ireland ceded her "medical" decisions to her family and physicians but found a sense of control in choosing "alternative" healers and in managing her state of mind.

Many patients attain another kind of control by finding some explanation for their illness, some meaning to it. Renée Fox reports: "The question 'why' was one that the patients of Ward F-Second frequently asked themselves and each other . . . ."[96] Arnold Beisser speaks for many: "My belief was that the universe was an orderly place, and there were cause-and-effect relationships that determined all things. I also believed that there was justice in everything. Good deeds were rewarded, and bad ones punished. Perhaps my illness was some form of justice. Perhaps I had done some terrible thing."[97]

Some of Fox's patients, like millions of others, found an answer to the question why they had fallen sick and hence won a measure of "control" in the consolations of religion.[98] One study of arthritis patients, for instance, found 44% of them used prayer as a means of achieving power over their disease.[99] A cardiac surgeon with AIDS put the issue in terms: "My dilemma was that I had to relinquish what I as a doctor prized most—control. . . . I had become God's patient, and he my heart surgeon, . . . trying to help me understand what he was going to do." The surgeon "spent a lot of energy trying to understand what this illness meant . . . . What had God said about it in his word?"[100]

Other patients find such explanations in their moral views, often by attributing to themselves a history of "'improper living or improper thinking.'"[101] Still others, particularly in an age when healthy living sometimes seems all morality demands, ask what principle of the healthy life they have traduced: "Behind it was the weight of the question I wanted so desperately to ask: I've followed all the rules of health and more, so how could this have happened to me?"[102] The search for meaning is, to be sure, not always successful, but meaning is a need widely felt. As Fitzhugh Mullan writes, "My plummet from youth and health to the depths of cancer must have been caused by something I had done . . . . [W]hat was it? What act of hubris had I been guilty of? What principle, what ethic had I offended by my behavior? What had I done wrong?"[103]

These moral explanations for illness can nurture a sense of control quite directly. Kathy Charmaz observes, "Ill people's 'should' recover often shades into 'merits' or 'deserves' recovery. A number of people . . . echoed this woman's comment: 'I really feel strongly that once this [illness and treatment for it] is over, that I've paid my dues with my health.'"[104] Charmaz thinks patients try to earn recovery by doing the "right things," and particularly by being good patients. They thus "atone[ ] for whatever prior failings or omissions for which they might have felt responsible" and "deserve to return to the activities on which their preferred identities . . . rest."[105]

Patients also reach for control by explaining their approach to illness. Their struggle with disease becomes the organizing principle of their lives. Thus Anne Hawkins' study of patients' memoirs notes that patients recruit metaphors to explain how they are handling their illness—military metaphors or the metaphor of a journey.[106] Arthur Frank observes that "[q]uest stories meet suffering head on; they accept illness and seek to *use* it. Illness is the occasion of a journey that becomes a quest."[107]

Patients may assert control through explanations that go beyond understanding their disease or their attitude to it and that instead interpret the meaning and purpose of their lives after becoming ill. Illness, particularly severe and chronic illness, can transform everything. For Reynolds Price, "The kindest thing anyone could have done for me, once I'd finished five weeks' radiation, would have been to look me square in the eye and say this clearly, 'Reynolds Price is dead. Who will you be now? Who *can* you be and how can you get there, double-time?' "[108] Hawkins writes that illness can be "so painful, destructive, and disorienting that it results in a counterimpulse toward creation and order. This counterimpulse is what Lifton . . . calls 'formulation,' a reparative process that deals with trauma by imagination and interpretation."[109] Thus his paraplegia taught John Hockenberry "that life could be reinvented. In fact such an outlook was required. The physical dimensions of life could be created, like poetry; they were not imposed by some celestial landlord."[110]

When we think about ethics and the ill, we think about clinical ethics, about the obligations doctors and hospitals have to patients and the responsibility patients have for their medical decisions. But for patients, especially the chronically ill, these questions often pale next to the larger question we all face—how to live a good life. Illness is not all of anyone's life, and illness does not obliterate—indeed, it often sharpens—the universal questions about the purpose and wisdom of one's life.[111] Answers to those questions can do much to reestablish a sense of control. Coping with disease can itself become a life-shaping challenge. As one patient glumly put it: "Illness has a seductive power, in that it bestows a life plan of sorts."[112] Serious disease makes extraordinary demands of courage and fortitude. But meeting them can give patients a sense of purpose and accomplishment—of control.

Some patients can make illness creative and productive, can emulate Oliver Sacks, who, Anatole Broyard thought, "reconciles afflicted people to their environment in such a way that they are not so much submitting to it in an impaired exchange as proposing a novel relation. He turns disadvantage to advantage."[113] This alchemy is hard. Flannery O'Connor put it nicely when she said she could only "with one eye squinted take it all as a blessing."[114] Nevertheless, squinting or not, surprising numbers of the sick find blessings even in the curse of illness.

For some patients, the blessings are direct, concrete, and practical. One man found, "You receive a lot of attention. You take a vacation from work. You have time to read things you have been putting off."[115] One woman commented of her lupus, "In addition to a healthier marriage, it encourages my writing, a creativity that would have remained suppressed as long as I worked full-time, an art form that allows me full expression of my feelings and thoughts. I am able to spend more time with the whole family, and I can concentrate some of my creative instincts on our home."[116]

Many patients go further and convert disease from menace to mentor. One woman "realize[d] that wonderful things would occur after the cancer experience as long as I had faith . . . ," for "cancer would always be a great teacher of mine which I would cease to fear and learn to respect."[117] For many, disease teaches a renewed and enriched sense of life's meaning. That meaning often lies in a deepened faith. A surgeon with AIDS wrote, "The more I immersed myself in the Word, the more I discovered that the coin of affliction has two sides. Every testing is also a hidden opportunity to show that our faith is real; more than that, to prove—to others as well as ourselves—that *God* is real."[118] And a Parkinson's patient affirmed, "Because I did turn to Him, God has furnished me with tremendous strength and has shown me how to creatively use my suffering to lead a meaningful life."[119]

Whether religious or not, many patients testify that illness has revivified their appreciation for existence: "The only changes are on the positive side. I no longer take things for granted, especially, just being alive. I appreciate things more. Every leaf and blossom and each rain drop has a meaning for me."[120] Illness particularly teaches patients how much they do and should cherish the love of their families and the affection of their friends: "My family is more precious to me with each day we are together and I savor every moment."[121] Illness also instructs patients about themselves: "[O]nce you face your own imminent death, reflection comes easy."[122] Through reflection, "[y]ou learn a lot about yourself."[123] Hawkins, for example, describes a patient who took from illness "a new perspective on life that enables her to see the difference between personal and societal goals. This understanding is itself a kind of 'rebirth'—a birth of the newly individuated self, perceived as radically distinct from the needs and pressures of the society to which it belongs."[124]

Not only can illness teach you about yourself. It can make you a better person. Physicians sometimes say illness makes them kinder doctors and wiser people. One commented ruefully, "If this kind of unexpected and traumatic experience can significantly increase the level of humility and sense of greater humanity in a physician, the experience is probably salutary."[125] Other patients learn other lessons. For example, "'I can honestly say that the cancer has made me a better, more tolerant person. I used to get upset and irritable about the most stupid things. Having breast cancer has put everything in perspective.'"[126] Patients have been inspired by illness to help other people, particularly people with their disease. Thus a lupus patient who tried to surmount his disease by treating it as an adventure wrote that that adventure "has been kept alive by my commitment to help and encourage others. Though I no longer feel the need for a support group, I like to attend so that I can aid others in need."[127]

One common way the ill feel sickness has improved them particularly speaks to our discussion of control. Patients often say their ordeal gives them "courage and strength to face other life crises."[128] As one wrote, "Crises improve one's ability to deal with helplessness, sharpen one's focus on important life issues, and result in a sense of accomplishment, once resolved."[129] In other words, by making patients stronger, illness ironically increases one kind of feeling of control.

One of Abraham Verghese's patients summarizes so enthusiastically so many of the ways illness can be considered an advantage that she deserves quoting at length:

"I have become a person I didn't know existed inside of me. I know I can make friends. I know I'm respected after people get to know me. And my heart is so full of love to give to them who need it. I'm so active in every organization I join. I'm now on the board of TAP! Can you believe it? An old country hick like me? I'm living my life to the fullest and thanking God for each day that I'm here. . . . So if anything, this disease has made me take a long look at how things were before I got it and afterward. I'm more of a complete person than I ever was." Here she pounded her right fist into her cupped left hand. "I set goals for myself that I'm determined to fulfill. I am somebody. I'm happier now than I've been in a long time."[130]

Whatever their content, then, explanations of their illness and of its place and their own in the world can give patients a sense of order, predictability, and meaning that serves some of the critical functions of "control." It even appears that this kind of control may have direct physical benefits, for "[i]t has long been noted in the study of pain that the meaning of an injury or its consequences for the individual dramatically affect the amount of pain felt . . . . [Individuals] search to find a meaning for the event; the meaning they assign to it determines their reactions and their ability to cope . . . ."[130a] Indeed, the control patients achieve through finding meaning in their disease can loom larger and last longer in the lives of patients than the relatively inconsequential kind that comes from the transient and perilous enterprise of making medical decisions. Making those decisions may simply fail to effect the kinds of control that will be crucial to many patients—like control over their minds and thoughts. "The old man, sick with an insidious internal disease, may laugh and quaff his wine at first as well as ever, but he knows his fate now, for the doctors have revealed it; and the knowledge knocks the satisfaction out of all these functions. They are partners of death and the worm is their brother, and they turn to mere flatness."[131] A sufferer from lupus expressed many patients' hope when she said, "You have little control over the fact that you have a certain disease, but you can control the way you respond to it, and that can strongly influence your ability to cope and to heal."[132] In short, for many patients "the paradox learned on the quest is that surrendering the superficial control of health yields control of a higher order."[133]

Illness is a physical crisis. But it is a moral crisis as well. Patients try to lead good and satisfying lives. They labor to vanquish the disabilities and disadvantages illness inflicts. This calls for virtues most of us would like to have in more abundance, particularly qualities of dignity, grace, courage, and perseverance. These are qualities that require self-command. For many patients, then, the central question of control is how to overcome fear and frailty, how to govern themselves. Triumphs in this struggle impart a sense of mission and mastery—of control—that runs deep. In short, there are many paths to the "control" people are assumed to require, and making medical decisions is only one. So people may crave control but still reject making their own medical decisions.

Ultimately, though, we need to put the search for control into yet deeper per-

spective: The brute and brutal fact, the central and insuperable fact looming implacably over the lives of the sick, is that for chronically or gravely ill patients,
control of the kind they most crave and require—of the kind whose absence is
felt most intensely and matters most—is exactly the kind they are least likely to
achieve. The control they most want is not decisional authority, or comprehension, or coping. It is control over their disease. It is a cure. And that control is the
most elusive of all.

Complexity: The Varieties of Medical Decision

*To Ivan Ilych only one question was important: was his case serious or not? But the doctor ig-
nored that inappropriate question. From his point of view it was not the one under consideration, the real question was to decide between a floating kidney, chronic catarrh, or appendicitis. It is not a question of Ivan Ilych's life or death, but one between a floating kidney and
appendicitis. And that question the doctor solved brilliantly, as it seemed to Ivan Ilych, in
favour of the appendix, with the reservation that should an examination of the urine give fresh
indications the matter would be reconsidered.*   Leo Tolstoy, *The Death of Ivan Ilych*

I have so far talked as though all medical decisions were the same and as
though patients' attitudes toward one kind of medical decision must be their attitude toward all. But this is false. "Medical decisions" is too compendious and diverse a category to be analyzed under a single principle. It matters where a decision is made, what kind of decision it is, what consequences it has, and who
contributes to it. A decision made in a hospital can vary critically from one made
in a doctor's office. A decision made with a long-trusted personal physician may
not resemble one made with an emergency room intern. A decision made by a
chronically ill patient may be quite unlike one made by an acutely ill person. A
decision to write a DNR order is not the same as a decision to do a nose job. A
decision to undergo a one-time procedure—like an appendectomy—has different
implications and contours from a decision to undertake a prolonged course of
therapy—like dialysis—that can be altered or halted *in medias res*. In other
words, here bioethics has again strayed onto the path of hyper-rationalism, of
substituting assumptions about human behavior for a sharp examination of its
complexity. This section, then, asks how medical decisions may differ.

    In the work of disaggregation we have not been helped by bioethics' paradig-
matic stories—cases like *Quinlan* and *Cruzan*. Both involved hopelessly ill, permanently comatose, young patients whose prognosis was uncontroverted and
whose decent and loving families wanted their life-support systems removed
after long and pained reflection. But those situations are unrepresentative not just
of most medical or any other decisions (for instance, both patients were comatose
and could not make medical decisions), but even of decisions at the end of life.
Howard Brody, for instance, astutely observes that "primary care settings [are] a
context typically ignored by medical ethics literature, but [they are] where the

majority of doctor–patient encounters occur." Likewise, he notes that "models of informed consent . . . typically take as the paradigm case something like surgery for breast cancer or the performance of an invasive and risky radiological procedure."[134] It is in just this way that, as Leon Kass comments, "today's approach to ethics abstracts still further from the rich context of our moral life by concentrating mainly on the *extreme examples.*"[135]

The predominance of these misleading paradigmatic cases also helps reveal how autonomy has attained so prepotent a place in bioethics. The autonomy arguments in *Quinlan* and *Cruzan* were especially appealing. Those young women and their families were particularly sympathetic, their plights were particularly wrenching, their interests were particularly strong, and their cases raised few real medical issues. There thus seemed little doctors could contribute to these decisions and much to be said for confiding them to the patient (through advance directives) or to their families. The danger is extrapolating from these comparatively rare cases to the ordinary run of medical decisions. The danger lies, that is, in assuming that because these cases might be readily understood in autonomy terms, *all* cases should be primarily analyzed that way.

The danger is not solely bioethicists'. It affects the general public, for the prominence of these paradigmatic cases misleads the uninformed and unwary about, for example, the range of decisions they make by signing advance directives. I recall a patient who was admitted to a hospital and was fast becoming unable to breathe. He arrived wielding an advance directive announcing his wish not to be intubated. A physician pressed him on the point and told him he would surely survive if, but only if, he allowed himself to be intubated for a few days. The patient expostulated that of course he wanted to be intubated, that his advance directive had only meant he did not want to be kept alive in a perpetual coma, to live like a vegetable. Such misunderstandings seem only too likely when so narrow a selection from so wide a range of cases occupies so prominent a place in the public mind.

In what follows, then, I will identify some of the principal lines of distinction within the category "medical decisions." My discussion will tend to show why patients might make some medical decisions but eschew others. I begin with the most obvious distinction, the one between "medical" and "nonmedical" questions. It is hardly easy to define "medical," but for our purposes a medical decision is primarily one about means and not ends. It is primarily a technical decision, a decision about what causes a particular disease, what symptoms reveal its presence, and what treatment will ameliorate it. A medical decision is a determination about whether someone has arthritis, about whether someone's high blood pressure can be controlled with a beta blocker, or about what side effects that drug might entail. A medical decision is the kind of decision medical training is primarily directed toward understanding. Doctors are therefore likely to make them better than patients.

A nonmedical decision is the residual category of decisions that are not medical. Every medical decision depends on a nonmedical decision, for medical decisions always promote an end which cannot be chosen by purely medical reasoning. Most commonly that end will be "health," or "normal functioning," or the closest approximation possible. Definitions of health and normal function are notoriously slippery, but despite the undoubted scope for disagreement, the goal will often be obvious, for there is a good deal of cultural commonality about what health means. In any event, nonmedical decisions are not technical, but rather are moral, religious, social, psychological, or even arbitrarily personal. And exactly because nonmedical decisions fall outside doctors' technical training, there are few strong *a priori* reasons to think doctors make them better than patients.

This distinction between means and ends, between technical and normative decisions, is hardly novel. Quite the contrary—it is at the heart of the autonomy paradigm. The distinction particularly helps make sense of that paradigm in cases like *Quinlan* and *Cruzan,* for in them, once the prognosis had been established there was essentially no further medical question to decide, no medical decision to make. Everything depended on the normative interpretation placed on the technical data.

The distinction between means and ends may help explain why some patients say they do not want to make their own medical decisions. They may regard "medical decisions" as quite different from the questions of withholding life support that were at stake in *Quinlan* and *Cruzan.* They may prefer that the technical issues in the former situation be handled by physicians; but they may wish to resolve what they see as the religious, moral, social, and practical issues the latter situations present. They may regard medical matters as painfully foreign but see choices about whether to live a merely vegetable existence as at least within their ken. Some evidence for this proposition lies, for example, in a study of patients of an HMO which found that they were more interested in making their decisions when they did not require medical knowledge than when they did.[136] And, for example, many of the patients I have interviewed wanted to decide what kind of dialysis to use (a decision which is often a matter of medical indifference) but never considered selecting medications to ingest, in whatever quantity or variety.

So informative is the distinction between medical and nonmedical decisions that one is tempted to say flatly doctors should make medical decisions and patients nonmedical ones. But this solution, though neat, fails. Patients may want, need, and be able to make at least some "technical" decisions. We have enumerated many reasons for this, and since they are the standard reasons autonomists advance, they hardly need repetition here. Let me mention two: First, patients who are chronically ill get to know their disease and their reactions to treatments for it well. They may thus become skilled in routine treatment decisions. In addition, such questions arise so regularly and inconveniently that the chronically ill cannot always consult a doctor and must make technical medical decisions.

Second, as autonomists have long argued, patients sometimes override technical decisions for nontechnical reasons. A physician might calculate, say, that a
patient whose kidneys had failed would be healthiest by the patient's own definition of health with a transplant. The patient might decide, however, that the risks
of surgical complications and the sequelae of severe rejection were too frightening to justify the benefits. Sometimes patients even seem surprisingly uninterested in "health." For example, the kidney patients I have observed often care
more about practical day-to-day problems than what might seem weightier issues, and I have virtually never found patients who, in choosing what kind of
dialysis to have, wanted to know how the choice would affect their chances of
morbidity or mortality. What they care about instead are questions like what they
can eat, how much they can drink, whether they can work, and how much time
they must spend sparring with their disease. In short, where patients feel strongly,
they are likelier to want to make even an apparently technical decision.

It is conventional wisdom that patients have these kinds of reasons to make
"medical" decisions. But it is also true that physicians may usefully contribute to
"nonmedical" decisions. Of course, doctors are expert about the facts necessary
for making nonmedical decisions. Thus people asked to decide whether to be
kept alive in a persistent vegetative state will often want to know the answers to
some technical questions, like whether they would feel pain. Less obviously, doctors may know how other patients experienced and thought about a choice and,
what is more, how they felt about their decision after living with the results. The
physician may thus see the normative issues more clearly than the patient. For
example, William Martin, the sociologist with prostate cancer who conspicuously wanted to make his own medical decisions, had a revealing conversation
with one of his doctors. The doctor had his own views about what Martin's values should be. He announced: "'Our three goals are survival, continence, and
potency—in that order.'" Martin thought that potency was badly misplaced in the
hierarchy. The doctor continued, "'Continence is an issue all the time. It's very
important.'" Martin "resisted his assertion for the moment, but knew he was probably correct."[137] Here, the doctor knew many patients who had suffered from
both incontinence and impotence and could draw some valuable, even if contro-
vertible, conclusions about which disability Martin would find more distressing.

The medical/nonmedical distinction, while basic and illuminating, is too simple in other ways. For example, significant decisions rarely fall neatly into either
category. They are rather analogous to what lawyers call "mixed questions of law
and fact." Breast cancer, for instance, is often cited as a disease which presents
patients with an important nontechnical choice.[138] But that choice is embedded
in an extensive network of technical problems.[139] Often the patient's goal—
perfect health—will be unattainable, and the patient must choose between several
treatments that offer varying levels of hope for reaching somewhat different
states of health. "So many tradeoffs, so much subjectivity. One trades the lessen-

ing of specific pains—here throat, chest, and spine—for mental dullness and headaches, nervousness and pouring sweats, bladder complications and bowel constipation."[140] So it will often be hard to disentangle means from ends, the technical from the normative.

The medical/nonmedical distinction is further complicated by the fact that it is only one of many axes along which medical decisions can be distinguished. For example, medical decisions can be divided according to how consequential they are for either doctor or patient; some are so trivial that a doctor or a patient may, in the great scheme of things, be indifferent to the choice of treatment. Even some substantial "medical" questions can be answered equally well in several ways. Kassirer and Pauker suggest that one explanation for the numerous situations in which experts "have different and strongly held opinions about the optimal treatment strategy" is that often "it simply makes no difference which choice is made. We suggest that some dramatic controversies represent 'toss-ups'— clinical situations in which the consequences of divergent choices are, on the average, virtually identical."[141] These are cases, that is, where differences between the expected utilities of the alternatives are not only "clinically unimportant, but [where] the error in the calculated utilities may well exceed the differences."[142]

In these cases, the patient may defer to the doctor's technical judgment and the doctor may bow to the patient's nontechnical preferences. For example, it has been the conventional wisdom that hemodialysis and peritoneal dialysis are medically equivalent for many patients. In such cases, questions that seemed to demand expertise dissolve into questions that can be decided according to the patient's preferences, however arbitrary or whimsical. While the question of dialysis modality may be medically inconsequential, it can be momentous to the patient for other reasons. For example, peritoneal dialysis is commonly performed at home, hemodialysis generally at a clinic. But many patients cannot easily go to a distant center for hemodialysis three times a week, several hours each time. In short, the choice of dialysis modality may matter little to the doctor and much to the patient. On the other hand, many patients doubt that choices are genuinely toss-ups, or that if they are toss-ups statistically, they are toss-ups for them personally. Such patients may be all too aware that medical opinion changes and that choices that look identical now may look different later. For these patients, the toss-up can be agonizing rather than easy and may seem to call more for experienced medical judgment than personal preference.

There is also a category of medical decisions patients do not regard as decisions because they seem to offer no real choice. The patient's kidneys fail, and earlier abdominal operations foreclose peritoneal dialysis. The patient is two or three years away from the top of the list for a cadaveric transplant, and no relative is a suitable donor. The patient will have hemodialysis or die. Few patients think this is a choice, and analyzing it in terms of autonomy may strike them as bitterly inapt. One sadly wise patient wrote me,

When I went into the doctor's office after the first round of chemotherapy and said that I couldn't do it anymore, couldn't take any more needles or IV's, is that exercising autonomy? I was saying that I was giving up; just let me die. I sure didn't feel very autonomous. I didn't feel as if either of the choices I saw available were acceptable. Saying "no," refusing treatment, is not really being autonomous, it seems to me. When I think of being an autonomous person, I think of being in charge of my life, determining things, making choices I want to make. When the only choices available are both negative, unacceptable ones, then I sure don't feel autonomous, in charge.

Another patient "had time to read all the grisly reports on whether or not to have open-heart surgery, whether it was really necessary, the continual debate on whether to 'bypass or not to bypass.' And yet, the fact of the matter was, what choice did I have?"[143] A doctor-become-patient put it flatly: "[W]hen you cannot walk and modern surgery offers an escape, there is no alternative."[144] Gilda Radner believed "oncologists have to tell you the worst possible side effects because they don't want to be sued. . . . There were a lot of other side effects, too, but since cancer kills you, you don't have much choice."[145] Another patient decided "rather lightly" to have radiation therapy and signed "extensive releases acknowledging the possibility of death, destruction, further cancers, and a host of other medical ailments and catastrophes" because he felt he "had no choice."[146] These cases are neatly summed up by Geoffrey Wolff. Told he needed a valve replacement to stay alive, he responded, "'What was to decide?'"[147]

The example of selecting a dialysis modality suggests another distinction among medical decisions—some are reversible and some are not. Where decisions are reversible and remediable, patients may feel more comfortable addressing even technical questions. Choosing dialysis modalities often falls in this category, since one modality does not preclude another, and it is often possible to switch if necessary. This, then, is another reason nephrologists may cede the choice of modality to patients, and the patient may comfortably make it.

Another useful distinction among medical decisions hinges on the patient's status. Some patients are more vigorous, more confident, or more experienced than others and may thus be better suited to handle decisions. For example, many chronically ill patients deal daily with their disease and treat themselves for it. They often become quite learned about how medicines affect them and quite shrewd about monitoring and dosing themselves. Diabetics, for instance, often discover just how they react to given combinations of diet, exercise, and insulin.[148] Many epileptics work out how to adjust their dosages of dilantin to achieve the nicest balance between seizures and side effects.[149] Asthmatics may become as well versed in managing crises in their illness as some emergency-room physicians.[150] As one patient says, "Parkinsonians have the edge on doctors, even neurologists, when it comes to understanding certain (but not all!) aspects of the disease. They also have the most comprehensive list of coping techniques. Doctors are limited to what they can observe, read, or speculate. The Parkinsonian acquires his knowledge from living with the disease day and night."[151] These are not trivial decisions, since mistakes can be costly, and even fatal; people die of insulin shock and asthma attacks. But such patients may confidently make them for several reasons. First, chronically ill patients develop mountains of experience. Second, the variation among patients is great, and a given patient will react differently to medication depending on the patient's circumstances. Chronically ill patients often become more expert at managing the recurring features of their own illness than anyone else can reasonably be. Third, patients must make many such decisions because often no one else can be there daily or in the crisis.

A related distinction is between one-time and repeated decisions. You can only decide once to have your appendix out. But patients who have undergone, say, cardiopulmonary resuscitation, or endoscopy, or blood tests may become more adept and assured in making decisions than patients facing the unfamiliar. Thus one physician-become-renal-patient found that "daily dietary decisions and taking of medication necessary to control high glucose levels and high blood pressure, or to prevent renal osteodystrophy, can best be carried out successfully by the knowledgeable patient."[152]

Another distinction among decisions concerns the time available to deliberate. The law of informed consent recognizes this distinction by creating an exception for emergency decisions, but the distinction is much broader than informed consent's narrow exception. Some decisions must be made in a few hours or a few days, and patients under such pressure may be inclined to rely on a doctor's advice or even decision. Other choices need not be made for years. Patients with kidney failure often wait several years before a cadaveric organ becomes available for transplanting, and during this time they not only can reflect on their decision but learn all about life on dialysis from personal experience and about life after transplant from the other patients around the dialysis unit.

Yet another distinction suggests why patients wish to make some decisions and not others, why they make some decisions satisfactorily and others less so. Some decisions present patients with many choices, some only a few. The more choices, the more forbidding the decision, since patients have more to learn and more complexity to subdue. This distinction is exemplified by the contrast between two patients anxious to make their own decisions—William Martin[153] and Barbara Creaturo.[154] Martin had prostate cancer and was given three choices: surgery, radiation, and watchful waiting. He read articles in medical journals and in periodicals like *Fortune* and the *Atlantic Monthly*. He talked with several doctors and with friends. He concluded there was some medical consensus in favor of surgery for a patient in his stage of the disease and that the risks of surgery were less distressing than he had feared. He could thus choose surgery with something like ease and assurance.

Creaturo, on the other hand, drowned in choices about treating her ovarian cancer. She consulted many doctors about surgery, chemotherapy, radiation, and immunological treatments. She contacted an advisory service that sent her "a single-spaced, six-page letter, chock-a-block with names and concepts and treatment programs that are dizzying in their number, their wildly exotic unfamiliarity."[155] This letter was accompanied by fifteen pages of computer printouts. Friends kept suggesting yet more programs and recommending books with yet more ideas. She could never find anything like consensus, particularly since she wanted the latest therapies. Because her alternatives covered such a welter of approaches, and because at her back she always heard time's winged chariot hurrying near, she could rarely make a well-considered choice, or one she remained satisfied with.

A final category of distinctions among medical decisions turns on the identity of the doctor and the patient and on their relationship. For example, someone walking into an emergency room for the first time has little way to know how knowledgeable, skilled, bright, thoughtful, empathic, or reliable the (ER) doctor is. Nor does that doctor have the time or means to understand the patient deeply. That patient may hesitate to entrust that doctor with decisions. On the other hand, a patient on dialysis for ten years with the same nephrologist and enjoying a sure rapport with and confirmed respect for him may cede virtually the whole burden of decision. (For that matter, the doctor may be more comfortable in allowing, or even encouraging, such patients to make their own decisions.)

If we are to understand autonomy questions in the fullness and complexity of the reality in which they occur, then, we need to disaggregate the various kinds of medical decisions and ask whether different approaches might fit different decisions. This is harder to accomplish in practice than to call for in principle. Much depends on context. A given procedure will raise different kinds of problems depending on the patient's medical and social circumstances. Further, "[m]ost cases are mixed cases, and we should not treat our classifications with too much respect."[156] Some medical decisions are not really medical. Some are not really decisions. Some will seem worth the trouble; others will not. Some decisions will be forbiddingly complex; others will become tiresomely routine. Patients will trust some doctors and not others. Some patients will virtually never want to make their own decisions; some patients virtually always will. The same patient may wish to make some decisions at some times but not at others. In short, it may be impossible to say that all patients want to make some kinds of decisions or that a particular patient always wants to make all decisions.

Conclusion

There's no rule so wise but what it's a pity for somebody or other.

George Eliot, *Adam Bede*

I argued in Chapter 2 that patients often decline to make their own medical decisions. I surveyed an expanse of evidence for that supposition, but I acknowledged it would seem counterintuitive to some of my readers. I therefore set about making such patients comprehensible. In Chapter 3, I proposed that the evidence was made easier to believe when one considered patients' reasons for making their own decisions. Patients may rationally conclude that someone else can make sounder medical decisions than they, that the burdens of decision are too onerous, and that they want help in maneuvering themselves into the right decision. In this chapter (Chapter 4), I have argued that the evidence that many patients want to delegate decisions becomes yet more understandable in light of several other factors. First, patients may want information (as they overwhelmingly say they do) without wanting to use it for making medical decisions. Second, some patients do not want "control," while others seek it through other routes than making medical decisions. Third, medical decisions vary greatly, and some decisions will be more forbidding than others.

At the same time that I have been presenting these multiple confirmations of my description of what patients want, I have begun to ask what patients do and should want. I have, in other words, begun to evaluate the principle of mandatory autonomy—the principle that patients should make their own decisions whether they want to or not. My explanations in Chapter 3 of why patients decline to do so provide a basis for gauging the reasonableness of that refusal. My arguments in this chapter provide further grounds for understanding patients and their duties. Among other things, those arguments suggest that what patients want, how they are situated, and what decisions they face vary enormously. Having thus looked at these aspects of patients' lives, we are ready to consider directly mandatory autonomy.

5

Reconsidering Autonomy
Evaluating the Arguments
for Mandatory Autonomy

It is only as a man puts off all foreign support and stands alone that I see him to be strong and to prevail. He is weaker by every recruit to his banner. . . . He who knows that power is inborn, that he is weak because he has looked for good out of him and elsewhere, and, so perceiving, throws himself unhesitatingly on his thought, instantly rights himself, stands in the erect position, commands his limbs, works miracles; just as a man who stands on his feet is stronger than a man who stands on his head.

Ralph Waldo Emerson
Self-Reliance

'Choices, choices,' he repeated to himself as he walked along the streets, now full of people all of whom seemed to be celebrating something. 'Too many choices. I don't like it. There must be more to life than choices. It would be ridiculous otherwise. But it seems to be the rule.'

Giorgio Pressburger
The Law of White Spaces

I have argued that law and bioethics have naturally but too easily assumed that all patients want basically the same relationship with their doctors, that they want the starring role in decisions about their own health, and that they want to play that part through "plans of action that have been formulated through deliberation or reflection, . . . [through] processes of both information gathering and priority setting."[1] However, I have contended that people react variously to the proffer of medical power, that many of them ignore it, and that perhaps many more fail to achieve or even to aspire to the elevated standards of research, deliberation, and reflection that law and bioethics posit.

My task, to put the point differently, has been to identify some of the anomalies the practice of Kuhnian normal science has uncovered in the autonomy paradigm. Principally, I have explored the disjunction between what the paradigm seems to want for patients and what many patients seem to want for themselves. I have argued that the empirical evidence of what those patients want—however counterintuitive it may seem to people who spend their lives studying, thinking, and writing about medicine, law, and ethics—paints a comprehensible picture of one reasonable reaction to illness.

But how should we respond to this empirical evidence? I cannot here resolve the whole range of ethical and legal issues raised by the presence of numerous patients who delegate their medical decisions. Such an enterprise exceeds the scope of this book, for it would require a full-scale reexamination of the autonomy paradigm, the legal doctrine of informed consent, and the structure of American health care. That enterprise would, furthermore, demand research into how patients make decisions that we currently lack and that it is one of my hopes to stimulate. Nevertheless, I want to begin discussing what the presence of so many nondeciders should mean for the principle and practice of autonomy and for a more textured and complex appreciation of bioethical problems.

Like an increasing number of commentators, I believe the autonomy principle has grown too monolithic and has come to be revered too uncritically. I want, then, to reconsider that principle by evaluating more directly what I have called the principle of mandatory autonomy. I have chosen that route because mandatory autonomy is the logical extension of more conventional ideas about autonomy and thus offers a window into autonomy's merits and hazards. In addition, mandatory autonomy may be becoming strong enough to warrant attention on its own merits. The mandatory-autonomy argument, we may recall from Chapter 1, holds that it is so vital for patients to make their own medical decisions that they should do so whatever their inclinations to the contrary. That position, I suggested, is supported by four kinds of arguments—the "prophylaxis," the "therapeutic," the "false consciousness," and the "moral." Each of these seems to me weighty. But each is crucially uncertain, flawed, and limited. To see how, we will examine them in turn.

The Prophylaxis Argument

Some [physicians are] impelled by necessity, some stimulated by vanity, and others anxious to conceal unworthy arts to raise their importance among the ignorant, who are always the most numerous of mankind. Some of these arts have been an affectation of mystery in all their writings and conversations relating to their profession; an affectation of knowledge inscrutable to all, except the adepts in the science; an air of perfect confidence in their own skill and abilities; and a demeanor solemn, contemptuous and highly expressive of self-sufficiency.
John Gregory, *Lectures on the Duties and Qualifications of a Physician,* 1772

The prophylaxis argument reasons that patients need to be encouraged to make their own decisions to prevent physicians from abusing their power. At the heart of the prophylaxis argument, then, is the belief that patients are weak, doctors are strong, and the weak need help against the strong. The patient's weakness is routinely described in forceful terms. The word "abject," for instance, has been deployed with some regularity and effect.[2] It is not news, I suppose, that physicians have power. Medicine is a profession, and members of professions have expertise clients need. Medical expertise is unusually valuable: a bad accountant can bankrupt you, but a bad doctor can kill you. Given the imbalances in skill and learning between doctors and patients, doctors will inevitably continue to wield power over their patients. What is more, physicians have incentives to dominate their patients: Socially, physicians bestride a hierarchical world, and patients who make their own decisions may disturb that social dominance. Psychologically, many physicians benefit from dealing with patients from the position of strength that the power to make decisions for patients gives them. Economically, doctors paid fees for their services can profit from telling patients which services to buy, and doctors in general enjoy the Jovian incomes that are supported by their near-monopoly position. Of course, not all physicians want or exploit these benefits, but they tempt doctors to make decisions without involving their patients, to ignore their patients' preferences, and even to do less than their best for their patients. Human nature being what it is, we may wish to structure medical care to dilute those incentives. And, it must be said, the ferocity with which organized medicine has defended its prerogatives gives wings to that wish.

So, doctors indeed have considerable power over patients. But patients too have powers. I do not wish to exaggerate them, but because they are rarely recognized, they will bear some attention. First, people set the terms of their relationship with their physicians by selecting them. To be sure, patients sometimes have little choice about prospective doctors, and all too often they have scant information about the choices they have.[3] But particularly in choosing a primary physician, patients frequently do have alternatives and do obtain information. Where the attitudes of doctors make a special difference—in, for instance, fields like obstetrics and gynecology—many patients search out doctors whose attitudes match their own. Eliot Freidson observes, for example, that

> the first visit to a practitioner is often tentative, a tryout. . . . The client may form an opinion by himself, or, as is often the case, he may compare notes with others— indeed, he passes through the referral structure not only on his way to the physician but also on his way back, discussing the doctor's behavior, diagnosis, and prescription with his fellows, with the possible consequence that he may never go back.[4]

Patients with chronic illness often have considerable experience with doctors, develop preferences about them, and make choices among them.[5] Patients referred to a specialist may ask questions about the specialist's merits. Finally, Anne

Hawkins observes that "[e]xtensive doctor-shopping" is apparent from the memoirs of "those who experiment with alternative medicine" and of those who "research and then 'shop' for state-of-the art cancer research protocols."[6] She mordantly comments, "We are a nation of shoppers, and ill people today often feel it appropriate to 'shop around' for a therapy they feel suits them best."[7]

Similarly, patients leave doctors who displease them. A 1976 study, for instance, found that 43% of the families interviewed had a member who had changed doctors without referral in the previous year.[8] Another study reported that 36% of the public have changed their doctors because they disagreed with them.[9] Some patients even revolt against what so many patients so much detest and resent—being kept endlessly, endlessly waiting, without explanation, without apology:

> After waiting an hour to see her obstetrician, Martha Zornow, a vice president at Viacom International Inc., fired the tardy doctor in favor of a more punctual physician.
> "I am a busy professional. I don't make people wait for me, and I don't expect to be kept waiting," she says. "Whenever I notice that kind of arrogance, I switch doctors."[10]

Such consumerist behavior appears with pleasing regularity in the memoirs of the sick, even those not corporate vice presidents. The following excerpt is typical: "I changed doctors, abandoning the specialist who was more interested in high-tech medicine and high doses of hormones than in taking care of the infection and talking me through my worries. I started seeing not a specialist but an ordinary gynecologist, Judy Schwartz, whose approach was both sympathetic and practical."[11] Some patients go from doctor to doctor to find one who is sympathetic or even competent. Eileen Radziunas, for example, struggled valiantly to obtain an accurate diagnosis of her lupus and encountered a parade of doctors who, she reports, cavalierly attributed her physical problems to psychological pathologies. Although she "wanted a competent caring specialist, someone I could work with effectively on a long-term basis," she was driven to "doctor-hopping."[12] After seeing a neurologist, for instance, she called one of her doctors "and told him the name of the medication [the neurologist had] prescribed. He told me that the neurologist probably suspected my problem was a simple case of nerves. With Dr. Dupont's endorsement, I refused to take the medicine, and decided that I would never see that neurologist again."[13] Finally, when memoirists give advice to patients, it is often in the same vein: "If you can't get your doctor to instruct you and to listen to you, look for another doctor."[14]

In my research among kidney patients, I have encountered many who knew what they wanted—and especially what they did not want—from doctors, who hunted resolutely for doctors who could provide it, and who discarded doctors who displeased them. One patient, a delightfully nice, marvelously sweet, and wonderfully conventional lady *d'un certain âge,* said to me mildly,

> I went to this doctor for a long time, and I know he was busy, but he began to not have time for me when I wanted to ask questions or wanted him to explain things—and this was during the process of my kidney rejection and of course there are a lot of things that you think about and you want to ask about—and he didn't have time to answer me. So I changed doctors.

Peter Schuck even suggests that "patients' bargaining power is not obviously or systematically weaker than that of consumers in products markets."[15] Furthermore, that power has in important ways been growing, since "corporate and governmental budgetary pressures are forcing the health care delivery system to change in ways likely to enhance the future power of consumers in the aggregate, if not also individually."[16] Not the least of these changes is the increase in the number of physicians as a proportion of the population and the decrease in the number of patient visits per physician, so that "[p]atients, rather than physicians, are becoming the party in short supply . . . ."[17] To be sure, many patients will not exercise the power these circumstances give them, but "[n]ot all patients have to be shoppers or assertive of their rights to make providers responsive."[18]

These developments may be teaching doctors and hospitals to be more solicitous of patients. They may, for example, help explain the experience of the lady I just described who left her doctor:

> I told the social director [she means social worker]. She asked me about him [the doctor] and what I thought about him, and I said, do you want me to tell you the truth? And she said, yes I do, and so I did. And she said, I don't blame you, I am glad that you told me. And even his superior called me at home to find out, and I told him, and he said that if there was any more . . . . And I said, well I had changed doctors. And he said, well that is all right, that is your privilege.

At some point in this process, the doctor the lady had left phoned her

> to find out why, and I told him why, and he said, he said he knew that it was his attitude, and he said he was sorry and that he was going to try to improve his outward demeanor. And he did, because they have had, they had several complaints about his attitude. Maybe he was just too busy, I don't know. I am sure it is a tough job. But when I went up there for dialysis, when my [new] doctor wasn't there he [the old doctor] would have to take over, and he came in and talked to me, and he was just pleasant and really nice.

I have been suggesting that patients are not powerless and that their power derives first from their ability to select and dismiss their doctor. Second, in dealing with the doctors they have chosen, patients have resources. They can announce their preferences about making decisions in general or about specific treatments, volunteer information, ask questions, and reject proposals. They can use all the devices for dealing with people that we all deploy in the encounters of daily life. As Molly Haskell unflatteringly puts it, in handling doctors we can be "shrewd manipulators. Instinctively, we try to ferret out and play on a doctor's vulnerability, present ourselves in a manner calculated to endear or, failing that, to intimidate."[19] Further, there are things doctors want from patients—like information and cooperation, like appreciation and admiration—that patients can withhold until they get what they want.[20] To put the point more broadly, patients are so strategically placed that often they "cannot but be brought into the decision-making work that needs to be done at the critical junctures (let alone during the minor episodes)."[21] Not all these techniques are optimal or easy, of course, but not all doctors are unresponsive to the better, easier ones.

Third, patients find allies in dealing with doctors. Most people discuss their illness, treatment, and doctor with family, friends, and fellow patients.[22] Those allies give patients perspective, information, and moral support. Those resources can also be gleaned from the many kinds of literature available from doctors, hospitals, associations, and bookstores, to say nothing of the Internet. These literatures range from informative pamphlets, through advice books on individual diseases, to the memoirs I have been drawing on (which are often avowedly didactic). There are, further, support groups, peer counsellors, patient advocates, social workers, and nurses who help patients manage not just disease, but doctors and hospitals.

Nor do doctors present a united front. Second opinions, for instance, are increasingly commonplace; third-party payors may even require them. Many patients see more than one doctor during their treatment. Medical disagreements—as to general approaches to illness and as to specific therapies—are common and help the patient locate doctors who present a range of real choice.[23] And while utilization-management programs in some ways weaken the power of patients, they offer them a well-informed ally in their efforts to avoid unnecessary treatment.[24]

Fourth, the temper of the times has changed in ways that permit and even prod patients to assert themselves in dealing with doctors. The world is less deferential than ever before. The bioethical movement has borne fruit, the authority of authority has withered, and the consumer ethos has infiltrated medicine. "Something has happened," Cassell writes, "to displace physicians from their previous preeminent status, something powerful enough to allow patients to express the common belief that 'doctors aren't Gods.'"[25] Roter and Hall believe that "the basic characteristics of the provider-patient relationship may be undergoing substantial evolution . . . ." They find "considerable evidence that patients are becoming more consumerist in orientation, and particularly [that] the new generation of patients is likely to challenge physician authority directly within the medical encounter . . . ."[26] In addition, the consumer-protection law that is the doctrine of informed consent has had its effects:

> The only way I could get my surgeon, a seasoned professional, to talk to me about the details of and alternatives to the operation he was planning . . . was to refuse to sign the consent form. In effect I denied his denial. We then had a long conversa-

tion. His knowledge and experience helped me, but this help came only after I had hit him with the only two-by-four a patient has.[27]

Fifth, the autonomist's standard reasons that patients are well situated and ought to make their own medical decisions suggest that patients are not un-equipped to handle doctors. For instance, the heart of the power imbalance between doctor and patient is the doctor's superior medical knowledge. But as Freidson notes, "this difference is neither absolute nor always of the same magnitude. In the case of those with chronic illnesses, for example, many have the time, opportunity, and motivation to learn a great deal about diagnosis, treatment, and 'management' of their particular complaint, and they become very active in their relations with doctors."[28] In brief, if patients have the insight, inclination, acuity, and energy to make their own medical decisions, can they not also cope with their doctors?

Finally, it is worth recalling that patients generally seem happy with the decisional authority they have. As the President's Commission noted, its survey found that "only 7% of the public reports dissatisfaction with their doctors' respect for their treatment preferences."[29] This is hardly proof that all is well in the power relations of doctors and patients, but it suggests those relations are not as entirely one-sided as autonomists sometimes seem to believe.

None of this, obviously, is to say that patients have achieved parity of power with physicians. It is to say, once again, that the world is a complicated place and that the picture so often painted of abject patients and omnipotent doctors is partial and misleading. It is to acknowledge the truth in Robert Zussman's conclusion that often a medical decision "is the result of a complex process of negotiation and mutual adjustment" among doctors, patients, and families.[30] Thus, despite the force of the prophylaxis argument, its factual basis is overstated and its conclusion overdrawn. And I have another concern about that argument. It suggests all patients should be encouraged to make decisions so that some patients will not be imposed upon. Individual patients who would rather not make these decisions may reasonably ask whether the social gain to be won this way offsets the disadvantage to them and people like them.

The Therapeutic Argument

I knew that blood had been drawn before I left the emergency room, but I was too befuddled to know what the result had been. I mumbled a question about what my pH had been and the resident asked my sister why I would ask such a question. She told him of my history of acidosis, and he immediately drew another sample, confirmed that my blood acid level was dangerous, and undertook corrective action. Regina Woods, *Tales from Inside the Iron Lung*

The therapeutic argument holds that patients should make their own medical decisions because they will benefit medically from doing so. This argument has several strands. The most speculative is the most technical—the psychoneuroimmunologic theory. There may be something in it, and certainly some patients credit it. However, "[a]lthough there is some evidence for each linkage, the theory remains relatively unsupported and largely unevaluated by comprehensive studies."[31] Thus, while I am not competent to evaluate it, I doubt it can presently sustain much weight.

A second, more substantial strand is Robert Kaplan's argument that because "patients are rational and they attempt to achieve better health outcomes by exercising personal control,"[32] maximizing control maximizes health. There is something in this argument, particularly for some kinds of patients. As I have said, many chronically ill patients (like those with asthma, diabetes, epilepsy, and end-stage renal disease) must manage their own daily care. Doctors provide basic information and direction, but often they cannot go far beyond stating rules based on general experience, while patients can (and commonly will) experiment to see how they specifically react to different treatments.

Kaplan's argument, however, is too strongly stated. For one thing, it depends on patients being solidly informed. In light of the factors we canvassed in Chapter 3—the extent of medical uncertainty, the opacity and unfamiliarity of the information presented to the patient, the patient's parlous condition, and the structural complexity of medical care—that goal must often be elusive. For example, extensive empirical research indicates that patients generally understand distressingly little about what they are told when their "informed consent" is solicited.[33] Some measure of the difficulties involved is suggested by the fact that "on average most estimates of patient recall are only about 50% of the facts communicated by the physician."[34]

Of course this problem of comprehension is not wholly irremediable, and solutions to it should be attempted. No doubt part of the trouble is the distrust, distaste, and even surliness with which some doctors have approached the law's—to say nothing of bioethics'—standards of informed consent. The empirical literature on how doctors talk to patients rests in important part "upon the findings of studies which suggest that practitioners restrict the flow of information to patients, often withholding critical facts about their diagnosis and treatment."[35] And no doubt another source of trouble lies in the factors that are regularly blamed for the problem: the poor training physicians receive in communicating with patients, incomprehensible informed-consent documents, and the primitive state of knowledge about how best to tell patients what they need to know.[36]

Nevertheless, these studies also suggest that patients will always face difficulties at the most primary level of decision—acquiring information. A number of the studies of informed consent have involved experiments in which people truly interested in communicating tried to fully inform people not operating under all the burdens real patients suffer. If success was elusive then, what must happen in more realistic circumstances? Furthermore, not all the structural difficulties that inhibit communication can be eliminated. For example, there will always be temporal and financial pressures in medical care which thwart communication, and they now seem to be increasing.[37]

Other reasons to doubt patients can be as fully informed as the autonomy paradigm demands lie with physicians. Most doctors are so affluent that they speak across a cavernous class gulf with most patients. Furthermore, I suspect that the people who are drawn to medicine and can master its science are not universally blessed with the intellectual and personal qualities needed to talk comfortably, comprehensibly, and patiently with the ill. Nor can claims for information always take precedence over the more exigent work physicians do.[38]

Ironically, doctors trying to inform patients can be impaired by their very expertise. I said in Chapter 3 that experienced physicians reason "intuitively." Klein explains, *"Intuition depends on the use of experience to recognize key patterns that indicate the dynamics of the situation."*[38a] Klein gives the example of nurses in a neonatal intensive care unit who could simply look at a baby and tell that it was becoming septic, sometimes even before tests could detect the development. Klein suggests that these nurses "reacted to a pattern of cues, each one subtle," that experience had taught them to associate with a septic infant.[38b]

The problem is that people who work "intuitively" may not know and thus cannot accurately explain how they think. "Because patterns can be subtle, people often cannot describe what they noticed, or how they judged a situation as typical or atypical."[38c] For example, Klein suggests that the neonatal nurses often did not consciously know what cues they were looking for and could not articulate why they thought an infant was septic: Thus while "[i]ntuition is an important source of power for all of us, . . . we have trouble observing ourselves use experience in this way, and we definitely have trouble explaining the basis of our judgments when someone else asks us to defend them."[38d]

The difference in the way experts and novices think also impedes communication by making it hard for the experts to understand how novices think. "Experts see the world differently. They see things the rest of us cannot. Often experts do not realize that the rest of us are unable to detect what seems obvious to them."[38e] The rest of us cannot do so because we lack experience. And there is no shortcut to experience.[38f] But doctors who do not realize how patients think will have trouble perceiving patients' mistaken assumptions and faulty reasoning.

These are not novel problems. They are the problems experts have always faced educating novices, that teachers have always faced educating students. Approaches to solving these problems have therefore been developed. Good doctors learn, for example, to describe recurring medical problems through analogies. ("Your heart is like a pump," one of the standard ones begins.) And doctors can try to discover what patients think by asking them questions.

However, these are approaches to solving the problems of communication; they are not solutions. In the real world of human doctors, human patients, scarce resources, and burdened institutions, these approaches find their limits. I remember one case with discouraging clarity. I was on rounds with an exceptionally conscientious attending, Dr. Knightly, who was exceptionally eager to involve his patients in their medical treatment. I—a lawyer, no less—was along to talk with the residents and medical students about the ethical problems they were seeing, which probably increased Dr. Knightly's already active inclination to get *real* informed consent.

The patient, Mr. Allworthy, was an elderly gentleman no one could help liking. Dr. Knightly was coming to believe Mr. Allworthy had multiple embolisms and an aortic aneurysm. Either ailment could be immediately fatal. The treatment for one seemed likely to exacerbate the other. But the dimensions of both conditions were still uncertain, as was Mr. Allworthy's ability to endure surgery for the aneurysm. Dr. Knightly and his flock had for several days been trying to decide what tests to perform to obtain better information and what treatments to provide until they secured it. The tests had risks, the treatments had risks, and delay had risks.

We entered Mr. Allworthy's room and said good morning. He said good morning and praised the fine breakfast he had been given. Dr. Knightly carefully reminded Mr. Allworthy of what he had been told on previous days and then tried to explain that day's situation and the current medical plan. Mr. Allworthy listened politely. Dr. Knightly asked him if he had any questions. Why no, he didn't. Did Mr. Allworthy approve of the plan? Why yes, what Dr. Knightly wanted to do was fine with him. Did Mr. Allworthy understand what his problem was? Why yes, I have thick blood.

At this point, Dr. Knightly gave up. Was he wrong to do so? Possibly Dr. Knightly could never have brought Mr. Allworthy to an understanding that would have permitted the kind of truly informed decision of which courts speak. But he could have given him a fuller understanding of his problem and that day's tests and treatments than he currently had. To do that, however, would have taken a good deal of time. Rounds for seven patients were scheduled for an hour and a half. Five of the remaining six patients had problems roughly as serious as Mr. Allworthy's. The only patient who seemed actively interested in what he was being told was the sixth, the one whose case was not serious. The rest would have taken as long as Mr. Allworthy to inform at all well. Of course, Mr. Allworthy's resident, not just Dr. Knightly, was responsible for keeping him informed, but Mr. Allworthy's case was changing significantly from day to day and even hour to hour, so the sorely busy resident faced the prospect of many prolonged and frustrating conversations. To make matters worse, it was Christmas, and the unit was short-staffed. It takes little imagination to guess what the resident replied when Mr. Allworthy said, "Whatever you fellows want to do is fine with me. I know you're doing your best."

Human communication, then, is notoriously difficult. It is especially difficult when people are separated by gulfs of experience and expertise. All these difficulties become crushing in the institutional settings of medicine. But even apart from all this, some things must always be hard for one person to tell another. Thus "[s]tudies of terminally ill patients, breast cancer patients, polio patients, and parents of mentally retarded children indicate that health professionals are sometimes reluctant to communicate openly in the face of tragic outcomes."[39] Even if patients are not in extremis, they wear the "lineaments," the "habiliments of sickness and affliction." They have been "stamped with the stigmata of patients, the intolerable knowledge of affliction and death."[40] They may evoke in doctors the emotions such signs evoke in us all, and those emotions can disrupt communication. Finally, there will always be doctors like Sacks' surgeon, "a decent, quiet man, professional and reserved; technically admirable," who was also so "uncomfortable with the realities of powerful emotions" that he could hardly talk with Sacks.[41]

For all these reasons and more, patients' memoirs seethe with horrifying stories about how badly—how abruptly, how indifferently, how cruelly—doctors deliver soul-shaking news. A modest example comes from Eric Hodgins, whose doctor suddenly told him, "'No useful therapy for that hand.'" Hodgins thought it was

> one thing to have reached an unhappy semiconclusion by yourself; it is quite another to be hit over the head with that same conclusion by a Man in White who is making an official statement and whose demeanor tells you he couldn't care less. This day I had sufficient gumption to say to this healer, "That's a pretty big capsule to ask a patient to swallow without a drink of water." The healer's answer was "Sorry"; with that he turned to the Next Case.[42]

Another patient recalled her doctor saying, "'The presumption is cancer.'" She commented: "Such brutal words, delivered in so neutral a tone, with no explanation and no expression of sympathy."[43] Another patient testified: "'I went down to the health department, and they just kinda, "OK, here, by the way you're HIV positive," poofed me out the door.'"[44] Reynolds Price was a patient at the hospital of the university (Duke) where he was a faculty member. Yet the "presiding radiation oncologist had begun our first meeting by telling me, with all the visible concern of a steel cheese-grater, that my tumor was of a size that was likely unprecedented in the annals of Duke Hospital—some fifty years of annals."[45]

Even where the gap between doctors and the laity does not exist, even where the resolve to be frank has been made, even where sympathy abounds, honesty can be hard to achieve. Consider, for example, Philip Roth's struggle to tell his father of his father's brain tumor:

> "You have a serious problem," I began, "but it can be dealt with. You have a tumor in your head. Dr. Meyerson says that given the location, the chances are ninety-five percent that it's benign." I had intended, like Meyerson, to be candid and describe it as large, but I couldn't. That there was a tumor seemed enough for him to take in. . . . It's pressing on the facial nerve, and that's what's caused the paralysis." Mey-

erson had told me that it was wrapped *around* the facial nerve, but I couldn't say that either. My evasiveness reminded me of his on the night my mother had died.[46]

As Roth comments sadly of the conversation, "Two minutes and I had learned to talk like a surgeon."[47] Later, Roth steeled himself to speak with his father about a living will. "But when I got there and discovered how depressed he still was as a result of the bathroom fall, I found it even harder for me to talk about the living will than it had been to tell him about the brain tumor the year before. In fact, I couldn't do it."[48] Only afterward, and only over the phone, was Roth able to have that conversation.

Finally, the life of a physician—like the life of a lawyer, a judge, or a teacher—is corrupting.[49] It requires self-awareness, dedication, and discipline to maintain patience, modesty, and solicitude when being constantly deferred to, relied on, and obeyed by subordinates and patients. And those virtues are abraded by the time pressures of medical practice, by the way practice makes misery routine, and by the monotony that eventually infects work of all kinds. To be sure, physicians are ethically obliged to strive to overcome this barrier to communication and all the others I have recited. But these barriers are so many and high that they will not always be scaled.

I have been arguing not only that it is hard for patients to acquire the information they need to make sensible decisions but that there are substantial impediments to ameliorating those difficulties. Confirmation of this comes from the fact that, as Peter Schuck notes, "problems with physician-patient dialogues . . . are not peculiar to the United States. They also appear in Canada, Europe, and Japan—countries whose organization of health care, political-regulatory structures, and professional culture and practices differ from ours in many fundamental respects."[50] This ominously implies that "these patterns are so deeply rooted in the psychology and structure of a physician–patient relationship as to be largely immune to change through legal doctrine or other exogenous factors."[51]

A standard response to this problem has been to urge that better training can teach doctors to communicate with patients well.[52] But since much of the problem lies in the personal qualities of many doctors, the personal qualities of many patients, and the aspects of medical practice I have described, I doubt that communication can be substantially improved by reforming medical education. I do not mean that nothing can be won, or that the experiment is pointless.[53] But I find my doubts well expressed in Judith Shklar's remarks about eerily parallel hopes of legal education:

> That changes in the curriculum are the answer to all public deficiencies is, of course, in keeping with the great American tradition of painless reform. Everything from the study of Chaucer to the pursuit of "social science" has been proposed to this end. What has not been shown, however, is that changes in the content of courses alter the social behavior and attitudes of students once they enter upon their professional life.[54]

As Holmes aptly wrote, "We learn how to behave as lawyers, soldiers, merchants, or what not by being them. Life, not the parson, teaches conduct."[55] In any event, the ever-expanding range of medical knowledge and the proliferating imperatives of specialization will always make time for teaching these arts scarce. My skepticism about reform through training swells to the bursting point when I read, for example, that we "must educate physicians not just to spend more time in physician–patient communication but to elucidate and articulate the values underlying their medical care decisions, including routine ones . . . ."[56]

Let me put my point in more familiar terms. Every semester I try to teach material no harder than that doctors often convey to patients. My students have all excelled in tests of general intelligence and aptitude to learn law. They have nothing to do but study. Even during the first year of law school, the pressures on them are trivial compared to those patients endure. I have been striving to teach well for many years. Yet as I read my blue books I am regularly chagrined at how easily even straightforward facts and black-letter law can be mangled in the learning. I emerge from every set of blue books with a fresh and chastened awareness that teaching and learning are both humblingly difficult.[57]

I have detailed the obstacles to informed decisions partly because cumulative evidence best demonstrates how forbidding they are and partly because judges and scholars tend to deprecate them. Observe, for instance, the court's careless confidence in *Canterbury v. Spence:* "So informing the patient hardly taxes the physician, and it must be the exceptional patient who cannot comprehend such an explanation at least in a rough way."[58] Even soberer commentators deprecate this problem. Jay Katz acknowledges that "[a]ll professions possess esoteric knowledge that, in its totality, is difficult to learn, understand, and master." But in response he says hardly more than that this fact "does not necessarily suggest . . . that this knowledge cannot be communicated to, or understood by, patients."[59]

The problem with the therapeutic argument is not just that patients often lack the information they need for rational decisions. It is that, unless "rational" is defined so generously as to render the term empty, patients are as irrational as the rest of us. Kaplan suggests "it is the *lack* of information and control, not the possession of control, that leads to irrational choice."[60] Well, so it can. But however superbly informed patients are, they can still achieve quite normal depths of irrationality. Kip Viscusi, for instance, argues persuasively that smokers not only know the health risks of smoking, they overestimate them.[61] E.J. Sobo reports that "[m]ost studies conclude that no significant relation exists between safer sex and the degree of AIDS or HIV knowledge people have . . . ."[62] Information is a necessary, but not a sufficient, condition for rationality because people reason badly and are swayed by nonrational drives and emotions.

The problem is not just "normal irrationality," but the special kinds of irrationality disease drives people to. Katz, for instance, deplores the magical reasoning patients succumb to. Eric Cassell analyzes the irrational—indeed, dysfunctional—reasoning the chronically ill sometimes use in coping with their disease and concludes that some of them, far from making themselves experts on their disease, become intellectual victims of it.[63] This is an argument we already know from my description in Chapter 3 of the ways patients make medical decisions. And it is an argument which can cripple the therapeutic rationale for mandatory autonomy.

When we think about patients and information, we primarily envision doctors telling patients what they need to know to make decisions. However, the stronger views of mandatory autonomy go beyond this, to imagine patients who independently search out information on their own. Such are, for example, the patients Korda met in his support group who "had become self-taught experts on prostate cancer" and who "had to tell *them*, the doctors, what was going on out there in the world beyond their own offices."[64] But this route will be barred to most patients. Medical journals baffle most of us untrained in medicine; reading them critically may be impossible. Judging by patients' memoirs, utter credulity seems to be the modal response. The attempt of one patient not a stranger to medical issues — she was a paramedic—is sobering. She spent two hours reading "without stopping about the treatment options available to me. My decision kept changing with each new piece of information I uncovered."[65] Ultimately, she retorted to the literature that if it were honest it would "'admit that you really don't know what I need—whether or not I should even have chemo, let alone which kind, for how long, which agents. All you can do is act on your hunches.'" Finally, she "slammed a book down on the table. The process of gathering information was like walking through a maze."[66]

A comparable, if hardly identical, problem—that of devising effective warnings for dangerous products—provides perspective. The quandaries begin, as Howard Latin suggests, with finding the right level of thoroughness:

> Many risks are complex and cannot be explained in simple terms; that is ordinarily true, for example, of drug warnings that describe a range of contraindications and possible health hazards. Attempts to give comprehensive descriptions of all risks and relevant circumstances would often decrease the clarity or impact of warnings about especially significant hazards and protective measures. Moreover, psychological studies show that many people are not adept at grasping crucial points in complex narratives. Other research findings indicate that the effectiveness of a warning is very dependent on the particular format selected, but exhaustive disclosure is incompatible with clear and vivid message formats.[67]

Unhappily, then, both too much and too little information can distort patients' decisions: "[I]nforming product users of every potential risk associated with intended uses and foreseeable misuses can be expensive, might deter worthwhile product uses, and would exacerbate problems of space and time constraints, ambiguity, and dilution of impact."[68] The problems continue with finding the right language: "Warnings often employ qualitative descriptive terms, such as 'hypersensitive' or 'allergic reaction,' that are vague and may not be intelligible to some users. A manufacturer's attempt to explain complex subjects concisely in lay-man's terms must often create ambiguity."[69] Even the right words, however, must be heard: "To conserve time and effort, people often rely on memory rather than rereading warnings and instructions every time they use products. Yet human memory is inherently limited and imperfect."[70] Finally, however lucid the infor-mation and however clearly heard, it may still not be heeded: "[U]njustified opti-mism is a common propensity in many, though not all, risk contexts. Overconfi-dence may sometimes result from ignorance about the full ramifications of the risk. . . . [O]verconfidence 'seems to arise from assessors' inability to appreci-ate how difficult or easy a task is.' . . . [P]eople often fail to realize how little they know and how much they need to know."[71]

In sum, the therapeutic argument for mandatory autonomy may in some ways be more persuasive than the prophylaxis argument. But like that argument, it is often overstated and carries us only so far. The therapeutic gains patients can make by involving themselves in their medical decisions are speculative and un-even. They are constrained by doctors' limited capacity to convey information and by patients' limited capacity to understand and analyze it. And as I intimated in my discussion of the multiple ways patients achieve a sense of control, some of those gains might be attainable in ways other than making medical decisions.

The False-Consciousness Argument

As examples of "false consciousness" taking the form of an incorrect interpretation of one's own self and one's role, we may cite those cases in which persons try to cover up their "real" relations to themselves and to the world, and falsify to themselves the elementary facts of human existence by deifying, romanticizing, or idealizing them, in short, by resorting to the device of escape from themselves and the world, and thereby conjuring up false interpreta-tions of experience.   Karl Mannheim, *Ideology and Utopia*

False-consciousness arguments are always hard to evaluate, for they hold that if people just were freed from some enslaving delusion, they would feel differ-ently about their world; that if they just saw their interests more acutely, they would want different things. But while that argument resists evaluation, it is not—in the medical context—foolish. Patients *are* often unfamiliar with their choices and *are* often uneasy making medical decisions. Doctors *have* encour-aged patients to be passive. Once accustomed to making decisions and liberated from doctors' discouragements, patients sometimes *do* come to appreciate their own competence and savor the benefits of shaping their own care.

But how far can you press patients to make their own decisions? How would such attempts be structured? How far can patients press themselves? One reason-able inference from the evidence I have mounted is that people have deep-seated reasons for not making medical decisions. It thus may hardly be possible to alter their attitudes about them. In addition, illness erodes yearnings for autonomy in stubborn, crafty ways. Oliver Sacks reports, "When I felt physically helpless, immobile, confined, I felt morally helpless, paralyzed, contracted, confined—and not just contracted, but contorted as well, into roles and postures of abjection."[72] Was Sacks just yielding to his doctors' demands for obedience, to socialization into the patient's role? Perhaps. But socially and medically he was scarcely helpless. He was a doctor. He was manifestly a person of independence, vigor, and confidence. He was cocooned by family and friends. As he understood it, his moral paralysis was tied to his physical paralysis. When the latter lifted, so did the former. He could then assert himself "because my world had enlarged—and so he [the surgeon], the system, the institution, could shrink, shrink into a reasonable and proper perspective."[73] In short, patients who resist making decisions might be immoveable. Even successful attempts to persuade them might, as the literature on control I reviewed in Chapter 4 suggests, cause unjustifiable distress. And even if patients can be cajoled or coerced into making their own decisions, reluctant patients may not make good ones. Autonomous decisions are conventionally thought likelier to be wise decisions, but that wisdom comes from the resources, attention, and energy typically devoted to autonomous decisions. Where decisions are not freely made, such assets may be only stingily supplied, and wise decisions consequently rarer.

Many of the problems with pressuring patients to make their own decisions are captured in this story of an English patient:

> When he asked me what I wanted him to do I was very upset. I mean he's meant to be the expert isn't he? How should I be expected to know what's the best if he doesn't? I thought it was cruel, I didn't know what to say. I asked him what he would do if it was his wife's X-ray and tests in front of him and he just said that what mattered was what I wanted. I don't think it's fair to say that to people like me who don't know much about illness and operations. In the end, I just asked my daughter who used to be a nurse what I should do.[74]

The false-consciousness argument is put into yet deeper doubt by Annandale's fascinating description of an "alternative" obstetrics clinic run by midwives committed to the principle that patients should retrieve control of birth from doctors. This clinic attracted, as one would expect, patients who wanted "control." In some important senses, they seem to have gotten it. But they seem to have gone less far than one would expect toward making medical decisions. Annandale concludes, "There would seem to be an ironic sense in which a trusting relationship between patient and midwife is similar in outcome to a relationship between patient and obstetrician where the patient's cooperation is gained on the basis of obstetrical dominance: both inhibit the patient's decision making role through the restriction of information exchange."[75] In short, we need to ask more rigorously how far the ambitions of autonomists can actually be accomplished and whether there are constricting limits to the ability even of eager physicians to endow patients with the fullest kind of decisional authority.

In sum, one difficulty with the false-consciousness argument is that it is hard to convince people that they "really" want to make their own decisions. Thus, my reaction to the argument is strongly shaped by the evidence about patients' preferences I surveyed in Chapter 2 and by the reasons for those preferences I canvassed in Chapters 3 and 4. As I review that evidence and those reasons, I am uncomfortable concluding that so many people so poorly understand their own situations, their own interests, and their own minds and that a few academics know those situations, interests, and minds so much better than patients themselves. This is not, plainly, an argument against resisting the often dismaying arrogance of doctors. Nor, of course, is it an argument against shaping the social structure of medical decisions to permit and even encourage patients to retain control over their own care. But it is an argument for caution and modesty, an argument against the arrogance of the critic.

The Moral Argument

There is no more ceaseless or tormenting care for man, as long as he remains free, than to find someone to bow down to as soon as possible. Did you forget that peace and even death are dearer to man than free choice in the knowledge of good and evil?
Fyodor Dostoevsky, *The Brothers Karamazov*

The moral justification for mandatory autonomy might take many forms. In Chapter 1, I said that a principal version of it derives from the duty of authenticity. As Friedman puts it, in our society of expressive individualism "the primary duty is to the self, and the primary job in life is development of this self."[76] The self is developed by making choices, for thus we discover and define the kind of person we truly are. This duty of definition is nondelegable. No one knows you well enough to understand how you should define yourself. No one else is responsible for you. And you cannot fairly impose such an impossible task on anyone else. These principles may be understood to require patients to make their own medical decisions. The syllogism is straightforward. All life-defining decisions must be made personally. Medical decisions are life-defining decisions. Therefore medical decisions must be made personally.

Many of my own doubts about the moral argument for mandatory autonomy spring from my reservations about some of the basic moral tenets on which it rests. This is not the place to undertake a thorough disquisition into these questions at their deepest level. My subject is the practice of autonomy, and I want to evaluate the moral justification for mandatory autonomy in terms of the effects it has on the ill. I will do so primarily by examining the call to independence. Mandatory autonomy makes independence basic. Without independence, free and self-defining choices are impossible. Independence is thus required by the logic of authenticity. Furthermore, potent strains of American thought have so much exalted independence and depreciated dependence that a strong duty of independence and a strong aversion to dependence have come to animate many aspects of American culture.[77] That duty and that aversion increasingly inform our understanding of the life of the ill. As the wife of one multiple-sclerosis sufferer asked, how "can a disabled individual function as an individual, and how can a disabled family function as a family, unless the dependency relationship is, as completely as humanly possible, eliminated?"[78] In this investigation of the fruits of the moral rationale for mandatory autonomy, therefore, I will concentrate on the call to independence.

Much of the appeal of mandatory autonomy arises from the ways independence can be a virtue and dependence can be dangerous and degrading. The ill have many practical reasons to dread and resent dependence. Dependence means being unable to do things for yourself and that some things, even important things, do not get done, since no one else has your incentive to do them. Franklin Roosevelt, for instance, was afraid his paralysis might prevent him from escaping a fire and that help might not come in time. Even when things do get done, it is only by dint of an effort that would be unnecessary if you could simply do them yourself. The dependent, then, live at the mercy of others, and others may disappoint. What is more, others may exploit their power to exact tribute from the dependent. And even if others do not abuse their power, how do the dependent know they will not? Apprehension insinuates itself into the hearts of the dependent, and propitiation seems the course of discretion:

> Dependence is the primary fact of illness, and ill persons act with more or less fear of offending those they depend on. It seems like a bad deal to express anger at someone who may soon be approaching your body with sharp pointed instruments or, if offended, may be slow to bring a bedpan, or who may be the only person one can say goodnight to.[79]

One multiple-sclerosis patient—Ernest Hirsch—thought with special care about dependence. He sums up many of these disadvantages when he says that in relying on people he felt himself

> trapped, at the mercy of the young man's will of someone less than half my age who will do what I ask of him whenever it suits him, who may or may not be on time, who may or may not willingly do what I ask of him, who may or may not possess a particularly agreeable temperament and to whom I have to give up my autonomy to suit his, rather than our mutual, convenience. Were I not afraid that he might abruptly take off before I could obtain a replacement for him, I would ask him to leave.[80]

Dependence born of illness also disrupts familiar routines and one's sense of the purpose of one's life. A housewife felt it "a real blow to me to have another woman coming into my home and doing the work I had always done for my family. It was almost unbearable for me."[81] A notably conscientious husband, father, and employee brooded about being "able to function in the world as an independent person without the constant aid of someone else to do this or that for me, to be able to do for myself," about "being able to support my family; about being able to be the role model for my son that I want to be; about being able to be a contributing, productive individual in our society . . . ."[82] As these comments suggest, patients who have become dependent do not just feel disoriented; they also begin to doubt their own worthiness.

Dependent people may not just feel less worthy, they may be regarded as less worthy. Social status partly depends on one's ability to control and improve one's world; dependence is associated with the disabilities of childhood. When Hirsch needed a young man to lift him from the floor, he found it "difficult to describe the feeling of helplessness, of inadequacy, of infantilism that a person experiences at such a time."[83] In addition, both the dependent and those they rely on live in a culture in which autonomy, independence, and self-reliance are pervasive, potent norms. "For the chronically ill particularly, failure to resume ordinary roles . . . is to permanently abandon the deeply held ideal of individual autonomy."[84] This abandonment will not win them admiration from those who care for them. As one doctor observed, "The dependent, complaining patient is considered weak, stupid, and generally less worthy than the independent patient,"[85] partly because "[p]atients who have neither the desire nor the intelligence to care for themselves require a great deal of constant attention if they are to do well."[86]

What is more, the dependent live uneasily with the norm of reciprocity that governs social life. "Parkinson's can be such a disabling disease that its victims all too often find themselves locked in the role of the dependent. It becomes tiresome, and mentally unhealthy to always be the one in need, and on the receiving end."[87] A woman with multiple sclerosis "couldn't imagine anything worse than being on the receiving end of someone's love with no way on earth to reciprocate or carry my fair share of the relationship."[88] The problem here is at least twofold. First, it can be hard to be a good friend to someone you depend on, since you may come to resent the power imbalance dependence can imply. It can also be hard to be a good friend to someone who depends on you, since you may come to resent the incessant and irritating requests dependence can necessitate and justify: The tyrannically demanding invalid is a familiar and tiresome literary figure. Second, dependent people risk violating the social obligation not to burden other people unduly and without reciprocating. It is for these kinds of reasons that one doctor-become-patient said, "The dependence was frustrating and even at times embarrassing. I had to ask for a lot more than others could comfortably provide. If they graciously did something extra for me I felt grateful, indebted, and embarrassed at being so needy. If they grudgingly or angrily acceded to my requests, I felt angry, trapped, and, at times, guilty.[89]

A number of these defects of dependence are illustrated by the reactions of a painter who was going blind. He wrote of walks with his wife:

> When we were in a decent mood, using Charlotte as a sighted guide was pleasant for both of us. When we were feuding, we both resented the inequality of the arrangement. I had to walk slightly behind her, thus being forewarned of approaching obstacles. I disliked being dependent on her pace, her choice of routes. When Charlotte stopped to look in a shop window, I, like a child without similar interests, had to stand patiently until she finished. At those times, she resented having to be my eyes, which made me somewhat fearful of where I was being led—into the crack between train and platform, an open manhole, under a bus?[90]

But dependence is even more perilous than I have yet suggested, for dependence can be psychologically and morally debilitating. It is an easy slide from the realization that you cannot do everything for yourself to the expectation that others will do everything for you. Dependence can conduce to weakness, lethargy, indolence, self-indulgence. Dependence carried too far becomes a betrayal of patients' duty to try to get well and to live lives as fulfilling and useful and good as they can. An example of this problem comes from the painter who was going blind. He wrote of his wife: "I wanted to be taken care of, read to, provided for. I wanted her to arrange for new lighting, to discuss my thesis with me, to give me advice on my counseling efforts. My blindness blinded me to Charlotte's needs: *she* wanted to be cared for, even by the likes of me."[91]

Disturbing and dangerous as dependence can be, the virtues of independence have their limits, and dependence has its attractions. Since the virtues of independence have become culturally central while the legitimacy and even the rewards of dependence are rarely acknowledged, I want to examine the pathologies of independence and the merits of dependence. This inquiry should lead us to see some of the ways the moral justification for mandatory autonomism can propel the ill too far along the continuum from dependence to independence. My concerns about the strong duty of independence and the sharp distrust of dependence that animate mandatory autonomy fall into two categories. First, those positions cast people back on their own limited resources just when they most need the succor and sustenance of other people. Perversely, those positions tend to distance the sick from the very people they should most readily turn to—their friends and family. Second, those positions promote an ethos which provides too little dignity for those forced into dependence.

Independence tends to increase the distance between people. The more independent you are, the less you need consult and be influenced by other people and the less they feel important to you. And as it has come to be culturally understood, the strong duty of independence seems especially prone to distance patients from those around them because it teaches them too well to be wary of threats to independence. It inculcates the attitude reflected by one of the women E. J. Sobo studied: "'When you're independent, you stand on your own two feet.

When I [find] a man that takes that away from me—you know, do so much for you till you feel dependent on him—I don't know if I would let anybody do that because I like being independent.'"[92] But what kind of intimacy is possible without dependence?

Intimate relationships threaten independence because intimates become involved in each other's lives. They discuss decisions with each other. They rely on and thus have power over each other, power to affect each other's choices. They may so influence each other that their decisions become inauthentic. We want to please the people we love, and we can often please them by choosing what they want rather than what we authentically want. The people we love have views and interests of their own that may not be—cannot be—wholly our own. So even the best of friends and the dearest of kin can impinge on our autonomy and our duty to ourselves. What is more, intimates may directly benefit from imposing themselves on us. This is, for example, the problem of "controlling" spouses or parents who gain satisfaction from dominating their children. The authentic person, then, should be on guard against the impositions of friends and relatives, should want "the courage to be who we were born to be, rather than what our families and significant others expect us to be," should have "not only the right but the obligation to be myself above all."[93] But can you be thus on guard without distancing yourself from your intimates? Does not being on guard require at least a suspicion, a wariness, that is at odds with intimacy?

To be sure, the strong duty of independence is not intended to distance intimates. And perhaps in principle it need not do so. But such distancing is the danger the strong view of independence presents, particularly when it moves from the pages of books to the practices of life. People share their lives with intimates by sharing decisions with them. They invite intimates in to decisions because they want help resolving hard problems and because they believe those intimates wish them well, have thought about their situation, can bring to bear insights they cannot, and thus will help them make better decisions. When intimates are excluded from decisions, they are excluded from a way of working with and helping each other that brings them closer together. In addition, people consult intimates about decisions because decisions affect intimates. Consultation not only allows intimates affected by a decision to contribute to it; it also acknowledges their interest and their importance. When intimates are not only excluded from decisions but are actively regarded as a menace to independence, these benefits of including intimates in decisions are lost. Worse, a disturbing distrust of intimates can develop.[94] Such a dynamic too easily leads to the situation of the AIDS patient some of whose "best gay male friends stayed distant, pretending that he was as self-reliant as he had always been . . . ." This patient "perpetuated that illusion—he was a stubborn, fiercely independent, proud man, who refused more than he accepted and eyed even friendly help with wariness and resentment."[95]

Furthermore, if dependence is indignity, how can the dependent not resent those they rely on? How can they not resent particularly their family and friends? Suzanne Berger's bitterness toward her husband could hardly be more scarifying.

> Then he hands her a white paper plate with a bright boiled hot dog stranded be- tween two slices of white bread. It is food . . . , but it is disgusting to her . . . . *That* she doesn't mention. Here's what she knows: she's supposed to feel grateful.
> Gratitude is expected, but . . . this *I* surveyed as *she,* feels like a dog that has been fed and must then lift moist eyes upward in thanks to its owner—the purveyor of food, the giver of small and large continual incessant kindnesses—must repress revulsion at the Dickensian meal. . . .
> The cosmic issue is that the previously autonomous person *would like to recip- rocate,* would like to perform all those "kindnesses" for her/himself. . . . Though no one is ever at fault, I know it is harder for the recipient—who should feel un- pinched gratitude and doesn't, and becomes knotted with subsequent guilt.[96]

But it is only gratitude to her husband Berger finds grating. She is rapturous about her appreciation for the people she pays to care for her:

> [T]he well-lit face of the other gratitude surfaces from the *freedom* to give it, and is always given beneficently. For me this kind was felt most intensely when the strong magical hands of physical therapists took pain away, however briefly. True, there is an exchange: there is consumer and formal provider of services, and healing is both the goal and (one hopes) the purchased product. All this is the tidy business part. . . . But no endless demand for appreciation oils the deal. . . . And so the grati- tude that flows from the exchange is gentle, unsullied.[97]

Berger's feelings are understandable. But they are not desirable, since it is hard to see how she can survive without her husband's help, since her husband seems not to have deserved her contempt, and since she will presumably want to reestablish good terms with him as she recovers. The question her observations raise is whether the strong view of autonomy and independence does not make it unnec- essarily hard for her to accept what her husband wants to give and she needs to take.

The duty of independence may weaken one's ties with intimates in another way. Intimate relationships are sustained by the familiarity, understanding, and affection intimates feel for each other. However, these sentiments are under- girded by duties, duties of mutual concern and mutual obligation that reinforce sentiments of affection and supplant them should they temporarily fail. The im- perative of independence lives in tension with these duties of mutual obligation, and can even corrode them. Those duties limit independence by obliging us to take other people's interests into account. In addition, those duties conflict with the principle of authenticity that animates the imperative of independence, since they are rules imposed from without, by "society," rather than assumed from within, authentically. As one patient particularly concerned with finding and being her "real self"[98] put it, she "was always afraid society was trying to put one over on me, which usually it was."[99] The strong view of independence, then, not only discourages people from including others in decisions, it also erodes the moral basis of relations between intimates by diminishing the extent to which people are led to feel responsible for each other. This is distancing as well, because responsibility for other people can promote a sense of closeness to them. And responsibility helps people care for each other and stay with each other in times of difficulty despite the costs of doing so.

The problem is not that the ideal of authenticity discounts the importance of relationships. On the contrary. As Charles Taylor observes, contemporary "culture puts a great emphasis on relationships in the intimate sphere, especially love relationships. These are seen to be the prime loci of self-exploration and self-discovery and among the most important forms of self-fulfillment."[100] But what we today expect from relationships is quite different from what the conventional wisdom that is now parched and withering hoped for. As Francesca Cancian writes, "[I]n the new images of love, both partners are expected to develop a fulfilled and independent self, instead of sacrificing themselves for the other person."[101] What Cancian calls the "independence blueprint" emphasizes "being self-sufficient and avoiding obligations."[102] This ideal represents a redirection of moral energies from a concern for others to a concern for oneself. "This is not to say there is an absence of generosity or love. . . . It is *relative* emphasis that is important here, and the point is that the individual will not only come first, he or she will have a social structure that will allow individual agendas to be accomplished."[103]

On the authenticity principle, this shift in the cultural rules that govern intimate relations is in everyone's ultimate interest, since "[d]eveloping an independent self and expressing one's needs and feelings is seen as a precondition to love."[104] As one patient wrote, "All love and caring expands from feeling it for ourselves first."[105] The duty of authenticity, that is, not only leads people to make better decisions for themselves, it leads to better relationships. If I am happy, I will behave in ways that make you happy. But I should not try to take your interests into account in making my decisions. Only you can fully understand those interests, and I should not want you to become dependent on me. In any case, we both entered the relationship hoping to find happiness, both of us should seek our own happiness within the relationship, and when the relationship no longer serves that purpose for one of us, it is effectively over and should not continue to bind either of us.[106]

I have been discussing in general terms the ways the duty of independence may affect people's intimate relationships. I now want to make this general argument concrete and bring us back to the specific question of medical decisions by investigating the effects that duty seems to have on patients. The logical inference from that duty—one reflected in the behavior of some patients—is that patients should base their decisions on what is best for themselves and that their intimates should do likewise. As one cancer patient put it, "In a contest between one's integrity—doing what's necessary for one's own essential well-being—and love for another, love must lose. This view might not be romantic, but I believe it's morally and psychologically sound."[107]

The strong duty of independence such comments embody finds more formal expression in the work of an influential set of critics of contemporary medicine. They are taken by a number of patients to be counselling the ill to fight off the impositions of their families and consider themselves first. Musa Mayer, for instance, writes of her discovery that many "theorists in the field of holistic health" believe "cancer patients possess certain psychological characteristics that make them particularly vulnerable to the disease. They are the 'nicest' people, the most patient of patients. They do not stand up for themselves, these studies claim, or follow their own dreams, but instead serve the needs of others."[108] Mayer believed that "refocusing on the self, so characteristic of cancer patients—and especially, I would venture to guess, of women who have cancer, because their traditional role as caregivers encourages them in the direction of selflessness, anyway—has often been referred to in literature as a 'benefit' of the illness."[109] Mayer tried to resist the threats her sense of obligation created for her and felt she had "made real progress. Surely, I was less given to caretaking than I'd been ten years ago."[110] But if caretaking is to be avoided, who is to take care of Mayer?

Jill Ireland, a movie actor and the wife of Charles Bronson, was personally counseled by one of the avatars of this view—O. Carl Simonton. Ireland told Simonton "how for a long time before my illness I had been driving myself, giving priority to duties and other people's problems, putting off the things I really wanted to do, simply not putting aside enough time for the quiet and solitude that I craved."[111] He admonished her, "'I'm telling you you are living a very unhealthful life-style. If you don't change it and start honoring yourself and taking care of your needs, you will die.'"[112] In the same vein, Rachelle Breslow came to understand that "repressing my needs and feelings for so long had caused the kind of cumulative stress that made me vulnerable to disease."[113] As she

> began to listen more and more to my intuition, I realized how little recognition I had given to my own needs, how much I had been living other people's lives and needs while neglecting my own. It had always been so much more important to please others than to please myself. In fact, it was downright mandatory to my well-being that I be needed by others. I had to live for others, no matter what the cost to myself. It took a life-threatening, catastrophic illness to force me to be attentive to my own needs, to go within and to listen to what I was all about.[114]

In short, these patients and their advisers believe families discourage patients from considering their own interests, interfere with patients' ability to make decisions, and exploit patients' concern for the people they love. Patients must be alert to resist these impositions and preserve their independence. It is this understanding of autonomy and of personal relationships that nurtures the view, some-

times found even among physicians, that patients should make decisions uninflu-
enced by their families. As one doctor (apparently an oncologist) said,

> Generally speaking, we feel the patient should make the decisions. Now, obviously
> family members should be present and should *hear* the information, but usually I—
> tend to reject—a family member—making the decisions for the patient. Because,
> ah, after all, it is still the patient that has to go *through* the treatment, or has to bear
> the results of, uh, of whatever the problem is. So in a sense, ah, that's very pre-
> sumptuous on her part, that she should be telling her husband what—should hap-
> pen, or telling the doctors how to treat her husband. . . . And, ah, you know, in—
> in pediatrics it's—it's usual for the mother to answer for the child. . . . But in
> adults, we generally reject that.[115]

So seriously do some doctors take this principle that they make themselves
guardians of patients' autonomy. For example, a doctor and nurse proudly describe their burn unit's practice: "When the diagnosis is confirmed, the physician
and other team members enter the room. Family members are not invited into the
room to ensure that the decision of the patient is specifically his own."[116]

This suspicion of the family's influence has also marked policy toward intrafa-
milial kidney donations. The Simmons study reports "a widespread skepticism
about the ability of an individual to make the major sacrifice of a kidney willingly and without significant regret later on. The perception is that family black-
mail and pressure will be pervasive and will be the major factor motivating the
potential donor."[117] Thus "Katz and Capron . . . have suggested societal policy
curtailing the use of related donors in transplantation because of relatives' basic
ambivalence and the possibility the donation will have negative psychological effects."[118] Yet the empirical evidence refutes these gloomy suspicions: "[T]he
comparison of nondonors and donors shows no difference between the two
groups in the proportions who seem to be 'black sheep,' no difference in the percentage subject to undue family pressure, and little difference in underlying self-
esteem and happiness."[119] And would it be bad if people felt pressure to donate a
kidney to a close relative?

This concern that families threaten patients' autonomy is not confined to medical people. As the Nelsons note, when the family surfaces in the bioethical literature, it may be treated dismissively and distrustfully: "While Buchanan and
Brock, for example, point out that 'the family as an intimate association is one
important way in which individuals find or construct meaning in their lives,' they
immediately go on to discuss mechanisms for safeguarding the patient from
being exploited by his next of kin."[120] When I ask patients who have assimilated
the autonomy principle why they should make their own medical decisions, I am
usually told, "Because it's my body." I am struck by how often this discourages
them from consulting their friends or family.

Even strong versions of the autonomy principle recognize a moral obligation that might reduce the distance between patients and their intimates—the obligation to communicate. Today self-expression supplants stoicism as a moral good. Patients have a duty to themselves to speak freely. They have a duty to their families to explain their situations and their feelings. And they have a duty to other members of the "'brotherhood of those who bear the mark of pain,'"[121] a duty "not just to work out their own changing identities, but also to guide others who will follow them. They seek not to provide a map that can guide others—each must create his own—but rather to witness the experience of reconstructing one's own map. Witnessing is one duty to the commonsensical and to others."[122]

One might expect this duty to communicate to counteract the tendencies that distance patients from friends and family. It is unclear if it does, but some clues may be found by examining patients' support groups. These loom ever larger in patients' lives, and many of the ill—like many of the well—value them.[123] They provide medical information, sympathy, and the assurance that one's experiences are not unique. Significantly, however, they intrude little on patients' independence. Robert Wuthnow, a leading student of support groups, finds they reflect an ethic that resembles the ethic undergirding the moral argument for mandatory autonomy. That ethic "suggests that we are ultimately responsible to pursue our self-interest and that each person, independently of others, must decide how best to do that. . . . It says that people should figure out their own lives, make their own choices, and suffer their own mistakes."[124] This duty has practical as well as normative bases: "Because each individual's experience and situation is unique, there can be no right or wrong interpretations."[125] Thus most such groups, Wuthnow found, have "explicit rules against members giving each other advice in the context of the group. Even telling a story about one's own experiences that is too obviously geared toward providing someone else in the group with a hint about what to do is frowned upon."[126] Wuthnow believes the "secret of the small-group movement's success is thus that it provides some sense of caring and community but does so without greatly curtailing the freedom of its members."[127]

Like Wuthnow, Bregman and Thiermann think support groups fit "with the model of autonomous individualism." They offer a "way to integrate 'cancer patient' or 'cancer survivor' into one's previously chosen identity. They can be joined and dropped out of at will." Like Wuthnow, Bregman and Thierman are impressed by the essential separateness of support-group members. From their reading of the memoirs of the dying and their families, they conclude that the existence of support groups suggests "the inadequacy of the isolated individual, however strong, wealthy, or well-supported by a family, to cope with illness and death alone." Bregman and Thierman believe the "mobile, affluent, and unencumbered" people "who seem most at ease in such groups—those who have had the chance to live out most completely the vision of the autonomous individual who is young and never dies"—have also "found this vision wanting at the time of illness and dying."[128]

Just as patients owe themselves a duty of independence that distances them from their intimates, intimates owe themselves a duty of independence that distances them from patients. Intimates are entitled to lives of their own, to seek the same psychological health and personal fulfillment, the same freedom from hampering commitments, that patients are entitled—perhaps obliged—to seek. Observe, for instance, the sympathy a patient with metastatic melanoma expresses for his wife:

> Lynne couldn't handle the total uncertainty of what was going on . . . . I tried to be as understanding and gentle with her as I could, but it was getting more and more difficult every day. She finally broke down and told me that she was sick of it, couldn't handle it, and didn't want to hear about it anymore. In fact she implied that if the spots kept appearing, indicating to her that I would die soon, she would have to leave because she was not prepared to deal with that. . . . I not only understood what she was saying and why, but I appreciated her leveling with me.[129]

This patient's wife was as entitled as he to find happiness, and if that led her away from him, there she should go. She had met the obligation of her relationship, since she had communicated honestly with him. As one student of contemporary culture says, "[O]ne can love most fully by deepening the honesty and communication in a relationship, even if the relationship ends as a consequence."[130]

A number of the ways independent patients can be distanced from their intimates are illustrated in Rosalind MacPhee's memoir of her struggle with breast cancer.[131] MacPhee believed that "[h]er decisions regarding her treatments [were] her own" and that "everyone should take responsibility for their course of action."[132] She was proud of her competence and independence. She said she had "tremendous support from my husband, daughters and friends,"[133] and she dedicated her book to her family. She recounted several parties her friends gave her and her friend Pat's encouragement. But it is hard to read her memoir without a saddening sense of how isolated she was in her independence.

That isolation began at the beginning. After discovering a lump in her breast, MacPhee told no one for a week, and then, still telling no one, saw her doctor. After he referred her to a surgeon, she told no one, even though "I felt cold and alone. And frightened."[134] She went home and read grim reports about cancer. Her husband entered the room, but she "thought only briefly of telling him about the lump I'd found. Since my childhood, I'd been used to dealing with things on my own."[135] After seeing the surgeon, she visited her "closest friend" and neighbor Deirdre but said nothing to her. Later, discussing an operation to biopsy the tumor, her surgeon said, "'If you would like to discuss this with your husband, or friends, you could call me with your decision.'" She answered, "'That's not necessary . . . . You can go ahead and book the surgery.'"[136]

It was only then she told someone about her disease. She selected her closest friend Deirdre, who replied, "'Roz, I don't need this right now.'"[137] After the biopsy, MacPhee immediately visited Deirdre to say she had cancer. Deirdre "didn't say anything . . . . . We drove the rest of the way home in darkness and silence, each staring out our separate sides of the windshield."[138] The next time they saw each other, they did not mention MacPhee's cancer. Finally, MacPhee told her husband and her two daughters. She also told her friend Pat, who encouraged her and offered to tell some of her friends. After this conversation, MacPhee "no longer felt as weary."[139]

Nevertheless, MacPhee primarily kept her own counsel. Several times she tried to learn about cancer by reading about it. But when she was selecting a treatment, she apparently discussed her choices only with her doctor. Conspicuously absent as a confidant was her husband, who floats vaguely and almost mysteriously in and out of the book. Eventually, MacPhee's best friend Deirdre casually announced she was moving twenty miles away, a decision which pained MacPhee. But she lacked language for justifying her reaction, and she even seemed to disapprove of it. Rather, she reasoned that "[m]y needs didn't jibe with her needs . . . ."[140] Her friend Pat consoled her and quoted a wise psychiatrist: "'Someone can't be what you want them to be—they just are what they are.'"[141]

MacPhee was a model of independence. No one made her decisions for her. But when she was frightened, she could not even turn to her husband for comfort. When her best friend abandoned her when she most needed solace, she had no resources even to justify her justifiable resentment. I cannot prove our evolving ideas about dependence and independence caused MacPhee's isolation, but it seems to me at least a plausible hypothesis that they contributed to it.

Suppose I am right and that the exaltation of independence and the depreciation of dependence distance patients from their intimates. Is this problematic? I think so, both prudentially and morally. Prudentially, it leads patients to deny themselves the rewards of dependence. Some of these are modest, homely rewards, the gifts of surcease of struggle, of repose, of cosseting and comfort. They are the gifts Stewart Alsop warmly recounts:

> I was dependent above all on Tish, and in a way that I had not been dependent on any human being since Aggie Guthrie took care of me when I was very sick as a little boy. I was dependent on Tish not only for edible tidbits, martinis, books, and the like, but for a sort of unspoken emotional sustenance—for the squeeze of a warm hand in a time of darkness and fear. In time, I got used to this sense of dependence, and I even came, in a way, for the first time in my life, to enjoy it.[142]

These comforts Katz appears to deprecate, but his very criticism of them suggests in its persistence and passion how pervasively they are felt and how gratefully they are valued.[143]

The exaltation of independence and the isolation of patients are also problematic because they foreclose the consolation of consultation and the insight, perspective, and reassurance it can bring. Many patients' memoirs bless these rewards. One patient, faced with a decision, "needed to talk to Eddie [her husband]. I needed to tell my fears to someone I knew would understand. His support had been constant throughout this illness. Maybe because our relationship began as good friends, living near each other in a small town, after 13 years of marriage we had the ability to communicate with each other as only close friends do. If I ever needed him, it was now."[144] A diabetic woman believed she had been "especially blessed with a husband that not only cares about me, but also cares about my 'problem.'" She considered herself "most fortunate. Over the years when problems with my diabetes have occasionally surfaced, my knight-in-shining armor does not turn his back on me saying, 'that's your "problem," you handle it!' No, he gently encircles me in his arms and says: 'This is our "problem" now. We'll handle it.'"[145] A woman deciding whether to have a heart transplant found comfort in her husband. She told him she thought the transplant would be a good idea. "'That's exactly the way I feel about it too, but I think it has to be your decision,'" he said sadly. She "looked at his face, so grim and concerned, 'No, it has to be *our* decision,' . . . and it was our decision."[146] Another woman wrote of her husband's struggles with cancer, *"With a few exceptions Phil and I have faced this challenge together, encouraging and caring for each other. He's made me happy. I feel I've made him happy too."*[147] This couple asked four other couples to help them make their medical decisions. "These couples struggled with us as we sifted through our medical choices. Their insights helped us avoid hasty or incomplete decisions. They were our liaison to the church and the broader community."[148]

The reverence some patients feel for the duty of independence leads them, I believe, to deny themselves other kinds of succor. For instance, several end-stage renal-disease patients I interviewed were loath to accept a kidney from a family member because of the loss of independence it might entail. One such patient said, "That was tough. That was one of the toughest things in my life was to ask for a kidney from one of them, from my siblings." I asked why it was so hard to ask. The answer was not that he did not want to impose on them, or that he feared they would refuse. Rather,

> I didn't want to ask them because . . . I knew that there might be strings attached. I didn't want to hear, say I got one from one of my sisters and I am at a party and I am having a glass of wine and they are saying, no, you have got my kidney in you, what are you doing? I didn't want to hear that. I had to come up with a way to ask them for an organ, but also with no strings attached. Granted they gave me life back, but I didn't want to feel guilty or have to worry about looking over my shoulder all the time. Because I had been living my own life too.

In fact, his siblings were longing to help him, with or without strings. He needed a kidney urgently, yet so exigent was his desire for independence that he might never have asked (as other patients did not). By asking, he acquired not only a kidney, but also the gratification of their reaction:

> So what I did was when I went to all four of them . . . . I hemmed, and I hawed, and I beat around the bush, and finally I just said, "Listen I am going through renal

disease. My kidneys are just about gone, and I need a kidney. Would you be willing to give me one with no strings attached?" And all of them—which really surprised me—just hugged me and said, "Why didn't you ask earlier?" and "What took you so long . . . ?" So it was unbelievable, the response I got from all of them.

Eric Hodgins learned much the same lesson: *"From time to time, now, I make tiny little discoveries. It is ridiculous to call them discoveries because most of the principles involved were explicitly stated in the New Testament, if not elsewhere. Put yourself, with trust, into a stranger's hands, and you will come out with flying colors—his colors."* But Hodgins too had to work his way to this realization: *"A certain surrender of pride is, of course, necessary. Why I went through all but what is left of my adult life confusing pride with self-respect, I don't know, but I did. If I still do, it is now to a lesser extent. What was the meaning of my bluff that it was up to me always to be self-sufficient—a bluff in which there is ample evidence I am far from unique?"*[149]

The strong duty of independence has yet further-reaching effects. When the patient insistently tells friends and family "it's my body" and repeatedly excludes them from decisions, they may reasonably respond by distancing themselves from the patient's concerns. One woman I interviewed, for example, regularly told her family not to meddle in her illness. Yet she cankerously resented their failure to volunteer a kidney when she needed one. She did acknowledge, when pressed, a tension between her two positions, but she had no way to resolve it. Similarly, one of the striking things about the story I told a moment ago was that, although the patient's siblings were longing to donate the kidney he longed to have, they felt obliged to wait until he asked before offering it.

Dependence has yet weightier virtues: It breaks down barriers between people; it nurtures intimacy. This was a discovery Arnold Beisser made when paralyzed by polio:

> My disability has shown me that I am not so separate from others, and I have come to see with increasing clarity that there is synchrony on all levels between people. We are neither as independent nor as autonomous as we have believed. The independence that I once prized I now realize was in part a luxury that I could indulge myself in because of self-deception. My eyes can deceive me into believing that I am separate from others, but when I admit awareness derived from other people's senses, I realize how closely we are related.[150]

His illness taught Beisser not just how he was related to other people, but how this relationship brought him and them nearer and bound them in ties of mutual interest, obligation, and concern: "Disability has forced me to see beyond the optics of the situation and to see how closely related I am to others. . . . Their fate becomes my fate. I must find ways of nurturing them, so they can nurture me."[151]

Similarly, Gerda Lerner reports that her dying husband, "whose losses were so total, brutal and final, was forced into dependence from the moment he entered the hospital. Everything now came to him through others. Instinctively, he grasped for every hand he could reach, transforming his increasing helplessness into a proud and giving acceptance of interdependence which enriched the giver more than the receiver."[152] The realization that dependence can be a gift to one's benefactors is also reflected in the comment of a lupus patient: "Dependency can call up the best in the person depended upon. That seemed to be true with Geoff [her husband], and it made me think that perhaps in normal life, I hadn't been dependent upon him enough. I realized that he liked the fact that I needed him, needed his complete support."[153] As yet another patient put it, *"It is blessed to receive."*[154] This theme of grateful interdependence is echoed by Donald Hall, who became so close to his wife "that I feel as if I had crawled into her body through her pores—and, although the occasion of this penetration has been melancholy, the comfort is luminous and redemptive. Every day she rubs my body, trunk and limbs; her hands knead my back, lift my head, pull my hair—and I feel, intensely, an interdependent fusing together of our bodies and spirits."[155] Thus Gerda Lerner came to believe that "[d]ependence on others can be an act of grace, an acceptance of our common human weakness. Acceptance of help without false pride is the last gift the dying can make the living. It is a handshake, a handhold, celebrating our mortality and our transcendence of it through kindness."[156]

These observations speak to a recurring concern about dependence—that it violates the norm of reciprocity and thus promotes unequal relationships: Even the ill can repay help—in the coins of sympathy, interest, companionship, appreciation, and affection. (Recall the blind painter whose wife "wanted to be cared for, even by the likes of me.")[157] They recompense their helpers simply by allowing them to obey the injunction to bear one another's burdens. These currencies may not suffice to pay the debt, but their value ought at least be acknowledged.[158] It ought also be acknowledged that thinking in terms of equality among intimates is only partly helpful. As Gillian Rose recognized, "There is no democracy in any love relation: only mercy. To be at someone's mercy is dialectical damage: they may be merciful and they may be merciless. Yet each party, woman, man, the child in each, and their child, is absolute power as well as absolute vulnerability. You may be less powerful than the whole world, but you are always more powerful than yourself."[159]

I have been suggesting that the devaluation of dependence is problematic for a related set of prudential reasons which we may summarize by saying that it deprives patients of guides and comforts just when they may be most needed. But the devaluation of dependence also is problematic morally because it tends to concentrate concern too exclusively on the patient. Patients are not the only ones affected by their medical decisions, and the other people affected may reasonably expect their interests and voices to be considered. Anyone the patient knows may be touched by a medical decision, and friends and family are likely to be, especially when they are recruited into service—often arduous service—tending the patient physically and psychologically.[160] For example, the mother of a young paraplegic asked his friends "not to let him drink" heavily with them because his drinking and debility made him "weak and sick the next day." She knew her son would resent her request, "but I felt I had no recourse. Larry couldn't seem to grasp the fact that it wasn't just his life, our whole family was all tangled up in the same web. The decisions, good or bad that one of us made, affected us all. If he died, a part of us died too."[161]

Little in bioethics acknowledges any claims except the patient's. The autonomy paradigm focuses on the conflict between doctor and patient and sides wholeheartedly with the patient. The rationales for mandatory autonomy only intensify that allegiance. This moral tunnel-vision may be due to the fact bioethicists have primarily wished to affect public policy and not to help patients think about their choices. The moral justification for mandatory autonomy does address those choices, but its concern is so much to preserve the patient's independence, so much to protect the patient from imposition, that it actively discourages patients from considering other interests.

It is true, as patients often say, that it is their bodies that are the object of their decision. But what happens to their bodies affects the people around them. It is true that the patient's interests may be greater than anyone else's. But a lesser interest is still an interest. It is true that we may understand and forgive the patient who, weakened by disease and ravaged by fear, ignores or infringes competing interests. But that should not set the limits of our moral aspirations for patients. Thus the Nelsons are quite right to remind us of the strangeness of the strong autonomist position:

> Is there any other area of human life where individual interests enjoy such a privileged position? Anything from changing careers to arranging an overnight business trip is ordinarily done in consultation with one's spouse or other intimates, since these people have a legitimate interest in the outcome. In medicine, the patient alone is presumed to have an interest—a power to veto or demand that is categorically different from anyone else's, no matter how deeply others are affected by the decision.[162]

It is not just that "families—anxious, needy, and easily swayed—are drawn into medicine's overwhelming commitment to patient welfare."[163] It is that patients seem almost to be regarded as having responsibilities only to themselves. One man asked his doctor how well the doctor thought he had handled his illness. The doctor replied, "'What the hell do you care what I think about how you reacted? I think a meaningful question for you to ask is not, Did I, Joel Solkoff, react well? That's a dumb question. A sensible question would be, When I reacted the way I [Joel Solkoff] did, did I get help where I needed it, when I needed it? You should be judging how I reacted to your reaction, not the other way around.'"[164]

In fact, patients' memoirs tell moving stories about the many concerns even desperately ill people have for their fellows. These concerns begin with consideration for those caring for them (for even if doctors and nurses provide a consumer service they are "just as human as the patient"[165]). Joanna Permut, who was quite capable of scolding her doctors, wrote,

> I was greatly indebted to such caring men, quite aside from the medical expertise they offered me. Consequently, I tried hard to be considerate as well as obedient, following my medical instructions to the letter. I had often seen my doctors exasperated over my condition when they could not help me. Dr. Gifford once said to me, "I really care about you. I don't like it when you don't feel well." Aware of their frustration, I tried not to call unless it was absolutely necessary. Often I had physical complaints but did not tell them because I knew there was little they could do.[166]

Simone de Beauvoir admired her dying mother's thoughtfulness for her nurse and her family: "In spite of the gravity of her condition she never varied from the careful consideration that she had always shown. She was afraid of giving Mademoiselle Leblon too much work. . . . She blamed herself for taking up my time. 'You have things to do, and you spend hours and hours here: it vexes me!'"[167] One woman found the feeling "of being a hopeless burden to your family is a terribly hard thing to overcome. Why don't I just die? is a thought that comes unbidden, but is often entertained in the minds of the chronically ill."[168] And a cancer patient deferred to her family when she noticed they were "worried about my doing too much, fearful that I was falling back into the old pattern of an over-programmed life, pushing my strength beyond a natural beneficial limit. For perhaps the first time, I accepted that their perceptions must carry more weight in guiding decisions about how to spend my time and still-limited energies. It is not fair to let them worry needlessly."[169]

Many patients consider the costs to others of their care. Acutely ill patients worry about impoverishing their families. The cancer patient I quoted earlier whose wife "couldn't handle" his illness said with sad resolve:

> If I am truly going to die, I think it would be more of a struggle than they could handle to rebuild to the financial level I want for them, and they are going to need those financial reserves to be able to maintain the quality of life that I have worked to obtain. How could I in good conscience spend all our reserves and risk losing everything they would need to live on, just to gamble on treatments that the odds are stacked against? It is true that I built up and earned those benefits, but I am not at all sure in my own mind that they morally belong just to me. If the high-risk treatment worked it would have been a great gamble, but if it didn't and there was nothing left for them, it would make their problems much greater and I just cannot risk that.[170]

One impecunious young tuberculosis patient "insisted that I be taken to the state sanatorium. No longer could I allow my friend to pay my hospital bills. . . . But I was feeling terrible that the county would have to pay my bill at the sanatorium."[171] Patients worry about more than their families' and friends' finances. I have, for example, encountered several patients who needed a kidney transplant but refused to allow family members—particularly children or grandchildren—to

be donors. Less concretely, but no less meaningfully, some patients soldier on because their families could not bear their loss. Robert Murphy "could not afford to
die yet. Beyond economic necessity, the family and all the people close to me
needed me alive more than ever, for, especially in my impaired state, I had to
symbolize for them the value of life itself."[172] The ill also worry about the larger
social consequences of their choices. One patient and his wife asked, "What right
did we have to consume enormous amounts of health care resources for a highly
risky attempt to forestall death?"[173] Simone de Beauvoir's mother apologized:
"'All this blood they are using on an old woman, when there are young people
who might need it!'"[174] Patients, then, can be self-abnegating, can be concerned
about the consequences of their choices for the people around them. There are
even social rules that recognize patients' duties to others. As Candace Clark observes, for example, we expect the sick to underplay their problems so as not to
overtax the well.[175] We also expect them, as Talcott Parsons wrote, to try to get
well. In short, illness may alter patients' duties to the people around them, but it
does not obliterate them. Illness may justify patients in burdening the people
around them, but not in ignoring what patients can do for those they burden. The
problem with the strong duty of independence is not just that it directs patients'
attention away from those duties, but that it even turns the people around them
into moral threats.

Let me put much of my argument about the strong duty of independence
somewhat differently. That duty lives in tension with what many patients regard
as the goal of their closest relationships. They aspire to incorporate their intimates' interests so much into their own that they become indistinguishable. Reflecting on her husband's fatal illness, Madeleine L'Engle said, "But if Hugh dies
first, would I ever be able to stop saying 'we' and say 'I'? I doubt it. I do not think
that death can take away the fact that Hugh and I are 'we' and 'us,' a new creature
born at the time of our marriage vows, which has grown along with us as our
marriage has grown. Even during the times, inevitable in all marriages, when I
have felt angry, or alienated, the instinctive 'we' remains."[176] For these patients,
the strong view of independence is a betrayal of their deepest relationships. As
Portia asks Brutus,

> Within the bond of marriage, tell me, Brutus,
> Is it excepted I should know no secrets
> That appertain to you? Am I your self
> But, as it were, in sort or limitation,
> To keep with you at meals, comfort your bed,
> And talk to you sometimes? Dwell I but in the suburbs
> Of your good pleasure?

There are patients who do not aspire to such a melding of interests, for it does
entail a loss of independence, does diminish autonomy. But I suspect it widely, if
uneasily, coexists with the ideas about independence and autonomy I have de-

scribed. Thus Joanne Lynn writes, "I, and surely some other patients, prefer family choice *over* the opportunity to make our own choices in advance." She wants to "have a community and family that is trustworthy about making choices," and she fears that advance directives "will prove an obstacle to a sense of trustworthiness."[177] Patients who tell me that their medical decisions affect their body, that those decisions are therefore theirs alone to make, and that they should therefore consult only their own preferences and welfare cannot fully account for those beliefs. When I say their decisions may devastate or delight their spouses, they eagerly agree, but they cannot accommodate that acknowledgment with their beliefs about making decisions. These patients may remind us of the Americans described in *Habits of the Heart,* who are "responsible and, in many ways, admirable adults. Yet when each of them uses the moral discourse they share, what we call the first language of individualism, they have difficulty articulating the richness of their commitments. In the language they use, their lives sound more isolated and arbitrary than, as we have observed them, they actually are."[178]

I have been arguing that one pathology of independence is that a strong duty of independence distances patients from their intimates. Another such pathology presents itself when people become dependent through no fault of their own. For such patients, the strong view of independence imposes an obligation which cannot be met but is culturally so basic that it can be neither escaped nor forgiven.

This problem has been aggravated by the rise to popularity of a theory Hawkins usefully summarizes. In it, "sick persons are understood to be responsible for incurring their illness, usually by their life-style, stress, or feelings of unresolved anger and depression, and they are also responsible for getting well again."[179] As Tim Brookes ruefully comments, "[T]he so-called 'wellness movement' has depicted health as a matter of will and of character, so being sick becomes a moral as well as a physical failure, and the more avidly we believe that we should be perfectly healthy, the more illness comes as a nasty surprise, a failure, an insult."[180]

This surprise is nasty partly because we have an unrealistic view of human independence in the ordinary affairs of life. The strong view of independence imagines and prescribes a degree of human independence that flouts reality. Most of us who live in industrialized societies have more freedom—political, economic, social, intellectual, and personal—than any mass population in human history. That freedom flows from the complexity and wealth of such societies, which give us an unprecedentedly broad palette of choices and unexampled resources with which to deploy them.[181] But still we live enmeshed in a web of dependence. We rely on our fellows to obey the norms that keep us from stealing from each other, breaking our promises to each other, and smashing our cars into each other. We count on government to furnish potable water, to make food safe, to maintain a currency, to protect property, and to provide for the common defense. In almost every vital aspect of our lives, we depend on the skill and knowledge of other people. Plumbers fix our faucets, mechanics repair our cars, farmers raise our food, teachers educate our children, pilots fly our planes, lawyers write our wills, mutual funds invest our pensions. They must do these things for us because we do not and cannot and do not want to know how to do them ourselves. "We sometimes, it is true, come across people not without nobility who find the idea of such dependence intolerable."[182] But dependence is an ineluctable feature of modern life, and one which brings its own freedoms along with its constraints, for it is this very division of labor which helps create modernity's astonishing range of choice.[183] Indeed, dependence is a feature of life in any period. Thus the blind Jacques Lusseyran asked of blind people who find dependence their greatest burden, "[C]an these sad blind point to a single individual anywhere who has not been dependent, even with his eyes, not waiting for someone else, nor subservient to better or stronger men or ones far away; not bound in one way or another to every living creature? Whatever the bond, be it hate, love, desire, power, weakness or blindness—it is part of us, and love is the simplest way to cope with it."[184]

An unyielding commitment to independence is unrealistic in an interdependent world. It is fatuous in the world of the sick, among people whose lives are transformed by their need for help. Yet "here in the United States, you have to be self-sufficient, by golly. You have to be independent. You cannot lose autonomy or the right to govern you own life." This "culture is particularly hard on hanging-in patients. It tells us to act strong and certain. Yet we live with uncertainty."[185] Janet James valued her independence "above all else."[186] How then could she endure multiple sclerosis? Gilda Radner was so "plagued" by the fact that "despite the war I was waging and my endurance, I couldn't control the outcome" that "if they found something I would really feel out of control."[187] How then could she cope with cancer? At best, adherents of this school must learn to be dependent gracefully and without undue regret. At worst, they condemn themselves to unremitting misery in dependence.[188] Surely it is better to accept Gerda Lerner's lesson: "Dependency is terrible only for those who live in the illusion of self-sufficiency and independence."[189] And surely it is better to learn the lesson multiple sclerosis taught Ernest Hirsch, that "while helplessness and dependency may have undermined self-esteem at the beginning of my illness, it seems to do so much less nowadays. It's as though I feel that my dignity can be maintained because it depends on my frame of mind, rather than on an external happening or situation. So long as I'm certain of my own worth, there's little that can be done to me which will spoil the feeling of value in which I hold myself."[190] For people who cannot be independent, then, obeying the strong duty of independence becomes not just irrelevant, but an encumbrance, and resignation and the rest and repose it offers become more rewarding than the bustling assertion and narrow inwardness of undiluted autonomism. "I lay awake all night on the train back to

London. I realized then that I had no obligation to improve my situation, that I didn't have to explain or understand my life, that I could simply let it happen. By the time the train pulled into King's Cross Station I felt able to bear it yet again, not entirely sure what other choice I had."[191]

Other readers of patients' memoirs have also perceived this problem with the strong duty of independence. Bregman and Thiermann say, "What we find significant in our accounts is how many of our protagonists reach a point where they cease to want to follow this [autonomy] model. A turning point in their lives comes as they recognize how an alternative path opens up an even deeper kind of blessing. Not in relation to doctors and hospitals, but in relation to a universe where surrender is wiser and truer than a never-ending struggle."[192] Similarly, Hawkins observes of one couple:

> There are difficulties in the transition from the controlling and self-reliant ideology of responsibility, which husband and wife had found so helpful during the phase of illness, to the gentler and quieter attitude of acceptance. The difficulty seems to arise from the inappropriateness of the healthy-minded mythos, with its aggressive, assertive, controlling sensibility, to the task of dying, which may be made easier by adopting what earlier generations referred to as "the passive virtues"—acceptance, surrender, and ability to let go.[193]

As Bregman and Thiermann say, "This is a difficult lesson for anyone to learn, and it is particularly vulnerable to becoming distorted into a plea for overall passivity, dependency . . . ."[194] But the lesson need not be so hard. The pains of dependence are intensified by the cultural overvaluation of autonomy, independence, and authenticity. We can establish a gentler, subtler understanding of what independence should mean, an understanding that acknowledges the limits and liabilities of independence and the truth that dependence has its moments and merits. Autonomism is Scylla, dependence Charybdis. The challenge is to sail safely between them.

I have been commenting on two pathologies of independence—the distance a strong view of independence promotes between patients and their intimates and the distress it causes the sick who are forced into dependence. These pathologies, of course, may spring from a misunderstanding of the true faith of autonomism. But they are at least the misunderstandings to which that faith is prone, the misunderstandings likely to arise in the translation from principle to practice. That independence has pathologies is not a reason to dismiss it from the catalog of virtues. But these pathologies seem common and serious enough to make the strong duty of independence undesirable and thus weaken the moral justification for mandatory autonomy.

I have been evaluating the moral justification for mandatory autonomy in terms of the central role it gives to a strong duty of independence. I want to close this section with several comments on that justification. One I have already made implicitly and now should make explicitly. In Chapter 3 I catalogued reasons patients might decline to make medical decisions. Insofar as these reasons are cogent, patients can hardly be obliged to do so. The duty to choose cannot be a duty to choose badly.

Another limit on mandatory autonomy arises from the difficulty—the impossibility—of being autonomous in all the areas of one's life. Even though American culture is moving toward according autonomy greater esteem, I suspect most people prefer to direct their attention and energies to those decisions they care the most about, can most affect, and can make best.[195] They delegate other decisions (albeit often with conditions and under some kind of supervision). They adopt a principle, then, of "selective autonomy." And why not? Was Isabella Stewart Gardner wrong to commission Bernard Berenson to choose art for her collection? Not, probably, if her goal was the best possible collection, or even the most enjoyable. Thus Gerda Lerner was helped to endure the long death of her husband by the advice of her dying uncle: "Focus on what is essential, he said. Don't thrash around. Save your energy, so you can give of it to others. Don't worry so much, don't fret and anticipate."[196]

Indeed, for many people in much of their lives, the problem is not the absence of choice, but its abundance. Peter Berger points out, "An essential element of modernization is that large areas of human life, previously considered to be dominated by fate, now come to be perceived as occasions for choice . . . ."[197] So, in modern life, "it is not so much that individuals become convinced of their capacity and right to choose new ways of life, but rather that tradition is weakened to the point where they *must* choose between alternatives whether they wish it or not."[198] As consumers, our choices have never been greater. We walk down an aisle full of breakfast cereals; national catalogs complete with local stores to sell us shirts and socks; we have to choose not only a long-distance phone company, but a cellular phone service and soon an electric utility. But these consumer choices are just the beginning. People make decisions about the most basic aspects of their lives. All affinities are elective. Your "lifestyle" is yours to select, your religion yours to reject, your family yours to define. Even commitments like marriage are "nonbinding," open to daily reconsideration. This proliferation of choice presses in on us, since "man's attention span is limited and . . . he can only tolerate a limited amount of excitement. . . . Social life would be psychologically intolerable if each of its moments required from us full attention, deliberate decision, and high emotional involvement."[199] This is why the "ideal of 'full participation,' in the sense that everybody will participate in every decision affecting his life, would, if realized, constitute a nightmare comparable to unending sleeplessness."[200] This is, Kierkegaard says, "possibility's despair," in which "possibility seems greater and greater," so that "everything seems possible, but this is exactly the point at which the abyss swallows up the self."[201]

In sum, the obligation to make all one's own decisions—to be fully autonomous in the strong sense—states an unattainable and unwise standard. Perhaps "[t]rue freedom entails constant struggle and anguish with oneself and with others,"[202] but any battle should be fought only where it is worth the cost and on suitable terrain. And that may not be the terrain of medicine, or even of disease. As Arthur Frank concluded of his ordeal with cancer, "The real question is not who is in control, but whether anyone is. One lesson I have learned from illness is that giving up the idea of control, by either myself or my doctors, made me more content. What I recommend, to both medical staff and ill persons, is to recognize the wonder of the body rather than try to control it."[203] And as Michael Kelly observes of colitis patients, "The sufferer's world is turned upside down by the symptoms, which come to dominate every aspect of life. There is very little by way of active resistance that he or she can do. The best way to deal with the illness is to let it take over, albeit temporarily, until a spell of remission begins."[204]

Patients who decline to make their own decisions may seem to be "avoiding responsibility" for them. I said earlier there *is* a psychological attraction to passing responsibility for hard choices to someone else. But ultimately people cannot escape responsibility for delegating authority. They are open to blame only if they attempt to deny that responsibility. And how much blame are they then open to? Even if people should maximize the times they personally make their decisions, I doubt the hour of illness is the moment to demand prodigies of choice. The world may be a moral gymnasium, but are agonies of exercise always required? Sufficient unto the day is the evil thereof. One gift the well can sometimes offer the sick is help in bearing the burden of responsibility for medical decisions.

Finally, though there is much to like and even admire in the model of life Isaiah Berlin eloquently expounds[205]—the life of the masterful chooser—his is hardly the only plausible position. Indeed, the saintliest lives in religions as various as Zen Buddhism and Christianity have often been esteemed lives emptied of any choice except the abnegation of choice: Not as I will, but as thou wilt.[206] One patient observed that a "great contemporary saint of the Christian church for whom I once worked said, 'Christians must learn to hold their blessings in open hands.' I assume he meant that Christianity at its highest—and at its basis, for that matter—is the art of relinquishment." She explained that "the first thing Christianity demands of its adherents" is "the giving up of the claim to oneself."[207] Berlin's position evokes respect for its sturdy, strenuous, and perhaps heroic quality. But even on this ground, his position is not clearly superior, for abnegation of choice demands its own strength, stamina, and fortitude. It is just those qualities I have come to admire in the patients I interview, qualities unrelated to whether the patient is an autonomist. In a mundane and conventional way, many—perhaps most—people live worthy and satisfying lives that are not centered on the exercise of informed, considered, rational choice. They go about their business doing what they have always done and what those around them do

without constructing "life plans,"[208] without scrutinizing themselves with professorial fascination, without Promethean struggles against constraints on their freedom. Perhaps they are open to William James' criticism: "His religion has been
made for him by others, communicated to him by tradition, determined to fixed
forms by imitation, and retained by habit."[209] But I doubt they are conspicuously
less happy or good than is given to most of us.

I have been examining the fourth rationale for the mandatory view of autonomy—the rationale that affirms that patients are morally obliged to make their
own medical decisions. Like all the rationales for the mandatory view of autonomy, it has much substance. But it is not an unmitigated good. To paraphrase
William James, "This practically amounts to saying that much that it is legitimate
to admire in this field need nevertheless not be imitated, and that [the duties of in-
dependence], like all other human phenomena, are subject to the law of the
golden mean."[210] Whatever duty of mandatory autonomy there may be, then,
varies from person to person, depending on all the kinds of factors I have
explored.

Conclusion

*But for all my talk about choices, I was afraid to make them, because choosing meant giving
something up.*   Paulette Bates Alden, *Crossing the Moon: A Journey Through Infertility*

In this chapter, I have found things to respect and use in each rationale for
mandatory autonomy. It is true, as the prophylaxis argument contends, that doctors have guild and individual interests which must be leashed. A strong principle
of autonomy is one way to do so. It is true, as the therapeutic argument contends,
that knowledgeable patients who make decisions sometimes can prevent medical
errors, and even lead themselves in the paths of health. It is true, as the false-
consciousness argument contends, that patients often underestimate their own
competence and find satisfaction in exercising it more vigorously. It is true, as the
moral argument contends, that people have responsibility for their lives which
may sometimes include a duty to make medical decisions.

That there is much to like in these rationales is hardly surprising, for they
speak to much that makes autonomy appealing. They speak to our dislike of
being buffeted about by people and organizations who purport to serve us. They
speak to our belief that God helps those who help themselves. They speak to our
realization that we are sometimes deceived into thinking we want less for ourselves than we do. They speak to our admiration for independence, vigor, and
self-command.

Nevertheless, each rationale contains only elements of truth; each of them is
partly false. Doctors have their guild interests, but patients have resources of
their own. Making medical decisions can be therapeutically beneficial, but not if

one is likely to decide foolishly. Patients can underestimate their abilities, but they are often quite shrewd about what they want to and can do. And while the supinely dependent patient does not cut an attractive figure, the strong version of independence which has become culturally so alluring is prone to its own pathologies.

In short, sometimes it may be wise for some patients to make their own decisions, sometimes it may not. Sometimes it may be a duty to do so, sometimes it may not. So even taken as a group the four rationales do not make a convincing case for mandatory autonomy. This is reasonable enough. Patients' lives and conditions are indescribably various, the normative questions the autonomy principle raises are complex, and we should not expect any single principle to resolve the problems patients confront. We should expect any attempt to analyze patients' situations to be tentative and equivocal, to vary with the facts of the case, and to change with changing circumstances.

What mandatory autonomy neglects, what the autonomy paradigm forgets, is how marginal autonomy can be in the concerns of patients. The sick often live lives that are harsh and arduous. They face life's ordinary problems cast into new and often dreadful forms by disease. They must wrestle with the dilemmas presented by the effort to cure or curb their illness. They must cope with the onerous moral problems instinct in all these efforts. They must decide how to treat their families, their friends, and their doctors. They must determine what responsibilities they have and to whom they owe them. They must consider what they should demand of themselves and what they may ask of others. To these questions the teachings of autonomism can have something to say, but those teachings are often less clear than we might wish, and less central than we might think.

Part of what is troubling about mandatory autonomy, what is troubling about the stronger versions of the autonomy paradigm, is the absolutist quality both take on. This is the besetting failure of American individualism—that it has trouble accommodating conflicting interests, that it extends itself beyond sensible limits. In law, this failing has produced a rights discourse that cannot find principled ways of setting limits.[211] In the broader culture, it has produced a moral language which cannot express the mutual obligation and allegiance people feel.[212] And I have been suggesting that a strong view of autonomy leads to a similarly unilateral and hence distorted view of how patients should behave. In that view, the moral attentions of patients are directed inward with little regard for competing claims, and "control" and independence become ultimate goods, goods whose diminution becomes intolerable.

The autonomy paradigm has triumphed on the field of principle partly because it embodies an ideal with rich contemporary appeal. The model patient is strong, competent, intelligent, aggressive, and self-reliant. The model patient asserts control over doctors and disease. The model patient tolerates no interference from family or friends. The model patient brings to medical decisions a well-considered life plan that is the product of long reflection on the kind of person the patient truly is. These characteristics have their merits. But they do not state all the virtues we might hope for, and they are conducive to some vices. They appear to relieve patients of the obligation to consider the interests of the people around them. They offer little help to, and even lead astray, patients who cannot achieve control and independence. They invite an overconfidence that borders on arrogance and distorts decisions.

Let me make these concerns more concrete with an example from a patient's memoirs. *Legwork* is the story of Ellen Burstein MacFarlane, an "investigative consumer reporter for a television station"[213] who contracted multiple sclerosis. MacFarlane presents herself as a model. She subtitles her book "*An Inspiring Journey Through a Chronic Illness*." She is "above all, very good at what I do."[214] She is indomitable. Despite her disease, "my spirit refuses to shut down . . . ."[215] She is "not one who sits back and lets things happen to me."[216]

MacFarlane insists she must be in control: "I am accustomed to setting my own limitations, and I will not allow the MS to take over. At forty-one, I am not only functioning—I am flourishing, personally and professionally."[217] But her insistence on control is hardly realistic. She asks her neurologist to tell her the best outcome she can hope for:

> "You'll be in a scooter or wheelchair for the rest of your life."
> "I will defy that," I exclaim.
> "You can defy it all you want," Labe [the neurologist] says with a hint of frustration in his voice, "but it doesn't change your condition."
> I am furious with Labe. He doesn't understand that I won't compromise.[218]

MacFarlane's belief that she must be in control helps lead her to make the medical decision which is at the center of her book. She reads an article in *New York* magazine about a cardiovascular surgeon named Dardik who

> claims his stress/recovery regimen, labeled Superesonant Wavenergy (SRWE), will correct imbalances in the immune system that cause such chronic illnesses as MS. Pendulum swings that are created by quickly raising and lowering the heart rate through exercise cycles eventually restore the body's equilibrium and banish MS as well as other chronic and fatal illnesses.[219]

Dardik's exercise program seems convincing to MacFarlane, and so does his personal assurance that "this is a cure and I will be walking within a year."[220] Nor is her confidence shaken by his demand of $100,000 in advance for a year's treatment. When her "mother and my other siblings balk at what seems like an exorbitant fee for an unproven treatment," MacFarlane is dismissive. "'Believe me,' I tell my mother and siblings, 'with the kind of investigative reporting I do, I'd be the first to know if Irv [Dardik] is pulling a scam. After all the liars and cheats I've exposed, I have built-in radar for this sort of thing.'" Her family can have nothing to say because only she knows what is best for her and because only "other chronically ill people . . . and I really know how Irv can help us. It is something so private, inside yourself, and by doubting, you only hurt yourself."[221]

On MacFarlane's account, Dardik not only denies her the attention he promised, he also fails to examine her before she starts his exercise program and deters her from getting help for what turn out to be concussions and a herniated disk. Nevertheless, she persists in his program. At one point, she feels better and concludes, "Clearly, Irv's program works!"[222] Her confidence in her judgment is unimpaired by her knowledge that multiple sclerosis notoriously comes and goes.

Her family learn to show "uncommon self-restraint by not expressing their thinly veiled skepticism about Irv."[223] They do occasionally offer some sound advice, to which her usual reaction is to say "that while I appreciate their concern and their desire to ease my pain, I am not a child and I am perfectly capable of making decisions about my health. I can't convince my family to stop telling me what I feel or to believe that I say exactly what I mean and will ask for help when I need it."[224] Her family urge her to get an aide to help her, but she resists, since it would mean "yet another loss of my independence and a further erosion of my self-esteem."[225] She resists partly because "the more power I lose in my body, the more important it becomes for me to keep control of my beliefs and decisions."[226]

Although her family may not make suggestions, MacFarlane feels free to call on them for money and services. They apparently paid Dardik's whole fee, and they cared for her often, particularly during several months of his treatment. And the consequence of her decision not to get an aide was that "at night the household help and my siblings pitch in."[227]

Perhaps MacFarlane's insistence on control and independence are as admirable as she suggests. But they are not harmless. Because of them she imposes on her family and the people looking after her. Because of them she rejects valuable advice and fails to take care of herself prudently. And because of them she makes and persists in a foolish and disastrous choice of doctors and treatments. My point is not that the virtues MacFarlane prizes are worthless. They are valuable allies in her struggle against debilitation. But untempered by competing virtues and a sense of moderation and even diffidence, they serve her badly.

6

Beyond the Reluctant Patient
Autonomy in New Times

The social relations to which the division of labor gives birth have often been considered only in terms of exchange, but this misinterprets what such exchange implies and what results from it. It suggests two beings mutually dependent because they are each incomplete, and translates this mutual dependence outwardly. It is, then, only the superficial expression of an internal and very deep state. Precisely because this state is constant, it calls up a whole mechanism of images which function with a continuity that exchange does not possess. The image of the one who completes us becomes inseparable from ours, not only because it is frequently associated with ours, but particularly because it is the natural complement of it.

Emile Durkheim
The Division of Labor in Society

I have stressed the difficulty of making medical decisions and the reluctance of many patients to undertake them. I have said some reluctant patients might make their own decisions if they realized that was possible and fruitful. But many patients have reasons for their reluctance, reasons that are substantial and should be respected. Finally, I have argued that while mandatory autonomism has plausible rationales, patients have no unvarying duty to make medical decisions. Rather, the question what role to take will often be problematic for all concerned, will vary vastly from case to case and time to time.

Then what is to be done? Ultimately, my purpose has been to analyze and not prescribe, to understand patients' lives and not order them, to unveil the world's complexity and not reduce it to governing rules. Social regulations—legal, professional, and cultural—are necessary. But my passion for proposing new ones is tempered by my apprehension of too-utopian an optimism about the ability of any rules to regulate conditions as various and confounding as doctors and patients encounter. Such rules must balance many interests that conflict and that therefore cannot be simultaneously served. Such a balance can only rarely be found: "Human nature invariably disappoints. Human institutions inevitably fail. In human affairs, to muddle through is to succeed."[1]

Nevertheless, the reader patient enough to have come this far deserves some hints about where my observations might lead. In this chapter, I offer them. I begin by asking what an ideal response to the variability of patients' preferences might be. My short answer is that that response would attempt to accommodate patients' differing tastes for autonomy, but that it would often fail. I then suggest that the bureaucratization of American medicine makes that response more problematic and raises questions about what kind of autonomy—and what kind of care—patients as clients of a bureaucracy might hope to find. Finally, I ask what patients might want of medicine besides autonomy and whether bioethics and the law might help them secure it.

Choosing Not to Choose

Life is not long, and too much of it must not pass in idle deliberation how it shall be spent: deliberation, which those who begin it by prudence, and continue it with subtlety, must, after long expense of thought, conclude by chance. To prefer one future mode of life to another, upon just reasons, requires faculties which it has not pleased our Creator to give us.
                                                                              Samuel Johnson

One of my primary themes has been that the world of the patient is insistently, irreducibly various. Chapter 2 demonstrated that patients' preferences about making medical decisions vary. Chapter 3 showed that patients' reasons for accepting or rejecting the power to make medical decisions vary. That chapter suggested that the circumstances and difficulty of medical decisions vary, that the lives of the sick vary, that patients' tastes for paternalism vary, that the ways patients make decisions vary, and that the ways doctors make decisions vary. Chapter 4 argued that people's appetites for information and control vary, that methods of securing control vary, and that medical decisions vary. Finally, the burden of Chapter 5 was that all these varieties of variety mean that no single rule about the wisdom and duty of making one's own medical decisions applies to all patients all the time. Sometimes patients should make their own decisions; sometimes they need not; sometimes they ought not.

There is an obvious resolution of this conflict between optional and mandatory autonomism: Some patients want medical autonomy, others do not. Both kinds of patients have exercised their autonomy in selecting the medical services they prefer; both should have what they want.[2] One may exercise autonomy by declining to exercise it.

This resolution of the contest between optional and mandatory autonomy seems to me essentially sensible and right. It is at base the resolution I work toward when I am a patient and would work toward were I a doctor. Its ideal is a flexible, individualized relationship between doctors and patients. In the best of all possible worlds, patients would select doctors who sympathized and worked well with their core preferences about authority to make decisions. Patients and doctors would arrange case by case who should make each decision. Often this process would be implicit, but it could demand the dialogue bioethicists often cherish such hopes for. Patients would ask themselves whether they would be better off practically if they made their own decision in a given circumstance and if they had some moral duty to do so. And in an ideal world, the people patients dealt with—especially family members and doctors—would help patients determine when to make their own decisions.

Nevertheless, this is not the best of all possible worlds, and this ideal of individualization is unattainable. Exactly because patients' views about making medical decisions are so complex and dynamic, it would be hard even with perfect information to match doctors and patients on that basis. Furthermore, that is not the only—or even the most important—kind of compatibility patients and doctors want. Nor is compatibility the only criterion patients use to select doctors, since patients also want qualities like competence. For that matter, patients cannot always pick their doctors.

In addition, the "dialogue school" of bioethics tends to forget that the quality of dialogues varies widely, even when the participants are willing. Applicants to medical school are not—perhaps cannot and even should not be—selected for their dialogic deftness. Such skills are rare, hard to teach, and prone to crumble under the pressures of practice: A good dialogue on these subjects demands participants who can listen to each other patiently, solicitously, and acutely and who can speak to each other delicately, wisely, and lucidly. Furthermore, if this model expects doctors to advise patients on their moral duty to make decisions, it may ask far too much. Doctors are neither selected for acuity in moral reasoning, nor does their culture promote it. As I intimated in Chapter 3, this is one serious limitation of doctors' ability to make good decisions for patients, and it similarly limits their capacity to counsel patients about who should make medical decisions.

What is more, a doctor who endeavors to implement the individualized model for allocating authority to make medical decisions faces no mean task. First, students of patients' preferences have generally failed to identify characteristics that are associated with a desire to make medical decisions.[3] One report typically concludes, "[D]ata from the present studies suggest little overlap between a variety of relevant personality measures and treatment preferences."[4] Thus a study of both cancer patients and the general public found that "[o]nly 14.8% of the variance in patient role preferences and 6.9% in householder preferences were accounted for by the predictor variables."[5] Analogously, another study concluded, "No patient characteristics reliably identified which patients want advance directives followed strictly."[6] In sum, "most of the difference among patients apparently is rooted within individual characteristics that are not captured by the variables measured."[7] Thus one observer commented that he had "witnessed first-hand and listened to many patients' accounts of their consultations with surgeons who have widely differing styles. These styles may range from old-style paternalism . . . [to] modern-day clinical glasnost. . . . It is surprisingly difficult to predict those who will be deeply distressed or those who will feel reassured and comforted by these different styles of consulting . . . ."[8] These data suggest that doctors may be hard put to identify patients who wish to assert their autonomy, that doctors will have fewer reliable clues to go on than one might think.

Furthermore, the structure of modern medicine increasingly frustrates ascertaining what decisional authority patients want. The bureaucratic organization of the hospital, the prevalence of specialization, and the rotation of physicians and other medical personnel, to say nothing of the mobility of patients, all inhibit doctors from knowing patients well enough to identify and understand their decisional preferences. These factors also mean patients and doctors must often be matched not just once but repeatedly. These developments in medical care and many more besides seem likely to accelerate and thus to diminish yet further familiarity with patients.

Of course, patients might simply be asked whether they want to make their own decisions. (Indeed, one group of empiricists believe they have developed a questionnaire which will identify people who do want to.)[9] Again, this seems sensible and right. But the question is hardly easy. Formulating, discussing, and answering it will often be complex and confounding. Patients themselves do not always know in advance what they want to know and what choices they want to make. Consider the contrast between two studies by Alfidi. In one study,

> he found that eighty-nine percent of patients who were informed of the serious risks of angiography, without being asked whether they wanted to be informed, "appreciated" receiving the information. . . . [I]n a later study in which he made disclosure contingent upon an affirmative response to an inquiry as to whether or not the patient wished to be informed of the risks of various diagnostic radiologic procedures, less than one-third of patients wanted to be told about risks.[10]

Even conscientious and self-conscious patients may be as baffled as Eric Hodgins: "When should a patient be submissive and when should he be obdurate? When is it wise to be dogged and when is it wise to give up? These are *the* questions when he confronts the various people who are trying, by their best lights and trainings, to help him, and I still do not have a clear idea of the right answers."[11]

Recall, further, how elaborately we could disaggregate the category "medical decisions" in Chapter 4. Patients may want to make some kinds of decisions but not others; to decide large, but not small issues; moral, but not technical questions; and so on. What is more, patients' desire to make decisions may ebb and flow, as the severity of their illness fluctuates and as they encounter the unanticipated: "Patients' preferences should be regarded as dynamic, not static. Whatever decision making powers they may forgo in acute illness they may reclaim as health is restored."[12] Chronically ill patients may want more authority over time, as they learn about their illness and their responses to it. In sum, if patients' preferences about making medical decisions are unexamined, complex, shifting, and ambivalent, it is hardly surprising, but significant, that the Strull study found that "[c]linicians were poor judges of patient preferences about decision making . . . ."[13]

Discerning and accommodating patients' preferences about making medical decisions becomes yet harder if one believes patients "want" to make their own decisions but have been deterred by the ethos of medicine from doing so or even perceiving their own preference. Such patients cannot simply be asked how they wish decisions to be made because that is exactly the question they misunderstand.

Even were these difficulties overcome, "the effects of interventions involving information and behavioral involvement . . . depend on the way they are presented and whether they enable individuals to satisfy their needs in that setting . . . ."[14] In clearer words, even if patients could be categorized as generally wanting or generally abjuring autonomy, much would turn on the particular situation in which they found themselves and on how the doctor dealt with them. For instance, some doctors might work well with patients who made their own decisions, while others might be less successful however earnestly they tried. Doctors, like patients, differ, and some doctors' personalities will better suit one style of patient participation than another. With one doctor a patient might seize the reins of decision; with another the patient might prefer to defer.

Finally, giving patients the decisional authority they want requires changing the behavior of many doctors. It means persuading them to do something that they would not otherwise do and that is not only hard, but requires delicate distinctions. While gross changes in behavior can be worked *en masse,* fine ones cannot be. People can usually follow the letter of a new rule, but its spirit is harder to capture. For instance, you can make hospitals have patients sign informed-consent forms, but not make hospitals provide timely, usable information. The following (edited) exchange between a woman with colorectal cancer and her doctor illustrates how formulaically new rules are often assimilated:

"Dr. Anderson. . . ." I started to cry.

"Have I said something to upset you?"

"Yes. I'm just not ready to hear all this. Can we do it another time?"

He started to make peculiar sounds in his throat and glanced about as if seeking help. "Well, goodness, don't you want to know the truth?"

"No. Not now. No."

"Yes . . . well, yes." He jerked out of the chair, nearly knocking it over. "I'll call Dr. Kelly and see when we can arrange another meeting." He drew his white coat around him and looking even paler than when he arrived, backed himself out, like a suppliant at a Buddhist shrine, into the corridor.[15]

Dr. Anderson was a physician who learned the first lesson of bioethics—tell the truth—too well. Basic principles are easy to teach; they are hard to apply delicately and judiciously.

In short, the obvious response to the variety of patients' attitudes toward making decisions is to accommodate each patient's preferences. But this is not easy, for those preferences are various, ambivalent, and fluid. Nor are they the only preferences we want medical care to promote. Doctors and patients have much to do besides pursuing the right level of autonomy for each decision, and those other things will often conflict with determining and implementing the right level of autonomy. Often, then, the costs of finding that level may exceed its benefits.

But there are even graver problems with the alluring device of according patients the autonomy they autonomously choose to have. There are, that is, problems with the practice of autonomy that arise from the changing structure of American medicine. To those problems we now turn.

The Autonomy Paradigm and the Bureaucratization of Medicine

Experience tends universally to show that the purely bureaucratic type of administrative organization . . . is, from a purely technical point of view, capable of attaining the highest degree of efficiency and is in this sense formally the most rational known means of exercising authority over human beings. It is superior to any other form in precision, in stability, in the stringency of its discipline, and in its reliability. . . . It is finally superior both in intensive efficiency and in the scope of its operations, and is formally capable of application to all kinds of administrative tasks. Max Weber, *Economy and Society*

Bureaucratic administration means fundamentally domination through knowledge. . . . This consists on the one hand in technical knowledge which, by itself, is sufficient to ensure it a position of extraordinary power. But in addition to this, bureaucratic organizations . . . have the tendency to increase their power still further by the knowledge growing out of experience in the service. For they acquire through the conduct of their office a special knowledge of facts and have available a store of documentary material peculiar to themselves. Max Weber, *Economy and Society*

Developments in the structure of modern American medicine are moving with tectonic power to alter our empirical and normative understanding of the world of physician and patient. The law and bioethics have imagined medical decisions as involving one doctor and one patient. Both disciplines have conceived their task as shifting the locus of decision from doctor to patient. This picture was always too simple; now it is badly anachronistic. Today, medicine is being organized, institutionalized, and bureaucratized, so medical decisions are increasingly made either in a bureaucracy or in a bureaucracy-rich environment. This further weakens the initially appealing solution of asking each doctor to establish with each patient the degree of autonomy the patient wants in each case.

In the modern world of medicine, a world of bureaucracy and economic stringency, we face a quandary. At the heart of our quandary lies this conflict: Patients vary, doctors vary, diseases vary, treatments vary, hospitals vary, and the lives of the sick vary. But legal rights, legislative and judicial principles, administrative regulations, institutional rules, social policies, and even cultural understandings depend on generalizations. How can the need to accommodate variety be reconciled with the imperative of generality? This is the question which will preoccupy us throughout this chapter.

The Rise of Medical Bureaucracy

A bureaucracy is a large organization which is hierarchically structured, meritocratically staffed, functionally specialized, reliant on the division of labor, intended to provide goods or services efficiently, and governed by rules. Bureaucracies increasingly dominate the delivery of medical services, just as they bestride the world in which we live. As Freidson writes, medicine is undergoing what

> might be interpreted as bureaucratization in Weber's ideal-typical sense, for [recent changes] are accompanied by an increase in hierarchical positions as health care organizations grow in size, records become more elaborate, specific standards govern the formal evaluation of more and more work, supervision in the form of evaluation of work becomes more widespread, and hierarchical positions of responsibility increase in number and variety.[16]

This bureaucratization is driven by potent forces which show no signs of flagging. A long-time engine of bureaucratization has been the demand for better medical care. That demand has evoked two responses which require more complex organizations. First, as medical knowledge has expanded, doctors have become more specialized. In a world of specialists, single doctors often cannot treat all an individual patient's ills, and any organization which wishes to do so must coordinate many specialists. Second, as medical technology has proliferated, medical institutions must hire specialists equipped to use that technology. Combined, these two trends have swollen the size and complexity of familiar medical organizations. Many hospitals, for example, were once small and informally run. Today, such a hospital cannot provide a full range of services. These two trends have not only led to the growth of familiar kinds of organizations; they have also prompted the creation of organizations that hardly existed before. Doctors increasingly organize themselves into large group practices, subspecialty practices, and clinics. They work for HMOs or urgent-care facilities. They join preferred-provider organizations and physician organizations (and even unions).

This brings us to the second engine of bureaucratization—economic necessity. More and more, medical organizations must expand to survive. Small organizations can muster neither the clients nor the capital to compete: "Competitive hospitals now offer a wide variety of new services to boost their revenues, from acquiring the latest medical technologies; to instituting helicopter transport services, free-standing ambulatory satellite clinics, inpatient psychiatric units, and home health care agencies, to establishing . . . non-health-care business . . . ."[17] The self-contained hospital struggles, and hospitals ally themselves with preferred provider organizations, independent practice associations, employers, health coalitions, HMOs, physician–hospital organizations, and insurance companies. Hospitals, even some charitable hospitals, merge and form chains, often large ones. Some for-profit hospitals have been organized into publicly held corporations of substantial size. Health-maintenance organizations have similarly expanded, even to the point of owning hospitals and outpatient facilities.[18]

Bureaucratization is impelled by yet a third force: Doctors and medical institutions are increasingly regulated by both public and private organizations, and especially by third-party payors. Governmental regulation has burgeoned as medical expenditures have reached 14% of the country's gross domestic product. As the range of medical activities has broadened and social expectations of medicine have deepened, private regulatory agencies like the Joint Committee on the Accreditation of Hospitals have insinuated themselves more thoroughly into the work of the organizations they supervise. Regulatory activities in turn stimulate organizational development. Thus the rise of malpractice law helped spur the growth of risk-management offices in hospitals. And as medical rationing becomes ever more plainly necessary,[19] the influence of regulatory institutions seems likely to heighten.

The fourth impetus to bureaucracy comes from the implacably rising costs of medical care. These have driven the institutions most centrally involved in paying those costs—the state and federal governments, employers, and insurance companies—to organize and act. They have encouraged some of the new forms of medical organization (like the HMO) and have tried to provoke more competition among health-care providers. They have also helped inspire the rise of other institutions (like utilization management organizations) intended to curb medical costs. Further, they have through incentives and direct pressure tried to get providers to control their costs.

Bureaucratization and the Locus of Medical Decisions

American health care, then, is moving impressively toward large and complex organizational structures located in elaborate and exigent organizational environments. In consequence, medical decisions are increasingly made "bureaucratically." Bureaucratization shifts decisions away from the patient, and in multiple ways. It moves decisions toward the doctor. But perhaps more significantly, it impels decisions away from the doctor toward the medical team, away from the medical team toward the organization, and away from the organization toward the system of institutions (not least the governmental agencies) that form the organization's environment. In short, medical decisions are being transferred not just from the patient, but also from the doctor, and even from the hospital. In this emerging world, the problem of patient autonomy takes on a new, and more implacable, aspect.

In other words, the problem is now and will increasingly be not so much that doctors think they know what patients need and impose that decision on them, but that medical decisions must be made and coordinated within a medical bureaucracy. Less and less does a single doctor collect and analyze all the data and recommend a treatment to a patient. More and more, diagnoses, prognoses, and proposals are formulated by a long series of people and teams, medical and lay, in a process in which the power to act is distributed around an organizational structure. As Anspach notes, "Organizations constrain the interaction in the medical interview; generate competing interests among professional groups; allocate resources to participants in decisions; influence the extent to which providers are oriented to the wishes of clients or colleagues; and . . . allocate different kinds of information to participants in medical decisions."[20] At its worst, the issue is not whether the patient is in charge, but whether anyone is: "There is no one person or thing in control. There is, rather, a hybrid, a powerful amalgam of heterogeneous elements, through which control is dispersed in intricate ways: dispersed over the entities performing the subtasks, and further complicated by the personnel's task of ensuring the tools' functioning in real time."[21]

The bureaucratization of medicine shifts decisions from patient to doctor for the reasons summarized in the second epigraph that began this section. Bureaucracies formulate decisions through formal and informal interactions staffed by technical specialists who are repeat players who know both their subject and each other and who are governed by the formal and informal norms of their specialty and institution. Lay clients are not readily integrated into this process—much less placed in charge of it—because they do not know the participants, the subject, or the norms. Thus, as Renée Anspach, for example, astutely shows, in hospitals as in other bureaucracies the bureaucrats tend to make their decision and then present a recommendation, take it or leave it, to the patient.[22]

The usual reasons clients are poorly placed to participate in bureaucratic decisions are aggravated by several features of contemporary medical organizations. For example, as medicine becomes more specialized and as attempts are made to tame costs, patients see doctors less often and paraprofessionals more often. This means patients have less access to the people best placed to influence their medical decisions. Hospitals have responded to the problem of patients lost in the bureaucratic maze by assigning employees relatively low in the hierarchy to speak for and guide them. But those employees *are* relatively low in the hierarchy, and creating new assignments for them rarely elevates them noticeably. A common response to this problem suggests that employees who spend time with patients should be better rewarded with status. But this seems unlikely, since such cosmetic efforts rarely alter the underlying structure of knowledge, skill, wealth, and power on which status ultimately depends. The dilemma is that, as in all bureaucracies, clients are generally best off working with the highest possible person, but this is costly, inefficient, and often unappealing to the higher-status experts.

The bureaucratization of medicine also drives decisions away from patients toward doctors by shifting doctors' orientation away from individual patients. This shift has two aspects. First, doctors' duty traditionally embodied the ideal of what Zussman calls "Hippocratic individualism," in which the doctor is single-mindedly committed to the interests of each particular patient. Zussman argues this commitment is put under crushing pressure when the physician also becomes responsible to an institution, as where a doctor whose patient needs intensive care is also the director of the intensive care unit and thus obligated to decide which of all the hospital's patients most needs the unit's only remaining bed.

This development is, typically, a blend of the welcome and the unwelcome. A recurring problem of American medicine has been the trouble it has in accommodating the conflicting interests of patients who are necessarily competing for limited resources. What Zussman describes might be a step toward such an accommodation. Yet the step is troubling because it weakens the doctor's ties with, and sense of obligation to, the patient. Thus, Zussman writes, "intensive care . . . is marked, perhaps above all, by a severe attenuation of the doctor-patient relationship . . . ,"[23] so that "all that remains are abstract values stressing the priority of individual patients."[24] Furthermore, this change probably occurs without the patient's realizing it or being able to respond to it.

The first aspect of the shift in physicians' orientation, then, moves responsibility from each individual patient and toward groups of patients. The second, related, aspect of that shift moves the doctor's orientation away from patients and toward the organizations which employ doctors, the subculture in which they work, and the profession to which they belong. Increasingly, doctors are hired, paid, and fired by organizations rather than patients. These organizations—profit and nonprofit alike—are increasingly driven by economic exigency.[25] And they are organizations over which patients often have only marginal influence, for any "large enterprise . . . tends to generate commitments to co-workers and subunits rather than to the enterprise as a whole, to separate employees from the customers or citizens affected by employee actions, and to operate on the basis of standard operating procedures that seem instrumentally rational even when they are substantively irrational."[26]

I have been suggesting that the bureaucratization of medicine propels decisions away from patients and that it does so partly by shifting doctors' orientation away from individual patients toward patients as a group and toward the organizations for or with which doctors work. This shift in orientation bespeaks another crucial shift in the locus of decisions—one away from the doctor and toward the organization. Increasingly, that is, doctors do not make decisions alone, and the decisions they make are shaped by the organizations for which and amidst which they work. Freidson, for instance, notes that

> in hospitals and other large practice settings, the authority of both the physician-administrator and the physician-researcher has become more extensive and definite and has become more binding on the practitioner. Formal administrative authority and formal cognitive authority analogous to "line" and "staff" authority in industry become much more definite, leaving rank and file practitioners with considerably less freedom of action than existed in the past.[27]

Medical organizations, that is, wield the authority of bureaucracies over bureaucrats. They determine doctors' employment, promotion, and income. They can harass them by assigning them the gloomiest offices, worst assistants, and foulest schedules. They can expose them to the condemnation and contempt of their colleagues. They can devise ingenious ways of giving doctors an economic stake in medical decisions. They can supervise doctors' decisions in more conventional ways. Freidson writes (perhaps a little prematurely), "Instead of being free to exercise their own clinical judgment, physicians become subject to systematic and formal review of their decisions by increasingly standardized criteria. . . . Instead of administering the affairs of their own practices in their own way, they become drawn into and dependent upon a highly rationalized and bureaucratic system of purportedly efficient management practices drawn directly from large business enterprises."[28]

In other words, *both* doctors and patients have lost some of their power to make medical decisions to the organizations of which they are increasingly a part. But those organizations themselves have had to cede power to the organizations with which they must work and to the organizations that supervise and regulate them. For example, third-party payors now realize they can only control costs by controlling medical decisions. Bradford Gray just hints at the dimensions of this problem when he writes, "More and more the services received by patients are not the result of a decision of a single person who is accountable to the patient but are instead the product of negotiations between providers and payers."[29] Third-party payors have intensified their long-standing practices of deciding which treatments they will cover and how much they will pay for them and of reviewing requests for payment after treatment has been provided. They press for second opinions. They demand that physicians get prospective approval of some nonemergency treatments and institute programs for monitoring continuing treatment. For example, "a primary care physician may be forbidden to order the costliest interventions without the approval of an administrator or of a consultant . . . . [M]ajor decisions such as selection of organ transplant recipients may be left in the hands of committees or a collectively constructed formula."[30] They employ specialized bureaucracies—utilization management organizations—to assist them in this work. In short, the various public and private "regulatory" agencies cast their nets so broadly that few doctors are not eventually caught in them. As Freidson notes, "even individual practitioners in their own offices are bound into reimbursement and review systems in which others become full-time specialists devoted to performing the functions of administration, evaluation, and sanctioning."[31]

The organizations that treat patients have ceded authority to the institutional environment another way. The bureaucratization of medicine has helped make it desirable and practical to establish standards for making specific medical decisions. Recent years have seen notable efforts in this direction, and, as Freidson observes, "standard classifications of complaints and diagnoses have been established, along with requirements that standardized techniques be employed for all cases falling within them."[32] This development has had considerable institutional support. The National Institutes of Health have sponsored conferences intended to develop standardized practices, and medical-specialty groups have increasingly tried to reach agreement about recurring medical issues. Similarly, "unlike the judgments made by individual physicians on the basis of their clinical experiences, the decision rules and criteria applied by UMOs [utilization management organizations] generally reflect some type of expert consensus and, in many cases, an up-to-date examination of the clinical research literature."[33]

Bureaucratization motivates these developments for several reasons. Like all bureaucracies, medical institutions need efficient decisions. Guidelines promote that goal. Like all bureaucracies, medical institutions and the organizations that regulate them want to reduce costs. Guidelines help identify the cheapest ways to provide adequate care and supervise its administration. Furthermore, medical institutions have an interest in providing good care and are aware of the defects in medical reasoning I charted in Chapter 3. As David Eddy argues, "No responsible institution can sit still while patients are subjected to serious interventions and costs fly, knowing that there is such a large random component to the decisions."[34] A principal institutional response has been guidelines:

> Practice policies and guidelines present a powerful solution to the complexity of medical decisions. They free practitioners from the burden of having to estimate and weigh the pros and cons of each decision. They can connect each practitioner to a collective consciousness, bringing order, direction, and consistency to their decisions. Practice policies provide an intellectual vehicle through which the profession can distill the lessons of research and clinical experiences and pool the knowledge and preferences of many people into conclusions about appropriate practices.[35]

With such hopes penned on it, the trend toward guidelines seems fated to continue. As Morreim notes, "insurance companies, HMOs, hospitals, and other institutional providers and payers are now compiling formidable computer databases that track diagnoses, interventions, costs, and outcomes, to serve as the foundation for guidelines by which to assess both the quality and cost-effectiveness of care."[36] Professional groups and government agencies of many stripes have called for and sponsored those guidelines. They have become the object of academic study. All this suggests that the authority to make medical decisions will continue to shift from individual patients and doctors toward the organizations that write, adopt, and implement these guidelines.

My point in describing the bureaucratization of medicine is not to prove that it is undesirable. On the contrary. Medicine is becoming bureaucratic for compelling reasons. Most obviously, bureaucracy is an inevitable part of delivering sophisticated, technological, large-scale medical services efficiently to many people. Furthermore, bureaucratization promises other advantages. For example, I have already suggested that the shift in doctors' orientation from individual patients to patients as a whole makes it easier to take broader social interests into account in making medical decisions.

The shift in doctors' orientation from individual patients to the organization as a whole may also have its merits. For example, bureaucratic organization and routine can motivate good work where a sense of obligation to the patient fails. As Daniel Chambliss writes, "There is only the institutional habit which substitutes for hope, which in many cases obviates the staff's pessimism or lack of interest. When standard procedure is followed, courage is unnecessary."[37] Similarly, Zussman comments that the sense of responsibility house officers are taught rests not on the doctor's obligation to a suffering human being, but rather on the bureaucrat's duty to other bureaucrats: "It is not responsibility of the sort stressed by attendings, based on abstract obligations to patients. Rather, it is responsibility to other housestaff, based on very concrete relationships and mutual dependence."[38] But the patient wins in the end, for "it is the peculiar genius of medical training that the implications of these two very different types of responsibility are often very much the same."[39] This bureaucratic duty, based as it is in the structure of medicine and enforced as it is by the doctor's peers, may in the end last longer than a general duty of benevolence enforced only by the receding echoes of conscience.

In some ways bureaucratization actually enhances patients' range of choices. Bureaucratization has increased competition and the advertising competition brings, and thus patients may find it easier to find out about the sources, nature, and cost of medical care. Furthermore, competition may help make institutions more responsive to what their clients want than many solo practitioners were. Specifically, medical organizations can be, and may see marketing advantages in being, a countervailing force against the paternalism of physicians, so that organizations may in some respects seek to enhance patients' ability to make their own decisions. Finally, some patients will be adept enough to use the multiple points of leverage bureaucracies provide to manipulate the system to get what they want. Anspach, for instance, describes the parents of a child in a neonatal intensive care unit who found "staff members [who] had previously been critical of some policies and practices in the nursery." These parents "mobilized these professionals' dormant concerns" in the parents' battle with other staff members.[40]

Nevertheless, the bureaucratization of medicine means both doctors and patients may be losing some of their ability to make medical decisions to the organizations which deliver medical care. How far, then, can patients practically be
integrated into the process of medical decision in a bureaucratic setting? The
classic bureaucratic (and legal) answer to such a question is to accord clients
"due process." But this solution is dubious.[41] A bureaucracy's clients are hobbled
by their technical ignorance, by their naiveté about institutional and professional
norms, and by their unfamiliarity with (not to say distance from) the other players. They are also impeded by their reluctance to assume the time-consuming and
wearisome burdens of a bureaucratic battleground. These impediments and the
discouragement they breed help explain the widespread failure of clients to accept proffers of due-process rights to participate in bureaucratic decisions.[42] All
these handicaps are exacerbated in the medical context by the factors we surveyed in Chapter 3 that deter patients from making decisions.

Another defect impairs the due-process approach to incorporating the client
into bureaucratic decisions, a defect we might call "bureaucratic formalism." The
temptation for a bureaucracy burdened with a troublesome requirement is to obey
its letter but flout its spirit. This has widely happened to informed consent:
Shortly before the operation the intern wearily presents the consent form, which
the patient mechanically signs. Thus are the rules followed, the law satisfied, the
hospital protected. Similarly, Zussman reports that "much of what appears to be a
decision about limitation of treatment is often better understood as the represen-
tation or dramatization of a decision."[43] The very emptiness of these forms then
persuades doctors the requirement is just more busywork concocted by an absur-
dist legal system. In this way, as Zussman rightly observes, "formal procedures
may become a means by which physicians withdraw yet further from intense involvement with their patients."[44]

Finally, even if the due-process response to the problem of the patient as client
were more successful than I think in bringing patients into decisions, we would
have to consider its costs, for it imports familiar problems of its own. They are
the problems of all bureaucracies, the problems of red tape, delay, routinization,
rigidity, and indifference. They are the problems which inspired Grant Gilmore's
mordant prophecy: "In Hell there will be nothing but law, and due process will be
meticulously observed."[45]

We are used to thinking about patients' autonomy as a contest between a doctor and a patient. Much of the reformist energy of bioethics has been devoted to
altering the terms of that contest. In the preceding section, I acknowledged the
appeal in the principle that patients should have exactly that degree of autonomy
they individually want, but I warned that that ideal would be frustratingly elusive. In this section, I have argued that it looks even more stubbornly distant in
the emerging world of medical practice, for in that world the locus of the power
to make medical decisions is shifting away from both doctor and patient toward

the medical bureaucracy. In an age of medical bureaucracies, the patient encounters structural barriers to the full-throated autonomy bioethics has longed for. And the standard solution to this problem—what I have roughly called due process—is both ineffective and expensive.

What do Patients Want? Bureaucracy, Bioethics, and the Depersonalization of Medicine

Hospitals, like other institutions founded with the highest human ideals, are apt to deteriorate into dehumanized machines, and even the physician who has the patient's welfare most at heart finds that pressure of work forces him to give most of his attention to the critically sick and to those whose diseases are a menace to the public health.
Francis W. Peabody, *The Care of the Patient* (1927)

[T]houghtful American physicians have been talking for over two decades about the importance of treating the patient as a human being, not a Case, or still more narrowly as a malfunctioning organ. Where all this talk is getting us, it is a bit hard to discover, and the hardest place to discover it is in the great American hospital, whatever its name. The American practicing physician may spend half his working hours in a hospital, yet he seems curiously unaware (or uninterested in) how his hospital behaves as an institution, particularly when he is not there. It does not function very well, and if there is a movement anywhere to rehumanize the American hospital, New York City is not its headquarters.
Eric Hodgins, *Episode: Report on the Accident Inside My Skull* (1964)

In the two preceding sections I suggested that achieving an optimal level of autonomy for each patient would be difficult under the conventional system of medical care and that the changing structure of American medicine is, and has for some time been, making that goal even more remote. In this section I want to consider that goal in yet another light. I have already examined bioethics' attempt to help patients make choices about medical care. I have said that many patients do not regard doing so as a first priority. But, what *do* patients want of their medical attendants? What future can those desires have in the emerging world of medical bureaucracies?

What Do Patients Want?

In my interviews with patients, I ask them what they want of doctors. Their answer is typically twofold. First, they want doctors who are learned, skillful, and effective. If patients do not make this answer, I ask whether competence is important, and they reply impatiently, "It goes without saying."[46] The second part of the answer to my question is the one patients almost always do make, promptly and passionately. They want someone who will care about them. They want a doctor with whom they can have some kind of human interchange. They want someone who will show them sympathy. As one of my interviewees said, "You know, you want them [doctors] to care about you, whether you live or die, and I think I have found that, here and in [X] Hospital because they just seem to—they are very caring about everything that happens to you. It is wonderful, I think." Or as another interviewee said, "They must have compassion."

Patients' memoirs put this point in many ways. One AIDS patient realized his doctor could not cure him, but could "be compassionate and understanding and make me feel he cared about my health."[47] One man chose to have his bypass operation performed by relatively inexperienced surgeons because they "were involved with me as a person."[48] A doctor with AIDS "learned that just as important as medical expertise and the proper use of new technologies is the ability of the physician to show legitimate concern, to be there during the bad times, and to provide hope even to the incurable."[49] One English doctor's patients thought him a good doctor "because he meets the deep but unformulated expectation of the sick for a sense of fraternity."[50] And an Israeli woman wrote of her husband's physician, "He was the ideal doctor, behaving like a *Mensch,* a human being, first and only then as a doctor, without thereby losing his medical stature."[51] In short, many memoirists join William Styron in conceiving "medicine to be a tender enterprise."[52]

Patients' memoirs overflow with gratitude for even modest displays of compassion. One lupus patient noted that the doctors at her hospital "seemed to combine knowledge with warmth and informality." She felt herself "privileged indeed to have such a share of their care and attention, and that was very important to me at this particular moment."[53] She valued one doctor because he "had a way of drawing me out—he gave just enough of himself to create a warm two-way relationship."[54] Another lupus patient praised a physician who "makes up for all those other doctors I dealt with along the way. He is so interested in the person, and demonstrates so much insight into the psychological problems of his patients.[55] Christy Brown liked his clinic because it had *"spirit* as well as efficiency, genuine human warmth as well as cold scientific precision. The people in the cool white coats have very warm hearts . . . . They are a set of human beings deeply and sincerely interested in the plight of another set of human beings faced with many huge problems . . . ."[56]

Similarly, a cancer patient admired her doctor's competence. "But what especially drew me towards him was that he made me feel my life mattered to him. When he looked at me, his eyes seemed to say, 'I want you to get through this.' I liked him. And I believed he had a sense of the individual catastrophe of cancer."[57] The much-afflicted poet William Cowper wrote gratefully of his physician, "I was not only treated with kindness by him when I was ill, and attended with the utmost diligence; but when my reason was restored to me, and I had so much need of a religious friend to converse with, to whom I could open my mind upon the subject without reserve, I could hardly have found a fitter person for the purpose."[58] Finally, when Geoffrey Wolf had ominous heart problems, his "cardiologist listened, and listened harder where other doctors had listened hard, and listened there some more. He was brisk; his hands were delicate; as he finished with me, he patted me on the head. I could have wept with gratitude for that gentle touch . . . ."[59]

Likewise, many ill doctors say how much they cherish human decency in their physicians and how often they find something else. As Robert Hahn notes in surveying doctors' accounts of their illnesses, "For several of these physicians, the reactions of their colleagues, both friends and strangers is [*sic*] a troubling surprise. When they are severely afflicted, many of their colleagues turn away; the afflicted physicians sometimes refer to this phenomenon as 'shunning.' They also discover that their colleagues often are not nearly as helpful as they might be."[60] For example, a doctor with AIDS found that

> [b]eing a doctor has not exempted me from feeling the coldness and indifference that medicine can give. I remember clearly when, soon after my diagnosis, my wife and I went to see an "AIDS expert." He sat behind his desk like a businessman discussing the markets, with no show of compassion or even concern for these two colleagues whose lives had just been shattered. He quoted studies and numbers but made no attempt to provide a bit of comfort or hope.[61]

Another doctor said what he "needed most, and did not receive from the medical profession, was a kind word of understanding."[62] Hahn adds that "while these physicians are often stunned at the responses of many of their colleagues, they are also occasionally gratified by the responses of other, exceptional colleague physicians."[63] As one doctor wrote gratefully of his physician, "His sense of succor was so spontaneous, generous, and accurate that it still astounds me."[64]

The absence of compassion scars many bitter pages of patients' memoirs. I have already related some stories about how brutally patients were told death was stalking them. But these stories only hint at the ulcerous memories that gnaw at patients. For example, Sue Baier tells the long and gruesome story of her travail with Guillain-Barré syndrome, a story infested by episodes like this:

> The next evening, Bill and I were still sharing our pleasure at my new forward step when Dr. Birmingham came up to my bed.
> "Well, you're off the machine," he said. "Now you need to start eating."
> Before I could react to what he was saying, he reached up to my nose, grabbed hold of the NG tube, and yanked it out brutally. A silent scream of pain and fear ripped through me. My eyes flew to Bill, pleading for help, but he could not move. He stood there stunned, anger and disbelief swirling across his face.
> "Now you'll have to eat," Birmingham said smugly, as he turned and left.[65]

When Ilza Veith went to have a carotid angiogram, the radiologist

> looked at me briefly and, with a short greeting, took hold of a fairly large syringe that he filled with a colorless fluid. Then he motioned me to lie back on the gurney, onto which my arms and legs were fastened with wide straps of cloth. Without any further words he positioned the needle of the syringe upon the carotid artery on the right side of my neck and, a second later, without an anesthetic or even a sedative or at least a warning of the forthcoming pain, he plunged the needle of the syringe into my neck. This extremely painful procedure caused me to wince, for which I was

scolded by the radiologist, who said sternly, "And now don't wince and don't moan and don't move even an inch." Immediately afterwards he pushed the plunger into the syringe, and again I moaned. . . . I felt as though my brain were on fire. The first injection was followed by a second and third, during each of which I was told not to moan. The repeated pain was incredibly severe, as was the frightening experience of believing that my head was on fire and ready to explode.[66]

Recriminations about medical callousness, crudity, and cruelty are not directed solely at doctors. The icon of nurses as angels of mercy and the catchphrase that doctors cure and nurses care hardly survive the buffeting nurses receive from their resentful patients. While some patients speak, with the warmest gratitude, of their nurses, others say "you learn very quickly in a hospital" that "the patients, by and large, are much more sympathetic and thoughtful and will go to greater lengths to help you than the hospital personnel."[67] Such patients tell stories of nurses who are lazy and indifferent, "closed and ill-tempered,"[68] self-important and petulant, bureaucratic and brutal. The paralyzed Arnold Beisser, ordinarily an easygoing and uncensorious man, testifies,

In one hospital, the first hour of the nurses' shift was spent in a detailed discussion of who would take coffee breaks when. Medications, patient needs, all other things paled in comparison. Sometimes people would literally leave you in midair in a lift to go on a coffee break, or leave you in some other awkward position, and just say, "It's my break time." They would often do everything possible to avoid helping me. What they did was done in a perfunctory manner. They seemed reluctant or grudging as they did things. There was a guardedness about them, fearing that they would be asked to do more than they were willing or able to do.[69]

And a physician tells how even doctors can be treated harshly by nurses when they become patients:

Within a few hours after my surgeon's visit, my pain gradually increased. At my request, my private-duty nurse asked the charge nurse to call the doctor. For over two hours the charge nurse put her off, convinced that I was a "crock." I was in severe pain and I began moaning. She continued to ignore it. I rang my call bell. No one answered. Finally, my husband went out to the hall pleading with the charge nurse to attend to me. She ignored him. I became desperate, crying and screaming, since the pain had become excruciating. My husband went out and pleaded again. Finally she barrelled into the room. "Doctor Brice," she exhorted, "I want you to quit moaning and quit manipulating. I have another patient in the next room moaning, and if you think you are going to get me to give you morphine or call your doctor, you are wrong." With that, she stomped out of my room.[70]

Eric Hodgins sums up the feeling of many—though certainly not all—patients when he quotes a lady of his acquaintance experienced in hospitals: "'Obviously, nurses become nurses because they are interested in suffering. But only some of them seem interested in relieving it: some others actually seem bent on intensifying it.'"[71]

Patients, then, want something of the personal in dealing with those to whom they turn for help in illness. Some of their reasons are therapeutic. They calculate that doctors who care about them will work harder to cure them and that kind doctors will try more alertly to avoid hurting them. But patients also want things as simple as sympathy. Candace Clark even argues that

it is often sympathy that people want rather than concrete assistance or advice about how to solve their problems. . . . I observed an elderly white woman hospitalized with a crushed hip. She told her nurse (and everyone who came within hearing range) that she had spent a difficult night. The nurse first responded by rearranging the bedding to try to make the patient comfortable, but the woman kept complaining. Next, the nurse offered advice: "If you just eat more and take your medication, you'll feel better." The patient's reaction was to repeat the details of her tortured night. Finally, the nurse responded, "I know how you feel." "Thank you for your sympathy," the woman said, and she immediately relaxed her taut muscles, wiped away her frown, and lay back on her pillow to sleep.[72]

While for many reasons and in many ways patients want some element of the personal in their relationship with their doctors, I do not think they expect or even always want doctors to be friends.[73] Patients realize that doctors have technical work to do and that their bodies are the objects of that work:

They handled my body the way I would have managed a broken stove or toilet. I wish to interpolate here something I think is important: I was handled by those men like a piece of meat, absolutely handled and manipulated, and not once then or in any other process that transpired in the hospital did I ever feel the slightest loss of dignity, the slightest loss of personality or worth, or the slightest loss or diminution of sex. Toward me, the woman, they were respectful and kind and as helpful as they know how to be. . . . [I]t was memorable because I was naked and helpless and marked up like a sacrificial calf for three hours and the three of us were alone. They were men of unblemished purity and it was, on the whole, a very nice experience spiritually.[74]

Patients generally understand that doctors are busy, that they have many patients, that they provide a service, and that friendship cannot be served up on command. But patients want doctors to know them, to care about them, to sympathize with them, to treat them gently, warmly, and well. This is no small part of what they expect from their doctors. All too often, it is something they do not find.

Bureaucracy and Impersonality

Changes in the nature of American medicine have created, and seem fated to accelerate, challenges to the vision of medical care I have just described. Bureaucracies are famously impersonal, and so it is unsurprising that the bureaucratization of medicine corrodes the model of the relationship between doctor and patient as a personal one. As one sophisticated patient wrote, "The hospital has all the features of a bureaucracy, and, like bureaucracies everywhere, it both breeds and feeds on impersonality."[75]

The impersonality of bureaucratic medicine flows from many sources. First, there is the impersonality of strangers. In today's medicine, patients and doctors may not choose each other, may not know each other, may not expect to see each other again. Far from choosing a doctor, patients increasingly choose an organization which then chooses (often-changing) doctors. Even where the doctor is in private practice and the patient is not hospitalized, the division of labor that increasingly characterizes medicine often sends patients to specialists they do not know.

Second, there is the impersonality of principle. Bureaucrats should treat similarly situated clients similarly, and similarity is defined impersonally. As Anthony Kronman writes, quoting Max Weber, "the bureaucrat's personal affairs—his own interests and feelings—must be excluded, insofar as is humanly possible, from the performance of his official duties; the ideal modern officeholder is one who rules '*sine ira et studio,* without anger or passion, and hence without affection or enthusiasm'."[76]

Third, there is the impersonality of efficiency. Part of what drives medicine toward bureaucracy is the need to contain costs, to provide treatment quickly and efficiently. Under these pressures and all the calls on doctors' time, it becomes a struggle to mount the effort Peabody commended:

> Here is a worried, lonely, suffering man, and if you begin by approaching him with sympathy, tact, and consideration, you get his confidence and he becomes your patient. . . . Once your relationship with him has been established, you must foster it by every means. Watch his condition closely and he will see that you are alert professionally. Make time to have little talks with him—and these talks need not always be about his symptoms. Remember that you want to know him as a man, and this means you must know about his family and friends, his work and his play. . . . Look out for all the little incidental things that you can do for his comfort.[77]

Fourth, there is the impersonality of the division of labor. The doctor is a specialist who mends bodies, or even a specialist who mends one part of the body. All else easily becomes irrelevant. This is a recurring complaint: "For a medical institution, the patient is an object to be processed in institutionalized ways and to be treated as a biomechanical entity. Patients are institutionally objectified: detached from their own lives and life stories, physically taken from their home settings, behaviorally managed as a conglomerate of discrete parts to be treated by different specialists."[78] Impersonality between doctor and patient can be promoted even by the effort to reduce the impersonality of the patient's relationship to the institution. Sometimes, a specialist in human relationships—a social worker, a psychologist, a nurse, a "patient advocate"—is assigned to deal with the more personal aspects of people's medical problems. Sometimes, people other than doctors, as well as pamphlets and videotapes, may proffer the information doctors cannot so cheaply provide. Such specialization, sensible though it is in many ways, reduces the opportunity for doctors to establish some personal contact with their patients and perversely distances the physician yet further from the patient.

Fifth, there is the impersonality of rules. Because bureaucracies must process large numbers of people in complicated circumstances, because they must efficiently coordinate numerous employees, bureaucracies are crucially governed by rules. These rules limit employees' discretion to accommodate special circumstances: The very function of rules is to reduce the need to notice and the authority to respond to the particularities of specific people. Thus the danger is that "[p]atients lose their uniqueness as individuals and become anonymous members of an abstract category or class."[79]

Sixth, there is the impersonality of rights. Individual doctors may resist thinking of their relations with their patients as structured by rights; bureaucracies are less reluctant. Indeed, the classic bureaucratic response to the client's desire to participate in decisions is a rights solution—to give patients formal claims against the bureaucracy. That is what administrative due process is all about. But such rights are both a product and a promoter of impersonality. Let me briefly explain why.

Bureaucracies are simultaneously removed from and responsible for their clients. This creates a tension which can be resolved in several ways, one of which assigns rights to the clients and therewith responsibility for their own welfare. This is partly a matter of human psychology. If I am responsible for you, there is hardly any limit to the demands you might make of me. But if you have rights to participate in the decision I am making, those rights establish limits to my duty to you. They allow me to say that, if you have been too foolish or feckless to use your rights well, that is your problem and not mine. Thus Zussman observes "that physicians may . . . become advocates of patients' rights in response to the impersonality of their relations with patients."[80]

Rights exacerbate the impersonality of the relations between doctor and patient in another way. Rights exclude me from affecting your choices. They thus distance me from you, for the less I can affect your behavior, the less involved in and concerned with you I am likely to be. This effect is intensified where I am excluded because I am considered untrustworthy.[81] Rightly or wrongly, but perhaps understandably, this seems to be how many doctors have responded to patients' acquisition of legal rights. Worse, the process is self-reinforcing: Trust wanes as relationships become more bureaucratic and less personal. This creates a call for rights. The rights solution further alienates doctor and patient because it distances them and because the doctor resents the distrust that motivated the solution. Furthermore, those endowed with rights often see a virtue in exercising them, simply because they are rights. This further lengthens the distance and exacerbates the distrust between doctor and patient, which in turn provokes demands for more rights to protect patients.

In sum, the increasingly bureaucratic structure of medical care aggravates in multiple ways the impersonality of a business that time and financial pressures already make impersonal. This is not all bad. The bureaucratization of medicine has merits, and impersonality is a cost of that process. Impersonality can even promote good medical care. Zussman, for instance, contends that (as bureaucratic theory would predict) impersonality permits a dispassion that leads to treating patients fairly and evenhandedly: "What might surprise us . . . is how little relevant the moral judgments of physicians and nurses are to life in intensive care. For the most part, the ICU staff neither demeans patients nor tries to reform them nor, most important, treats them differently on the basis of such judgments."[82] Impersonality also frees doctors to become absorbed in treatment: "Only because the housestaff do not know or think of their patients as full people can they think of the medical care they provide as a 'physiology experiment.' Yet, at the same time, thinking of care as a game, a puzzle, or an experiment allows the housestaff to maintain a level of energy that operates in the interest of the patient."[83] Finally, depersonalization allows doctors with disagreeable patients to concentrate on the intellectual challenges they pose, thereby offering them competent, if not compassionate, care.

Nevertheless, the bureaucratization of medicine has thwarted an end patients hold dear, dearer perhaps than control over medical decisions—solicitous personal care. This is unsurprising; that is what bureaucracies do. My next proposition may seem less obvious, for I want to suggest that, like bureaucratization, modern bioethics lives in tension with the goal of personal medical care.

Bioethics and Impersonality

Traditional medical ethics embodied the ideal of a personal relationship between doctor and patient, a relationship governed, mediated, and protected by the principle of trust. Patients were supposed to confide themselves to their doctors' care because doctors were supposed to be trustworthy. Doctors were supposed to be trustworthy because they were committed to a system of professional ethics that put patients' interests first, because doctor and patient shared a culture and beliefs that made them comprehensible and loyal to each other, and because doctor and patient were joined in a personal relationship which as such made moral demands on the doctor. The personal relationship between doctor and patient was thought rewarding to the doctor and therapeutically beneficial to the patient not just because the patient appreciated the doctor's interest, but because the doctor learned about and came to cherish the patient. As Francis Peabody wrote in his classic article,

> The good physician knows his patients through and through, and his knowledge is bought dearly. Time, sympathy and understanding must be lavishly dispensed, but the reward is to be found in that personal bond which forms the greatest satisfaction of the practice of medicine. One of the essential qualities of the clinician is interest in humanity, for the secret of the care of the patient is in caring for the patient.[84]

Doctor and patient, in short, were supposed to be linked by a "personal bond" made possible by their membership in some kind of community. It was this personal bond which made plausible the paternalism we now distrust, deplore, and even despise.

Bioethics has centrally asserted the autonomy of patients against the paternalism of doctors. Thus bioethics has been deeply skeptical of the old model of the relationship between doctor and patient and the personal bond it envisioned and advocated. To be blunt, bioethicists have doubted that doctors will be trustworthy, for doctors have individual and guild interests that are not the patient's. Bioethicists have further doubted that doctor and patient share the commonality of belief, the community of values, that might make medical paternalism more understandable. Bioethicists continue their critique of the personal bond between doctor and patient by pointing to the inequality in power between them, an inequality that inhibits free and genuine personal relations. Finally, bioethicists argue not just that the personal bond is illusory, but also that as an ideal it is pernicious, for it lures doctors into paternalism and patients into acquiescence.

In other words, bioethics' view of doctor and patient embodies yet another source of impersonality. This source draws on some powerful cultural currents. Not least is the belief that in a modern, pluralist society, people of differing and even discordant cultures, experience, and belief are brought together. Their differences shape their natures and separate them in ways they cannot overcome. To make society possible, people must be tolerant, for their differences are essentially unbridgeable. People, then, do not know each other because they cannot know each other. Doctors should not make decisions for their patients because they cannot enter into their patients' minds and hearts well enough to understand their lives, their wants, or their beliefs.

In response to this critique, bioethics has sought to rein in physicians' power. Not least, it has advocated limiting the doctor's role. The old model left that role relatively open-ended: The personal element in the tie between doctor and patient meant doctors might be confidants, advisors, even friends. The emerging model, on the other hand, prefers to treat the doctor as essentially the provider of services for hire. The relationship is not personal; it is commercial. It is not open-ended; it is defined by its function. It is not ordered by custom; it is established by negotiation. In short, Maine's famous dictum—"that the movement of the progressive societies has hitherto been a movement *from Status to Contract*"[85]—may usefully be applied to the emerging relationship between doctor and patient. As Bradford Gray comments, "we have steadily moved from medical care relationships based on status (with open, unbounded obligations, as among family or neighbors) to relationships based on contract (with mutual obligations legally specified)."[86]

Bioethics not only constricts the doctor's role; it expands the patient's. For in the place of trust, bioethics puts rights. As Zussman says,

> if the close personal relationship between doctor and patient has become a thing of the past (if indeed it ever existed at all), it has been replaced by a relationship organized around different principles. In particular, in the absence of a personal rela-

tionship—in the absence, as it were, of trust—the doctor-patient relationship has been reorganized around principles of patients' rights.[87]

It is the patient who has the authority and even the duty to define the relationship, to make the decisions, to call the doctor to account. The doctor's power is constrained by the patient's rights; patients are endowed with rights to protect them against the doctor's depredations. Doctors must not infringe the authority of rights holders; rights holders must be alert to such infringements.

The new model has not obliterated the old. Personal sympathy and professional duty still overcome the distance between doctor and patient. But the view of the therapeutic relationship as a commercial one, the image of the patient as a skeptical and abused consumer, the doubt that doctor and patient share cultural understandings, the resentment of medical imperialism, and the rights language bioethicists deploy all stimulate distrust between doctor and patient and thus erode the personal bond between them.

Even admirable doctors and decent patients can readily become mired in distrust. Few experienced patients have not been affronted by rude, callous, and incompetent doctors, have not heard woeful tales from family, friends, and fellow patients. Patients have every reason to be anxious for good care and little way to assure themselves they are getting it. All this gives patients plentiful reason to worry. When those reasons are amplified by the lessons of consumer activism and assertion, distrust becomes easy. Consider, for example, an article in *Newsweek* entitled "When Your HMO Says No: How to Fight for the Treatment You Need—and Win," which begins,

> Chances are your HMO wormed its way into your life by becoming a world-class loafer. Doing nothing is a key attribute of a successful health plan. Withhold an MRI from a patient with a headache, and presto! A plan saves $500. Keep the parents of a howling 9-month-old from visiting the emergency room, and an HMO's expenses fall by $300. . . . The fact is, just saying no helps your HMO charge your employer a nice low price—and still turn a profit.[88]

Doctors bring their own anxieties to the examining room. Few experienced doctors have not been assailed by rude, belligerent, and demanding patients, have not heard woeful tales from their colleagues. If people are vile to you when you have been civil or even kind to them, you begin to wonder whether civility and kindness are worth the effort and sense of personal exposure they cost. All this gives doctors reasons to protect themselves from unpleasantness and criticism. When those reasons are amplified by the feeling that their profession is under perpetual attack from "advocates" for patients and that their patients distrust them on entering the room, graciousness wilts.

I do not mean that bioethicists set out to destroy the personal element in the relationship between doctors and patients. However, the bioethics movement attacked aspects of the old norm that supported that element and substituted principles that threaten it. In doing so, it has found an unexpected ally in doctors. Bioethics is commonly seen—by doctors as well as bioethicists, by participants as well as observers—as the antagonist of the medical profession. But the duties bioethics would impose—to share information and defer to the patient's autonomy interests—and even the distrust bioethics nourishes have advantages for doctors. They transfer a weight of decision from doctor to patient. They make it easier for doctors to distance themselves from patients, to shed the psychic and moral burden felt by doctors who comment, "'If you are involved with the patient, you're going to become emotionally drained and burn out very soon,'"[89] or who say,

> "The hardest thing you do in medicine is making the decision for a patient and accepting the responsibility of the outcome. That really is a pretty big burden. That is the hardest thing to do, when you talk someone into doing something and it goes wrong. I would love a patient who, I know it is hard, is as informed as I am. . . . People who you have to push a little bit, they are the ones who say, 'Doctor, make the decision.' I find it to be the hardest."[90]

Thus, "[w]hether because of fear or because of indifference, overwork, or diffidence, physicians may be prepared to abdicate responsibility for some decisions to patients. Giving patients information, they have discovered, may be easier than withholding it."[91] This development may help explain bioethics' successes in changing the relationship between doctor and patient.

In sum, the traditional ideal that envisages a personal relationship between doctor and patient has, however inadvertently, been eroded by two forces: the bureaucratization of medicine and the bioethics movement. Both forces impel us away from a personal relationship and toward a contractual and bureaucratic one. It is contractual because it is more essentially a business relationship and because the parties' duties and authority are stipulated more precisely and loom larger in their minds. The relationship is bureaucratic in that it exists within an institution, or at least within a context surrounded and shaped by institutions. It is increasingly bureaucratic in the sense that the primary relationship is between the client and an institution (a hospital, a clinic, an HMO), not between two individuals. Both contractual and bureaucratic relationships are relatively impersonal. They are governed by rules articulated with some specificity. They assume no more commonality of interest and culture than is necessary to accomplish the goals which gave rise to the relationship.

The impersonality of modern medical care arises out of much-desired developments—out of advances in medicine's methods and structure and out of bioethics' victories over medical imperialism. The impersonality born of bureaucracy exists and persists because we know no other way to offer complex and sophisticated medicine to millions of people. In other words, we cannot serve one desire of patients—efficient medical care—without disserving the other—personal medical care. The impersonality nurtured by bioethics may not be what patients want, but it is understandable and perhaps ineradicable. Doctors *are* selling their services. They have *not* always deserved their patients' trust. Where a relationship has grown impersonal, patients may be foolish to rely on a personal bond. Further, these developments are part of a larger trend toward impersonality in modern life that springs from a pervasive need to coordinate the affairs of strangers among whom trust is missing. Freidson is quite right, then, to conclude that, regardless of good intentions, "patients will often be treated as objects rather than as individuals, and that care will become routinized."[92]

Thus the emerging world of medicine presents us with an old question in a new incarnation. It is the problem of the doctor–patient relationship in its many aspects beyond those addressed by the autonomy paradigm. This relationship, of course, was the subject of much traditional medical ethics. Unhappily, medical ethics as they were too often understood and "the doctor–patient relationship" as that phrase was too often deployed were polluted by professional groups like the AMA, which used them to defend their crassest guild interests against even the gentlest rebukes and feeblest reforms. But that misuse should not deter us from rescuing this important problem from the disrepute into which it has fallen or from searching for the optimal balance between the personal and the efficient, between solicitude and paternalism.

One of my themes has been that bioethics needs to examine the realities of illness and medical care. I have concentrated on one of those realities—the preferences of patients, particularly of patients who are reluctant to make medical decisions. In this section, however, I have looked beyond the reluctant patient to descry the shape of our emerging world, a world in which the autonomy paradigm has become the conventional wisdom, in which medical services are increasingly shaped and provided by institutions. In this world, the patient's relationship with the doctor has, like many relations of modern life, become less personal and more contractual, structured more by rules and rights than temperament and trust. Responding to these changes will be challenging, for the things patients want for themselves conflict with each other and with the conflicting things we want for them. In the next section, however, I will speculate about at least one direction bioethical thinking might profitably take.

From Consumer Choice to Consumer Welfare

The mundane must be respected. . . . So if we are to accomplish good in the world, I think it will be less through single, dramatic acts of moral courage than through relatively unglamorous, unnoticed lifetimes passed in (properly designed) organizational routines. . . . People don't live only in bright visible moments of decision; they live, and die, and work in the ordinary everyday world.   Daniel F. Chambliss, *Beyond Caring*

Those are merely the skills of human sympathy, the skills for letting another creature know that his or her concern is honored and valued and that, whether a cure is likely or not, all possible efforts will be expended to achieve that aim or to ease incurable agony toward its wel-

come end. Such skills are not rare in the natural world. What else but the urge to use and per-
fect such skills on other human beings in need could drive a man or woman into medicine?
What but a massive failure to recognize one's stunted emotions before they blunder against
live tissue—that and an avid taste for money and power? . . . Maybe we have the right to
demand that such a flawed practitioner display a warning on the office door or the starched
lab coat, like those on other dangerous bets—Expert technician. Expect no more. The quality
of your life and death are your concern.   Reynolds Price, *A Whole New Life*

I began this book by saying that we live in the time of the triumph of autonomy in bioethics. As a matter of principle, that triumph has been overwhelming.
As a matter of practice, it is less overwhelming, but at least doctors have become
less autocratic, and patients have more of the latitude many of them want to govern their own treatment. Nevertheless, we may have reached the point of diminishing returns on the autonomy paradigm in bioethics. As I have argued throughout this book, many patients have reasonably declined to make their own medical
decisions. As I argued in the first section of this chapter, helping each patient toward an optimal level of autonomy is undertaking a long, hard climb. As I argued
in the second section, changes in the structure of medicine may be making it like
scaling Everest. As I argued in the preceding section, patients want things from
medicine besides autonomy. In light of all this, where should reformist energies
now be directed?

The Limits of the Consumer-Choice Model

If we ask patients what they want from physicians, we hear two things: competence and kindness. These answers pose an awkward challenge to bioethics.
They raise questions about what role bioethics can play in the continuing reform
of American medicine. What do bioethicists know about medical competence?
How can that favorite tool—the law—promote it? What can anyone say about the
virtue of kindness, or how to secure its increase? The role of bioethics in medical
reform in general and of these questions in particular is complicated by the
movement of American medical care toward bureaucratization and rationing—
forces which place what patients want from doctors at some risk—and by the fact
that bioethics itself has helped promote an impersonality patients appear to regret. What, then, can bioethics contribute to the problem of the patient as client to
a bureaucracy?

In answering these questions, we may usefully think of bioethics in terms of
the principles of consumer protection. Bioethics has primarily advocated the
model of consumer choice. That model seeks to allow consumers to choose the
products they prefer by assuring them the information they need to make choices
and by insisting they be given what they chose. Thus, for example, merchants
may be required to reveal the terms under which they sell goods on credit so that
customers may evaluate what they are offered. Once the customer has chosen a
purchase, the merchant is held to the terms agreed upon. In short, the consumer-

choice model attempts to let customers make successful decisions by mandating a market that, in the economist's sense, works efficiently.

Conventional bioethical reform may be understood along these lines. The doctrine of informed consent is intended to provide patients the information they need to make wise choices that express their preferences. Patients must become consumers knowledgeable enough to make sensible decisions, and those decisions are given more binding effect by, for example, the threat of informed-consent suits and various provisions for advance directives.

The consumer-choice model makes a good deal of sense, but it rests on some fragile assumptions. It assumes human preferences differ so much people should make all purchasing decisions for themselves. It assumes engaged and energetic purchasers. It assumes purchasers can practically be given—in useful form—all the information they need to make wise decisions. It assumes people's preferences are clear and strong enough to drive them to analyze and act on the information they receive. And it assumes a market that responds efficiently to people's purchasing decisions.

Of course consumers do not always get what they want even in relatively efficient markets. Consumers long said they wanted fuel-efficient cars with seat belts and airbags, yet those cars remained scarce. Such disappointments occur partly because the assumptions of the consumer-choice model are demanding and frequently not fully met. Consumer's preferences are often undeveloped, weak, and conflicting. Making and implementing decisions costs consumers both time and trouble. Decisions are painful, and many people dislike and resist making them. For all these reasons, consumers often fail to use effectively the information the law labors to supply them. Finally, sellers do not always respond rationally to the market's incentives.

All this is no less true of making medical choices than buying cars. My arguments in this book put the assumptions of the consumer-choice model in medicine systematically in doubt. Many patients delegate their medical decisions because they doubt their capacity to make good ones, lack the vigor to do so, and even wonder whether they fully appreciate their own interests. The information patients need to make decisions is opaque and hard to convey in useful forms. Patients' preferences are often inchoate and ambivalent and thus too feeble to drive patients to make decisions. And the market in which patients act responds to internal and external forces which make it unresponsive to consumers. In short, so many assumptions of the consumer-choice model are so little applicable to medical decisions that we may be hitting the limits of its usefulness.

These doubts find some confirmation in an important recent study, the Study to Understand Prognoses and Preferences for Outcomes and Risks of Treatments, more conveniently known as SUPPORT.[93] SUPPORT investigated over nine thousand seriously ill patients in five prominent teaching hospitals during four years. Doctors were given reports on their patients' prognoses and were told their patients' feelings about CPR, the treatment of pain, receiving information, and advance directives. Specially trained nurses promoted communication among patients, their surrogates, and their doctors. Put succinctly, SUPPORT revealed "no significant change in the timing of DNR orders, in physician-patient agreement about DNR orders, in the number of undesirable days [patients experienced], in the prevalence of pain, or in the resources consumed."[94] The study did not alter patients' preferences about DNR orders, their communication with doctors, or their satisfaction with their medical care. Only 15% of the doctors discussed the information they had received with their patients (or with people acting on the patient's behalf). In short, despite an elaborate and costly program designed, in part, to increase patients' participation in medical decisions, remarkably little changed.

SUPPORT does not speak directly to all the assumptions of bioethics' consumer-choice model. Nevertheless, this ambitious and impressive research confirms the fruitfulness of the questions I have raised about that model. SUPPORT followed the model in trying to increase the communication between doctor and patient so both could make better decisions. But what is striking about the study is that, despite a commitment of resources unlikely to be matched, much less sustained, in the dullness of daily life, the SUPPORT instantiation of the model failed to produce statistically significant benefits.

What are we to make of this unsettling negative? To put the point simply, a strong reading of the study challenges the usefulness of remaining fixated on consumer choice. Efforts to implement that model have not been wasted—they have helped spur changes in medical attitudes which are making doctors' behavior more tolerable to contemporary American norms and are allowing more patients to make medical choices. But SUPPORT does raise doubts about the profit of sustaining the consumer-choice model at its present preeminence and exclusivity. SUPPORT does seem to confirm the doubts I have expressed throughout this book about how far the law and bioethics should make the autonomy principle so much their central concern. In short, it is time to ask how far the consumer-choice model can continue to improve the lives of patients.

Part of the reason for the failures reported in SUPPORT probably lies in the SUPPORT authors' explanation—that patients, strangers in a strange land, accommodate themselves to local custom. But I think the reasons run much deeper, into the factors I canvassed in Chapter 3—into people's sense of their own competence, into the vigor with which sick people can exert themselves, even into questions about where people's sharpest concerns and deepest interests lie. In short, SUPPORT and my arguments raise the possibility that the consumer-choice model may at some point confront strong resistance not just from the structure of medicine and the imperialism of doctors, but in the hearts and minds of patients. One legitimate response to such a suggestion is to say we must fight on however long it takes because the principle of autonomy is too vital to compromise. But if the reasons patients decline to make their own decisions are as potent as I have supposed, such a battle is hardly an appetizing prospect.

The Consumer-Welfare Model: Competence

What, then, is to be done? Our analogy to consumer protection suggests one answer. The consumer-choice model has long been supplemented with what we may loosely call the consumer-welfare model. When the market failed to deliver fuel-efficient cars with airbags quickly enough, we created regulatory incentives for them. Similarly, it may now be time for bioethics to accelerate a shift that seems already to have begun—away from patient choice and toward changing the medical-care system so that it delivers a better product. To put the point provocatively, it may be time to think about giving patients what we think they want, but have not been able to secure for themselves. We might even consider giving patients what we think they would want if they thought about it.

Let me make the suggestion less wickedly. Perhaps we should redirect our attention away from the procedures by which medical decisions are made and toward their substance. Bioethics has historically looked to the former, partly because it was supposed to lead to wisdom in the latter. Common sense has been thought to suggest that if patients had good information, they would make good, or at least satisfying, decisions. But my explanations of why patients decline to make their own decisions, my description of the way they make them, and the SUPPORT data raise doubts about how far the procedural approach improves decisions or even patients' satisfaction. If these doubts are well founded, one alternative is to look directly at those decisions and try to improve them.

SUPPORT suggests yet another reason it may be more fruitful to change what medicine does rather than to increase patients' autonomy. SUPPORT was conducted in notably bureaucratic settings. That is where many critical medical decisions are now and increasingly will be made. But our experience with bureaucracies shows that giving clients an authoritative voice in them can be implacably difficult: Often the cure for the ills of bureaucracy is more bureaucracy. Thus it will often be better to deliver the "right" service in the first place. That way, patients will at least by some standards be better off, for if the standard is well chosen, it will reflect what a large majority of patients want. To put the point differently, the rise of medical bureaucracies means patients need help in coping with them. Leading bureaucracies to make "good" decisions in the first place is one way of providing it.

How might we move in these directions? One approach is to build on a development I have already mentioned—the movement toward writing and implementing guidelines. Guidelines represent one of the likeliest ways of making the world better for patients by improving the medical and bioethical decisions that affect them, for guidelines can sharpen medical decisions by promoting consensus among experts about how to treat common conditions. Much of the work of writing them has been technical, work only experts wholly understand and can perform. Bioethics may, however, usefully encourage this work. In addition, some guidelines can be improved by making them more responsive to what patients want and to the bioethical issues they face, and here bioethicists may have contributions to make.

I argued a moment ago that the bureaucratization of medicine makes well-considered guidelines more desirable. It also makes them more effective. Bureaucracies tend to standardize decisions, to push them upward, and to fear unpopular policies. Guidelines are ready-made policies a bureaucracy can easily adopt. Because they should have been carefully developed and have attained some professional and public approbation they will seem relatively safe. And not only do bureaucracies need such guidelines, they have mechanisms for enforcing them. In short, because bureaucracies need policies and can enforce them, guidelines are likely to be more widely adopted and used in the age of medical bureaucracy than ever before.

Let me make my proposal more concrete by suggesting examples of areas in which guidelines might be useful. SUPPORT, for instance, notes that a troubling number of dying patients suffer a disquieting amount of pain. Yet doctors have been notoriously slow to exploit progress in pain management, and many of them undertreat pain. As Reynolds Price bitterly comments,

> [I]n the technological paradise of medical America, I was left to sit and bear central pain with whatever resources my solitary mind could summon in its torpid drugged state. And that was the plight of a man who'd been lucky enough to acquire nineteen years of free education, a man with compassionate and decent doctor-friends and with a better-than-average lay knowledge of medicine.[95]

Paul West proffers similar testimony: "Pain is often enough of no interest, like steam rising or vapor. I keep meeting people whose pain has gone untreated, or whose loved ones have had their pain untreated, which is to say unrecognized, unaccepted, unfelt."[96] Given the extent and gravity of this problem, it might be more rewarding to look directly to ways of getting doctors to treat pain more aggressively than to try to do so indirectly by increasing patient choice.

Another example of what I have in mind is the progress that has been made and still needs to be made in encouraging physicians and patients to use medical screening. It is commonly thought that American doctors screen too little. Recent years have seen efforts to persuade them to use particular screens more widely, but much remains to be done. For instance, Pap smears are widely considered a useful way of detecting cervical cancer early. It is now more ordinary than before for doctors to offer them to their patients, but doctors still seem to do so less routinely than is desirable.[97] Such screening is a particularly desirable arena in which to follow the consumer-welfare model, since the problem is not patients making the wrong choices, but doctors offering no choices.

As my last example suggests, a number of the successes of the kind of program I am proposing come from the area of women's health. There lay and professional criticism has helped lead to reevaluations of a number of medical practices and to changes in the incidence of some of them. This process has, for example, apparently reduced the frequency with which caesarian sections, radical mastectomies, and hysterectomies are performed and increased the frequency of some kinds of screening.

We are already seeing progress toward the kind of guidelines the consumer-welfare model calls for in just the area SUPPORT treats—end-of-life decisions. For example, through processes like the social discussion of cases from *Quinlan* and *Cruzan* we seem to be moving toward a cultural consensus that patients in persistent vegetative states should not be kept alive. And under the rubric "quality counts more than quantity," we—the public, patients, and doctors—are moving toward a reluctance to treat dying patients in the aggressive way SUPPORT implicitly criticizes.

Indeed, much consumer-welfare reform has already been conducted in consumer-choice guise. In recent decades, the dominance of the autonomy paradigm has led reformers of many kinds to put their case in terms of patient choice. This partly reflects a whole-hearted belief in that goal. Nevertheless, I doubt the principle of autonomy is always the strongest motive. Rather, reforms are often driven by substantive views about how patient choices should be resolved. For example, *Cruzan* is only nominally about patient choice; its abiding lesson is about the undesirability of keeping people in a persistent vegetative state alive. Criticism of the overuse of CPR is not so much about involving patients in writing DNR orders as about sparing them the cruelty of futile attempts to keep them going for a few more weary hours. The criticism of doctors' haste to do hysterectomies and reluctance to do Pap smears is at least as much directed at the perils of both attitudes as at women's autonomy.[98]

In sum, guidelines show promise in a number of kinds of areas. They are an attractive vehicle for consumer-welfare programs for several reasons. First, they can help doctors make better decisions: They give specialties an occasion to ask how a disease is presently handled, to expose the assumptions behind current treatments, to explore alternatives systematically, and to establish measures of quality. They help doctors monitor and evaluate the flood of studies in which journals are awash and to draw inferences about treatment from them. They should thus help protect patients against the tendency of busy people to fall behind the most recent research and the tendency of most of us to prefer the familiar and comfortable to the novel and discomfiting. They should also protect patients by directing doctors toward kinds of care it has not been advantageous for them to offer—care which is less interesting intellectually or less rewarding economically. Furthermore, the process of writing guidelines permits bioethicists and patients as a group to participate in formulating policies and to inject into them the voice of the patient. Finally, guidelines provide a standard against which performance can be judged.

Guidelines have a second attraction as part of a program of consumer protection: Although they have so far been directed at doctors, they may also help patients who want to make medical decisions. When numbers of people regularly make challenging decisions, social patterns and institutions commonly emerge that help them deliberate by establishing customary answers. Alan Wolfe thus writes, "When people make decisions, they tend to look not to a mathematical formula to determine what is to their best advantage, but to what others do, to what they have traditionally done, or to what they think others think they ought to do."[99] Social institutions embody the experiences and preferences of those "others," and "by the very fact of their existence control human conduct by setting up predefined patterns of conduct, which channel it in one direction as against the many other directions that would theoretically be possible."[100] As Bernice Pescosolido observes,

> [P]eople do not have to solve each problem anew or even understand the logic of old solutions; much human behavior is habitual, predictable, expected, taken-for-granted, and recurrent. . . . Cultural routines, which form the basis of much day-to-day action, are largely acquired through association, "produced" through interaction, and dependent to a large extent on affective reactions . . . . Affect underlies "acquired instinct" allowing people to sense what they should do without necessarily knowing why . . . , to tap an "embodied history" . . . where much of the "cultural heritage of reasoned action" is stored . . . , and to continually build for themselves a tacit dictionary, a font of experience and information, which makes the unfamiliar familiar.[101]

There are probably already social patterns patients seek to and do rely on in facing medical decisions and resolving bioethical dilemmas. Such patterns help people confronting recurrent but difficult questions by memorializing solutions to problems, solutions which have become socially so deeply ingrained that they seem natural and comfortable.

Part of what this means is that patients benefit from knowing what the consensus of expert opinion is, what patients' common experience is, how most of them made a particular decision, and how satisfied most of them have been. For example, a patient considering a kidney transplant might rather learn whether the average nephrologist would decide to have a transplant instead of continuing with dialysis and to learn whether the average patient chooses a transplant and is glad afterward than to hear that in X% of transplants a new kidney lasts Y years with Z% complications.

Another virtue of guidelines as an embodiment of social experience is that patients making decisions need a default position, a choice to fall back on if they cannot decide. Furthermore, people deciding on patients' behalf may find a default position useful in two circumstances. Surrogates trying to determine what a now-incompetent patient would have done and families and doctors trying to interpret an ambiguous advance directive may be helped by knowing what most patients would do. (Analogously, courts interpreting an ambiguous will commonly ask what similarly situated testators ordinarily do.)

This defense of guidelines offends strict autonomist principles, which require doctors to be neutral in presenting patients with alternatives. This neutrality is supposed to reduce pressure on patients to make any particular decision and to increase pressure on them to make their own decisions—to be autonomous. Guidelines have no such effect. Rather, they deliberately channel patients in one direction rather than another. But this hardly leaves patients helpless. Lurking within autonomism is an insufficiently noticed tension. Autonomists want to confide decisions to the people affected by them. Autonomists therefore must believe those people will make wise decisions. But autonomists are so delicately sensitive to the ways decisions might be influenced and thus distorted that one wonders how much faith they actually have in people's judgment. Influence may in fact not be undesirable. But even if it is, autonomists underestimate people's ability to resist it.

I would even argue that guidelines improve decisions, not just by stating the best current substantive answer to a medical question, but by helping patients make better decisions procedurally. Many people find that firmly stated advice, far from corrupting their thinking, clarifies their preferences. Max Lerner, for example, "had to learn how to resolve the often conflicting advice from my array of doctors and consultants." He commented, "'If I want to hear someone's opinion,' said Goethe, 'it must be expressed positively; I have ambiguity enough in myself.' I was in the realm of conflicting judgments and values. I needed the input to resolve my own ambivalence and end in decisive outcomes."[102] For many people it is being confronted with a mass of unordered choices that muddles thinking and even discourages thought. Guidelines provide a starting place for deliberation. They offer a position to criticize. As Walter Lippmann wrote, conventions— embodied experience—

> are as necessary to a society which recognizes no authority as to one which does. For the inexperienced must be offered some kind of hypothesis when they are confronted with the necessity of making choices: they cannot be so utterly open-minded that they stand inert until something collides with them. In the modern world, therefore, the function of conventions is to declare the meaning of experience. A good convention is one which will most probably show the inexperienced the way to happy experience.[103]

Guidelines may improve the quality of medical decisions in a third way—by helping doctors and patients comprehend each other. Guidelines, that is, coordinate social understandings. As Martin Krygier writes, "There are many social situations where our decisions are strategically interdependent [with the decisions of other people] . . . . [I]n such situations, *norms* will be generated which provide 'some *anchorage;* some preeminently conspicuous indication as to what action is likely to be taken by (most of) the others.'"[104] Social institutions serve people's need to understand and predict what other people will think and do so that they can readily and safely deal and cooperate with each other. Patients, then, will be aided in making decisions if they understand the assumptions of their doctors, and vice versa. Guidelines help create, disseminate, and promote common and thus predictable assumptions.

Let me illustrate this last point with a problem in structuring medical decisions. You are a nephrologist. Your patient faces accelerating kidney failure and will soon die without dialysis or a transplant. The patient is competent. You must describe the patient's prognosis and choices. Do you include "no treatment"—i.e., death—among those choices? If so, how do you describe it? As obviously not in the cards? As no more or less desirable than the others? As a choice patients not infrequently make that should be taken seriously and that can offer a "good death"? What if the patient seems likely to do well under treatment but immediately refuses it? Should you simply acquiesce, or press the patient to reconsider? If the patient perseveres in refusal, should you recruit the family to dissuade the patient? Which of these courses most respects the patient's autonomy? Which promotes the best decision? Which will the patient prefer? Which will the patient understand?

This case and these questions raise, I think, the question of whether doctors should simply "provide the patient with facts about the diagnosis and about the prognoses without treatment and with alternative treatments,"[105] of whether doctors can and should play so neutral a part. I suspect that in the circumstances I have posited (approaching kidney failure but no other medical problems) most patients would greet the "no treatment" alternative—death—with alarm. Most patients will rely on the conventional assumption that a doctor's first commitment is to the patient's life. Most patients will know that people in the situation I have described overwhelmingly choose to live and that they can live for some years on dialysis or with a transplant. These patients will wonder why, at this early stage, their doctor thinks they should consider dying. They will shudder at the grim news their doctor must be concealing.

The problem here is that doctor and patient have different assumptions. The doctor wants to present all the alternatives neutrally. The patient thinks the doctor values life too highly to lightly propose surrendering it. The misunderstandings caused by the disruption of such social assumptions are illustrated by one study that observed that "[p]hysicians often seemed too ready to concede patients' 'right to refuse' rather than to recognize the clinical problems that lay at the bottom of the refusal (*e.g.*, poor or inconsistent communication) and to take steps to remedy them. The disinclination of physicians to encourage patients over time to accept the treatment in question often left patients confused as to the validity of the original recommendation and, by implication, the competence of their physician."[106]

My point here is not so much to specify what role a doctor in this case ought to assume. Rather, it is to explain the necessity of constructing and sustaining social institutions that ease decisions and help doctors and patients understand how decisions are to be made. Nevertheless, I am inclined to think that the conventional assumption about the doctor's role that patients bring to these decisions probably should be retained. For one thing, such deeply rooted social beliefs are hard to extirpate. For another, they helpfully simplify the doctor's role. As Thomas Schelling writes, "It must be hard enough to be a good physician without being lawyer, clergyman, ombudsman, referee, and family counsellor or family arbiter, and it may help both patient and physician and their relation to each other to have the physician unambiguously devoted to the patient's life and comfort."[107]

Guidelines, I have argued, may improve medical decisions by offering doctors expert guidance, by providing a starting place for patients to think about their choices, and by providing a background of common understandings for both doctor and patient. Guidelines have yet another virtue: They offer a vehicle for the expression of broader social interests. Where medical decisions are made solely by a patient, or by a doctor, or even by the two together, such interests do not readily enter the calculus. Yet the social customs and practices surrounding medical decisions affect us all. We all have an interest in shaping those practices to serve broad social goals.[108] We all have, for example, an interest in eliminating unnecessary medical costs because medical insurance spreads them throughout the population. Guidelines are only one step toward solving this problem, but they can remind doctors and patients of the social consequences of their choices and can mold the assumptions that guide them.

We all have another interest in the customs and practices surrounding medical decisions. Any decision must be made against the background of assumptions that have substantive connotations. Even complete neutrality—were such a thing possible—would seem to suggest that all possible choices are legitimate. These background assumptions help shape the process and substance of medical decisions. Because we will all be patients, we all may want to shape those shaping influences before they catch us unaware.

Let me provide one brief example of some of what I mean. The brunt of much contemporary reform activity has been to elevate the "right to die" to the status of an accepted social institution.[109] As several people have recently noted, such a reform does more than increase patients' choices. It also creates a social environment instinct with social pressures. Schelling, for instance, comments,

> The right to depart this world at least raises the question whether the decent thing wouldn't be to discontinue being a burden, an annoyance, an expense, and a source of anxiety to the people in whose care a dying person finds himself. My disability is

a burden we share as long as no alternative is available; it is a burden of which I can relieve you if the option of dying is known to be available.[110]

Robert Burt even suggests that too single-minded an emphasis on the doctor as the servant of the patient's autonomy can corrupt the doctor and disserve the gravely ill patient:

> [W]hen the patient requests death from a doctor schooled in this new regime, the danger is that the doctor will comply with great rigor and haste, and even moralistic self-righteousness. He will do so in order to keep intact the rigidly separated roles prescribed for each, in order to reassure himself that he is not the patient, to reassure himself that he does not feel the terror and pain the patient feels, to reassure himself that he will not die because it is only the patient who will die.[111]

In short, all of us have an interest in controlling the pressures we may feel in making life-or-death decisions—pressures from family, friends, and doctors. Guidelines provide one of the few means of doing so.

Bioethicists may ask whether what I am proposing is "bioethical" work. Insofar as guidelines have ethical implications, the answer is yes. And since few medical issues do not have ethical aspects—questions of rationing, of how human goods like life and health should be weighed against one another—the answer will often be yes. Nevertheless, guidelines will often raise primarily technical issues bioethicists will have little to say about. Pain control, for example, presents some ethical questions, like the relative value of freedom from pain and clear-headed consciousness. But the core problems of pain control are technical: How do you do it? What drugs will work? What alternatives to drugs are worth exploring? In any event, however, the principal question should not be "what should bioethics do next?" but rather "where should reform energies next be directed?"

I have been advocating movement toward a consumer-welfare model of medical reform, a model that looks to the substance of medical decisions and not just to how decisions are reached. But what is truth? said jesting Pilate. How may we know a good choice when we see it? Faced with a hopeless prognosis and a pain-filled prospect, one person will soldier on to the bitter end, another will hasten to it. Faced with breast cancer, one woman will prefer a mastectomy, another a lumpectomy. Faced with kidney disease, one patient will opt for dialysis, another for a transplant.

The point can be made more emphatically. I have insisted on the variety of patients' preferences. So how can I favor any approach that does not enhance sensitivity to that variety? I do believe patients' preferences vary mercilessly. I do want doctors and nurses, hospitals and HMOs to be alert to and accommodate those differences. But as I said earlier, there are limits to the precision with which this can be done. Furthermore, social policy cannot be established and implemented one person at a time. It is made by locating areas of commonality and implemented by finding broadly useful changes that respect dissenters as fully as possible.

Three factors make it plausible to use guidelines to look for ways of accommodating the need for generality with the need to honor individual differences. First, I am not proposing that we coerce or deceive patients into what we think is good for them. Rather, I want to develop social consensus—where that is possible, as much as it is possible—on recurring medical and bioethical questions. Crucially, these would not be positions patients had to accept. They would instead be well-thought-out answers to standard medical and bioethical problems. Any patient could reject those answers, but they would be there for patients and doctors to consult, and they would be the default solution where patients would not or could not act. Guidelines might direct people toward one answer and make it seductively comfortable, but they would not compel it. Guidelines thus represent a compromise between the dangers of coercion and the sense of disorientation and abandonment people may feel when venturing into a foreign and disorganized set of issues.

Second, while patients' preferences vary, and while the variation is sometimes great, there are also many areas where it is small. While at the borders there can be considerable disagreement about what "good health" means, there are also wide areas of agreement about its core content. Even in the United States, and even today, powerful elements of cultural commonality continue to shape views about health, as about other basic subjects. In addition, many medical decisions do not involve the kinds of moral, social, and psychological issues which deeply divide people. For example, few patients wish to suffer pain. True, susceptibility to pain differs. True, patients may disagree about the trade-off between reducing pain and maintaining alertness. But most of the time for most patients, reducing pain is an uncontroversial good.

Third, guidelines of the kind I propose might themselves make patients' preferences on some issues less variable. As I argued in Chapter 3, people often have no preferences about their medical care before they become ill, and what preferences they have are often inchoate, ill-formed, and insubstantial. Instead of pre-existing illness, patients' preferences develop as they learn what it is like to be sick, as they interact with family, friends, and doctors, and as they see new problems with new eyes. Further, the preferences they develop arise from and are molded by prevailing cultural attitudes. The effort I am proposing may influence the cultural attitudes that in turn shape patients' attitudes, so that the norms that develop will seem agreeable to many patients.

The real question, it seems to me, is not whether norms will shape medical decisions. Shape them they will. The question is what their nature will be. There are effectively guiding norms now, as SUPPORT implies. Such norms can hardly be prevented from developing and from affecting the way we see the world. I find it hard to imagine many recurring decisions of importance where people are neutrally presented with an objective range of choices and make decisions free of social practices and pressures. The question is not whether norms should structure medical decisions, but how those norms should be criticized and improved. Some of the informal norms we now have may be as satisfactory as contemporary knowledge can make them. But many of them have not been systematically thought out or implemented. Often they simply reflect the individual practices of physicians. The process I envision would take advantage of the contemporary trend to develop protocols for managing recurring problems that reflect the best current thought, that expose medical assumptions and reasoning to professional and public criticism.

It is desirable to structure medical care so patients are as involved as they want to be. That is what the consumer-choice model does and is right to do. But we need to ask where to put reformist energy, and that model may have done much of what it can for us. It may thus be time to experiment with a consumer-welfare model. Writing guidelines that improve the quality of care patients receive and that give them guidance in making medical decisions is one way to start. But SUPPORT suggests a cautionary note. It is harder to change human behavior and norms than we think. "And enterprises of great pith and moment with this regard their currents turn awry and lose the name of action."

The Consumer-Welfare Model: Kindness

In the preceding section I argued that guidelines offer a means of moving from a consumer-choice toward a consumer-welfare model in securing for patients something they uncontroversially want—competence. In this section I will propose that a similar device offers hope for progress toward another central patient desire—kindness. To be sure, there is less urgency about using the consumer-welfare model to secure kindness than to secure competence. Unkindness wounds; incompetence kills. Furthermore, consumer choice should work better when the goal is kindness than when it is competence, since patients can better evaluate the former than the latter. Even the bureaucratization of medicine—which in so many ways fosters the impersonality many patients dislike—can promote something like kindness if medical organizations perceive they cannot attract patients without it.

Nevertheless, many patients passionately resent the way their doctors (and nurses, and orderlies) treat them, and being treated better matters to them. One small measure of this lies in what I noticed while making excerpts from patients' memoirs. I started out to learn how patients make medical decisions. I increasingly asked why patients resist making them. But in the end my largest category of notes was about how patients wanted doctors to treat them, and within this category the most common were those bespeaking patients' desire for something of the personal in their relationship with doctors.

Let me put the point a little differently. I said several times that what matters most to many patients is not the grand but the quotidian, not maximizing autonomy but living life day to day. The proposals in this section continue in that vein, for they suggest modest changes in doctors' behavior that can make major differences in patients' lives. As one doctor found, becoming a patient

> made me more aware of some aspects of medical care that, although seemingly trivial from the physician's perspective, are terribly important from the patient's perspective. It is what we would call "the little things," like being left waiting indefinitely in the X-ray room . . . . The abuses and mistreatments toward patients that troubled me as a physician now infuriate me as a patient.[112]

The problem, then, is that patients feel their care is too impersonal. The consumer-welfare model calls for giving patients what they want—kinder care. If this means assuring patients that doctors and nurses are genuinely motivated by deeply felt concern, that they truly empathize and sympathize with their patients, and that they will manifest those feelings at every turn, the effort is hopeless. Insight and concern are fragile plants, and they wither easily when they must be mustered routinely for every person, however boorish and belligerent, who comes along.[113] And many patients merit more sympathy than should be demanded from any stranger. Furthermore, one can rarely transform doctors' characters. People are much what they will be by the time they enter medical school, training cannot induce lifelong kindness, and little about the practice of a profession—particularly about the practice of medicine—transmutes technicians into great souls.

Happily, few patients expect doctors to be saints. We all treasure our encounters with warm, thoughtful, and kind people, but we know them to be rare. So what ought we expect from doctors? At least, not to be treated badly. (First, do no harm.) This may seem too banal to be worth saying, but the stories I recounted earlier are about more than indifference—they are about callousness and even brutality. Beyond not being treated badly, we should expect to be treated considerately. That consideration need not spring from the depths of doctors' souls. Elemental good treatment may not demonstrate deep human sympathy, but it evinces a basic level of concern and respect.

The problem is to devise ways of inducing ordinary people to behave well; in this case, to treat their patients decently. One might imagine many approaches to this problem.[114] Let me discuss one. Inveigling people to behave well habitually, even against their inclinations, is a problem societies have pondered throughout history, for it is the problem of manners. Manners are not principally about making bad people good (although that may be their by-product). They are about instilling the habit of acting in ways that are at least inoffensive and at best solicitous, generous, and gratifying: "Assume a virtue, if you have it not. / That monster, custom, who all sense doth eat, / Of habits devil, is angel yet in this." No one should expect all doctors actually to like all their patients, genuinely to share all their troubles, and truly to consider all their feelings. But one can expect them to act so they seem to entertain those feelings. The goal is civility, not authenticity.

What does civility mean between doctors and patients? I will propose a series of rules which, if followed, would go far toward making patients feel doctors cared about them in some personal way. These rules are intended to be easy to follow; as much as possible they describe concrete things doctors can do with little calculation or effort. They are drawn from my reading of patients' memoirs and will be illustrated with examples—good and bad—from them. They are arranged roughly in the order they might arise on a first meeting between doctor and patient.

Rule 1. Do not keep people waiting. One of the things patients bemoan most frequently and fiercely is the interminable waiting they are repeatedly forced to endure:

> We sat and waited and already we understood perfectly the ritual of waiting. The life of the patient is more than anything else spent in that way, time parceled out into little packages of sitting around, staring unobtrusively, making small talk, glancing at magazines. Waiting for doctors, nurses, bureaucrats, for tests and results and meals, waiting for companionship to arrive.[115]

A cancer patient explained his anger at a doctor who was almost two hours late for an appointment: "I felt that, if I was asked to be someplace at a specific time in order to get started on a program that was as important as this one was to me, the least I could expect was that the doctor be there on time too."[116] Patients are not just kept waiting for appointments, but also for test results. One doctor with tuberculosis found his "periods of greatest apprehension were the intervals after taking a gastric specimen for culture, and also after each roentgenogram. Parenthetically, let me plead for prompt reports from physicians to their patients. The periods between tests are tolerable; waiting for the reports is an agony."[117] Another patient regretted that many of her tests "took as long as a month to schedule, and then there was another wait for the results. When you lie awake crying all night, every night, with penetrating pain throughout your body, a month can seem like a year."[118]

Waiting cannot always be prevented—tests take time; emergencies cause delays. But so many patients are so often kept waiting so long it is hard to believe patients have been considered during scheduling. They certainly have been ignored in clinics which schedule all their afternoon appointments for the same hour. Or in the story of the mother of a patient awaiting a kidney transplant:

> Well, we just seemed to be waiting for that person with those bloody forms for hours and hours. [After the person came and they were signed] we just sat there. Nobody said, "Why don't you go home" or anything. I think we sat there until three o'clock in the afternoon. Somebody kind of just shut us off and let us go. Finally I just said, "I don't know why we don't go home, do you?" and she [the patient's wife] said, "I don't think they'll even miss us."[119]

That these incidents are often unnecessary is suggested by the happy reports of patients who have visited clinics that try to schedule patients so they need not practice "the infinite patience of the ill, whose lot it is to wait in the antechambers of laboratories and doctors."[120]

Making people wait unnecessarily is rude because it causes them to waste time, reduces them to miseries of boredom, and lays on the lash of uncertainty. What is more, "monopolizing others' time by making them wait reflects and reinforces power differences."[121] It makes obnoxiously clear who waits on whom and whose time is valuable. Therefore waiting should be minimized whenever possible, and when it cannot be, the reasons should be explained and apologies offered. Even airline pilots sometimes manage to do this. Its importance to patients is indicated by the story of a woman who had been kept waiting. "I had gotten more and more upset and angry, and strangely, I felt I would cry. When I'd finally gotten in, I announced that we had to discuss how long I had waited before we could talk about anything else. Dr. Kuneck wasn't defensive and was appropriately contrite. He said he'd feel exactly as I did, which defused me, though I still wanted to cry."[122]

Rule 2. Respect privacy. This particularly means not barging in on people who are not ready to receive you. One patient commented appreciatively,

> My best emblem has come to be what Obeid did on my last visit. Ever courteous, he ushered me into his office after the half-hour physical examination, during which he expressed pleasurable surprise at how calm and steady my heart was (one of its good days). After a while, he went out and, when he returned, knocked at the closed door. He *knocked on his own door,* paused, then came back in. He not only knew how his patient felt among the polished wood and the models of the heart. The prefect of the beam that sees through you, and interrogates you, had looked the other way for once, giving my ghost a chance to collect its wits.[123]

A doctor with ulcerative colitis had less happy experiences: "Social boundaries, professional boundaries, personal boundaries were repeatedly subject to thoughtless violation. Doctors walked into the bathroom to examine me on the commode. . . . I wanted a modicum of privacy, respect, and control."[124] But privacy means more than knocking on doors. It means, for example, letting patients be as fully dressed as possible. Patients' disgust at hospital gowns is notorious, but the problem runs even deeper. For example, Leon Kass reflects my own observations when he deplores "a group of (male and female) doctors and medical students stand[ing] around the bed discussing its occupant, oblivious to his profound discomfort at being left there stark naked and uncovered . . . ."[125]

Rule 3. Introduce yourself to strangers. Gillian Rose was in an ICU with cancer when she found that "[a]n unknown man, dressed in brightly coloured sports clothes (it was a Sunday), was bouncing up and down beside my cot. He enquired breezily, 'How are you, young lady?' Through the haze of pain, I replied with outrage, 'How dare you call me "young lady,"' and demanded that the intruder introduce himself."[126] The expression "you have me at a disadvantage" aptly captures the problem here. Rose did not know who the intruder was, so she did not know how to treat him. The intruder knew who she was, and had started a conversation in which he knew what was going on and she did not. Introductions are especially needed in hospitals where many different medical people with many different motives (but, to the patient's eyes, much the same dress and gear) approach the patient. Failures to introduce oneself are particularly troubling when they mislead patients, or at least keep them from raising awkward questions. Patients are often, for example, unable to tell which visitors to their bedside are caring for them and which are there for their own education or curiosity.[127] This problem reaches its nadir when medical students do not introduce themselves but leave the impression they are doctors or, worse, introduce themselves as "student doctors" or even "doctors."

Not only is failing to introduce oneself discomfiting; introductions can express solicitude and respect. A particularly generous demonstration of this comes from a lupus patient.

> "Joanna? This is Dr. Gifford. You're scheduled for a consultation with me this week and I just wanted to call you and introduce myself. I know you're probably scared. I hope very much that I can help you with your problems, and I'm looking forward to meeting you." Stunned, I did not answer him immediately. Finally I managed to thank him. When I hung up the phone I was still in shock. Did doctors really make phone calls like that? Were some of them truly that kind and sensitive?[128]

Rule 4. Grant other adults the same courtesy in titles you accord yourself. Gillian Rose's story about her intruder illustrates another common grievance—doctors who address patients by their first name while calling themselves by their last name and title. "Hello, Sally. I'm Dr. Smith." is often justified on the grounds that patients regard first names as friendlier than last names. If this is the principle, why is it "Dr. Smith"? A patient who was the daughter of a physician recognized how demeaning this practice is. She wrote that such doctors don no

> mask of egalitarianism, preferring a clear-cut one-up, one-down relationship. Addressing the patient—solely because he is a patient—by a first name serves this purpose perfectly: It defines, at the outset, the role that individual is expected to play, and vice versa. It thus recreates the relationship between an adult and a child—the one dominant, intelligent, and important, the other submissive, unintelligent, and unimportant.[129]

As one journalist remarked acidly, the doctor "expects your gratitude (and your fealty, suggested by his demand that he be referred to at all times by the honored title of 'Doctor')."[130]

Rule 5. Take the time you need to talk to the patient. Norman Cousins, a tribune of the patient, wrote, "Time is the one thing that patients need most from their doctors—time to be heard, time to have things explained, time to be reassured . . . . Yet the one thing that too many doctors find most difficult to command or manage is time."[131] Patients' memoirs speak with gratitude bordering on disbelief of doctors who took time for them:

> The doctors I consulted were incredible too. Each one made himself or herself available over a weekend and, in three cases, while they were out of town at the same convention. Dr. Figlin was more than willing to set up a conference call with Joni and me at 7 in the morning from a hotel where he was vacationing. "How long do we have?" I asked him. He answered, "As long as it takes."[132]

The vehemence with which patients resent being brushed off is captured by an anecdote from a study of heart-attack victims. His doctor asked Mr. Stein

> if he was having any pain. Mr Stein had had pain the night before and wanted to be sure to express it clearly so the doctor would realize it was a different kind of pain than he had been having previously. He paused to construct his answer but the doctor began to step away and Mr Stein thought he would leave before he could answer. So he lunged at the doctor and held him by the lapels of the jacket. Mr Stein then said to him if he wanted an answer he would have to wait a moment. Mr Stein reported that after this incident, his doctor seemed more patient and spent more time with him.[133]

As these comments suggest, patients want time with their doctors partly because they think it will lead to better care: Time is needed for doctors to collect adequate information from patients and to provide them adequate counsel in return. Time is also a matter of politeness. Someone who rushes a conversation implies that you are not much worth talking to. So patients want time and resent its denial. But time is what doctors often lack. The doctors I know work exceptionally hard, as hard as the lawyers I know. The bureaucratization of medicine can increase the demands on doctors' time, if only because it takes longer to make decisions in groups than individually and because bureaucracy multiplies paperwork. Furthermore, programs to reduce medical costs often attempt to use the time of highly paid people like doctors more efficiently by rushing them along from patient to patient. Nevertheless, physicians can at least recognize how much their time means to patients and do what we all do when we have too little time to talk to someone but regret it. For example, the way doctors approach patients affects patients' perceptions of physicians' attitudes. A surgeon turned patient commented,

> Bill is the kind of doctor you can't help liking. Even though he has a very busy practice, he never makes you feel as if he were in a hurry. When he comes into the examining room to see you he sits down, stretches out, and acts as if he had the entire afternoon to spend with you. It's an attitude you don't find in many doctors.[134]

In short, this rule asks more of doctors than the other rules because doctors' time is scarce and precious. But no one has more control than doctors over how they spend their time, and there are things doctors can do to lessen patients' distress about being ignored, hurried, and brushed off.

Rule 6. Listen, and seem to listen. This is another rule that speaks both to competence and to kindness. Doctors must gather much of their diagnostic information from talking with patients, which cannot be done well without listening closely. And few things suggest indifference like not listening to someone you are talking to. Both these concerns are reflected in the following observations:

> I found Dr. Z difficult to deal with. He seemed to question us at several places, as though he did not believe us. He seemed indifferent to our questions. Instead, he lectured us about CML and bone marrow transplant.
>
> If only Dr. Z had taken time to listen to us! Instead, he kept telling us we needed to make a decision about bone marrow transplant. We had already decided to attempt a bone marrow transplant. Our question was where![135]

This rule and Rule 5 are among the most difficult to apply because they require judgment. Doctors need to discover what is worrying patients and to take their histories, so patients need to be allowed to talk. But left to their own devices, many patients will roam and ramble. In short, doctors need to acquire information as politely as possible, and always with at least an appearance of attentiveness.

Rule 7. Say "please" and "thank you." Few rules are more elementary to good manners. And few rules are more easily followed and even made habitual. Saying "please" and "thank you" displays a desire to be polite, which itself implies a concern for the people one is dealing with. What is more, doctors who do so assure patients and remind themselves that the patient is not the doctor's vassal to command. Patients notice and value this consideration. One woman "liked the low-key way [her doctor] approached things: not, 'Now, we're going to do so-and-so,' but 'If you don't mind. . . .'"[136] Another woman said appreciatively that her husband's doctor "never complained about my calls to him at home and, in fact, with unfailing courtesy, never neglected to thank me for having phoned."[137]

Rule 8. Express sympathy when you deliver bad news. It is usually rude to ignore the suffering of someone you are talking with. That is why it is polite to offer sympathy, commiseration, and condolence. Even the cops on *NYPD Blue* routinely say "I'm sorry for your loss." But patients' memoirs recount time after time when doctors not only fail to accompany the grimmest news with any note of concern, but show the baldest indifference. I have already described several of these incidents, but a reminder may be helpful. A mild example comes from Arthur Frank, who was told he had "massive tumors. The physician added nothing to his abrupt statement. He would send a report to my family physician; that was it, not even a goodbye or good luck, just over and out."[138] Yet more horrible is the story of an Englishwoman:

I felt terrible; I was scared stiff and shaky and really embarrassed lying there on the examination couch with just this flimsy gown that didn't cover me right up. He came in with a couple of young doctors, and oh I was so ashamed, the way he examined me—I've got such big breasts you see. He just didn't seem to act as though I was there and kept talking to the others about the difficulty in knowing what to do with big breasts. I asked him what was wrong with me. He said 'You must realise it's cancer; we'll have you in next week sometime' and walked out. I've never felt so confused in my life. I was terrified—I'd got cancer, I didn't know what they were going to do for it, I was angry, embarrassed and didn't know what on earth to do.[139]

It is often said doctors should empathize with their patients.[140] True empathy seems to me too much to demand every time frightful news must be delivered; its emotional burden would be crushing. But some expression of regret and concern is required by common courtesy, and it is not much to ask.

Rule 9. Return your phone calls. Patients often find it infuriatingly difficult to reach their doctors. The following story is all too typical: "The surgeon had not called with the results of the bronchoscopy several days after he had promised to be in touch with us. Bill and I called the hospital repeatedly, but none of the people who had been involved in that strange operation ever seemed available to come to the telephone or inclined to return our calls."[141] Even doctors who become patients can have trouble getting their phone calls returned: "For the next two days I tried to call his office to speak with him. My calls were never answered."[142] The reasons doctors should return phone calls hardly need be stated: Patients may have important information to convey, and patients are entitled not to be ignored.

Rule 10. Think about the effect on your patients of what you do and say. The first nine rules generally can be followed almost mechanically. But guidelines of that sort cannot state all the duties politeness imposes. This tenth rule states the general principle from which the rest follow and from which other obligations may be inferred. If obeyed, it would, for example, go far toward abating patients' sense of doctors as aloof and arrogant. As one observer commented several decades ago of the way doctors treated parents of children with polio: "In general, the behavior of the parents in these encounters may be characterized as eager, deferential, and subordinate; that of hospital personnel, especially the doctors, as brusque, noncommittal, and superordinate, even at times—or so it appeared to parents—condescending or indifferent."[143] If vigorously and imaginatively followed, Rule 10 could lead doctors to the thoughtfulness patients cherish, like that of the doctor whose patient (herself a doctor) thought him exemplary because he "eased the pain of many transitions with his warnings" about what to expect next.[144] More modestly, it might help doctors avoid inadvertent cruelty. One patient, for example, tells of a friend whose doctor asked him, " 'What *was* your profession, Mr. Burke?' When his wife, Vee, objected with, 'What *is* his profession?', the doctor replied, 'Well, you *are* an optimist.' "[145]

At the least, Rule 10 should dampen doctors' tendency to absent themselves psychologically from seriously ill patients. Patients' accounts of this tendency are disturbingly common and similar. Reynolds Price: "My presiding oncologist saw me as seldom as he could manage. He plainly turned aside when I attempted casual conversation in the halls; and he seemed to know literally no word or look of mild encouragement or comradeship in the face of what, as I later learned, he thought was hurried death."[146] Arthur Frank: "I always assumed that if I became seriously ill, physicians, no matter how overworked, would somehow recognize what I was living through. I did not know what form this recognition would take, but I assumed it would happen. What I experienced was the opposite. The more critical my diagnosis became, the more reluctant physicians were to talk to me. I had trouble getting them to make eye contact; most came only to see my disease."[147] Even a physician: "Having made the diagnosis, the doctors seemed to avoid me as much as possible . . . ."[148] And yet another physician: "My surgeon's soul could not reach back. Frequently, when he came to see me, he would not look at me. His gaze would often avoid mine to wander toward the window or the television. I yearned for him to sit for a minute, hold my hand, give me some reassurance. He never did. . . . The sicker I became, the colder he became, and the more death loomed in our minds."[149]

Patients clearly and rightly feel doctors should heed minimum standards of courtesy, should acknowledge their patients' human distress, just like anyone else. As Reynolds Price said, "[S]urely a doctor should be expected to share— and to offer at all appropriate hours—the skills we expect of a teacher, a fireman, a priest, a cop, the neighborhood milkman or the dog-pound manager."[150] As a doctor-turned-patient said, "I wish that some of my doctors and nurses could have opened themselves up to the empathy in themselves that I have received from such widely diverse people as neighbors, grocers, flight attendants, and dog trainers."[151] In short, doctors "may not wish to become too involved or identified with patients, but there is no way of dropping out of the species . . . ."[152]

In this section, I have asked what the future of medical reform should be in a world where the autonomy paradigm has less and less that is fresh to offer and where medical care is more and more organized bureaucratically. That question forces us to balance the need for broadly applicable policies with the irreducible variety of patients. The answer I have explored—one of many possibilities— posits that patients can be helped toward some of what they want from medicine through what I have called the consumer-welfare model. This model asks for identifying subjects about which many patients agree and for instituting social norms that guide doctors and patients in their decisions. Finally, I have proposed several areas where guidelines for substantive medical decisions might be instituted, and I have identified ten rules that might improve the way patients are treated.

7

Conclusion

Grau, theurer Freund, ist alle Theorie
Und grün des Lebens goldner Baum.
Johann von Goethe
Faust

In this book, I have argued that the law and thought of bioethics rest too easily and too often upon a set of hyper-rationalistic assumptions about human nature. These assumptions allow bioethicists and lawyers to see patients as essentially similar, as responding to the same drives and as thinking and acting in the same ways. These patients are taken to want control not just of their health, but of their medical treatment, and to want to effectuate that control by assembling all the relevant information about their medical condition, assimilating those data, subjecting them to rational analysis, applying a carefully developed set of personal beliefs to them, and, finally, deciding what treatment is best for them.

Real people are stubbornly more complicated than this model supposes. Some people may behave as autonomists imagine, but an imposing number of them act quite differently. Their desire for information is more equivocal than the model assumes; their taste for rational analysis is less pronounced; their personal beliefs are not as well developed, relevant, or strong; and their desire for control is more partial, ambivalent, and complex. Especially, many people do not hunger to make their own medical decisions. I have argued that much empirical evidence supports this conclusion. I have also proposed that these people have substantial reasons for forgoing medical decisions, reasons which make it more plausible that they truly wish to forgo them.

This much seems to me reasonably clear. The harder question is what, if anything, to do about it. Now that the principle of autonomy has won so commanding an intellectual and moral victory, now that the law has installed an armory of devices to promote patients' autonomy, bioethicists and lawyers need to undertake the grubbier but rewarding work of asking what people actually want, how they actually behave, and what changes are actually possible.

But that is only a start. We also must work out how to respond to those desires, deeds, and possibilities. I have tried to demonstrate that this question, too, is complex, for we need to accommodate people who aggressively want to make their own medical decisions, people who think they do but really do not, people who think they do not but really do, and people who aggressively do not. We will ultimately have to accept that no solution can accomplish all we want it to. But I have tried to show that one part of the solution should be an effort to structure services to accommodate the many ways the sick respond to their illness and that not all the sick respond by wanting to make their own medical decisions.

I confess I have made this suggestion with some trepidation. That trepidation arises out of the knowledge that sides have been chosen in the bioethics wars, and that for the more passionate of the adversaries he that is not with me is against me; and he that gathereth not with me scattereth. The fiercer autonomists can too easily take my reflections on the reluctance of many patients to make their own medical decisions as a condemnation of autonomy as a legitimate goal of bioethical policy. This would be an egregious misreading of what I am saying. It is certainly true that I criticize overweening claims for autonomy and that I believe there is much we should cherish beyond autonomy. It is true that I see problems in the practice of autonomy that others have not remarked. It is true that I doubt that law can bring about a new Jerusalem in the lives of doctors and patients. But none of this seems to me a betrayal of the belief that patients are free men and women.

It would equally be a misreading for doctors to use what I am saying to justify paternalism. (Paternalists want friends; autonomists want enemies.) Perhaps all professions are not conspiracies against the laity. But they are all invitations to arrogance. It is hard to train yourself in a specialty for many years, to learn a powerful new way of thinking, to have clients come to you for help and advice, to compare your understanding to your clients', and to have your clients, your employees, and your colleagues defer to you without coming to believe that you are better than most of the world and that it would do well to accept your guidance. The medical profession may be particularly susceptible to this temptation. Doctors are trained and often live in surprisingly insular environments. Many of the doctors who populate that environment are oddly bitter people who feel unappreciated and even beleaguered by the world in general and by people— bioethicists and lawyers not least among them—they perceive as their attackers. These doctors may wish to read what I have written as a justification for returning to palmier days when doctors were respected and not questioned. I can see nothing in my ruminations on the relationship between doctors and patients that confirms such a reading.

In the end we all need to learn the lesson of modesty. Even while we have crusaded for patients' autonomy, that goal has gradually begun to slip away from us, as changes in the structure of medical care have distanced it from us. In the very course of seeking that goal, we may have impaired our ability to seek other goals we value, like the kind of personal relationship between doctor and patient so many patients seem so much to want. I have suggested we should begin to think less exclusively in terms of consumer choice and more in terms of consumer welfare. I believe there is good work to be done here and that informing our bioethical thinking with an understanding of how the world works will richly reward the effort. But I offer no vision of the millennium, for here as everywhere we face warring wants, clashing interests, and conflicting goals.

Notes

This book is written for a perilously varied audience, including lawyers, doctors, bioethicists, and sociologists. Each of their disciplines sports its own style of citation. I have chosen the lawyer's style, not just because I am a lawyer and use legal sources not well cited otherwise, but also because the lawyer's style I use— that of the *University of Chicago Manual of Legal Citation*—seems to me superior (more informative and easier to use) to its legal and nonlegal competitors. In any lawyer's style, the volume number of a journal precedes the name of the journal, the page number on which the article begins follows the name of the journal, the number of the page on which a quotation appears follows the number of the initial page, and the date concludes the series. Thus 92 Annals of Internal Medicine 832, 834 (1980) is a citation to a quotation that appears on page 834 of an article that starts on page 832 in volume 92 of the *Annals of Internal Medicine* and that was published in 1980. For brevity's sake, I have abbreviated the names of three journals. I refer to the Hastings Center Report as "HCR," the Journal of the American Medical Association as "JAMA," and the New England Journal of Medicine as "NEJM."

Acknowledgments

1. In addition, some of the material in the Introduction and Chapter 2 appeared in an early form in Carl E. Schneider, *Bioethics with a Human Face,* 69 Indiana L J 1075 (1994).

Introduction

1. The reader may have noticed my use of "patients." That word defines sick people in relation to their doctors. I dislike this, for I am broadly interested in how people who are sick handle illness. However, I use "patients" to avoid the clumsiness of the alternatives. I should also say that by patients I mean only physically ill adults. I have excluded children and the mentally ill from my research because they raise questions of competence which exceed this book's scope.

2. Carl E. Schneider, *Lawyers and Children: Wisdom and Legitimacy in Family Policy,* 84 Michigan L Rev 919, 932–37 (1986).

3. Idem at 932.

4. For a criticism of social science as hyper-rationalist, see Amitai Etzioni, *The Moral Dimension: Toward a New Economics* (Free Press, 1988).

5. For criticism of legal hyper-rationality, see Carl E. Schneider, *State-Interest Analysis in Fourteenth Amendment "Privacy" Law: An Essay on the Constitutionalization of Social Issues,* 51 Law & Contemporary Problems 79 (1988); Carl E. Schneider, *State-Interest Analysis and the Channeling Function in Family Law,* in Stephen E. Gottlieb, ed, *Public Values in Constitutional Law* 97 (U Michigan Press, 1993).

6. Howard Brody, *Stories of Sickness* 144 (Yale U Press, 1987).

7. 42 USC §§ 1395cc (f) 1396a (w).

8. Daniel F. Chambliss, *Beyond Caring: Hospitals, Nurses, and the Social Organization of Ethics* 6 (U Chicago Press, 1996).

9. Irving L. Janis, *The Patient as Decision Maker,* in W. Doyle Gentry, ed, *Handbook of Behavioral Medicine* 327 (Guilford, 1984).

10. For a survey of those criticisms, see Ronald C. Kessler, et al, *Social Psychology and Health,* in Karen Cook, Gary Fine, & James S. House, eds, *Sociological Perspectives on Social Psychology* (Allyn & Bacon, 1994). For explorations of human rationality in making decisions, see Daniel Kahneman, Paul Slovic, & Amos Tversky, *Judgment Under Uncertainty: Heuristics and Biases* (Cambridge U Press, 1982). For an examination of the emotional context of decisions, with special attention to medical patients, see Irving L. Janis & Leon Mann, *Decision Making: A Psychological Analysis of Conflict, Choice, and Commitment* 16 (Free Press, 1977). On the social context of one kind of medical decision, see Bernice A. Pescosolido, *Beyond Rational Choice: The Social Dynamics of How People Seek Help,* 97 American J Sociology 1096, 1106–7 (1992).

11. For a particularly good treatment of the tendency of modern bioethics to abstract problems from their human and social reality and to think hyper-rationalistically about them, see Leon R. Kass, *Practicing Ethics: Where's the Action?,* 20 HCR 5 (Jan/Feb 1990).

12. AMA Judicial Council, *Ethical Guidelines for Organ Transplantation,* 205 JAMA 89 (1968).

13. Arthur L. Caplan, *Informed Consent and Provider/Patient Relationships in Rehabilitation Medicine,* in *If I Were a Rich Man Could I Buy a Pancreas? and Other Essays on the Ethics of Health Care* 245 (Indiana U Press, 1992).

14. Ezekiel J. Emanuel & Linda L. Emanuel, *Four Models of the Physician–Patient Relationship,* 267 JAMA 2221, 2225 (1992).

15. Renée R. Anspach, *Deciding Who Lives: Fateful Choices in the Intensive-Care Nursery* 38–39 (U California Press, 1993).

16. 28 American Sociological Rev 55 (1963).

17. Idem at 61.

18. Idem.

19. *Order Without Law: How Neighbors Settle Disputes* (Harvard U Press, 1991).

20. On this literature, see Robert H. Mnookin, et al, *In the Interest of Children: Advocacy, Law Reform, and Public Policy* (W.H. Freeman, 1985); Carl E. Schneider, *Lawyers and Children: Wisdom and Legitimacy in Family Policy,* 84 Michigan L Rev 919 (1986); Richard L. Hasen, *Efficiency Under Information Asymmetry: The Effect of Framing on Legal Rules,* 38 UCLA L Rev 391 (1990); Carl E. Schneider, *Social Structure and Social Control: On* The Moral Order of a Suburb, 25 Law & Society Rev 875 (1990); Carl E.

Schneider, *Rethinking Alimony: Marital Decisions and Moral Discourse*, BYU L Rev 197, 203–9 (1991); Lynn A. Baker & Robert Emery, *When Every Relationship Is Above Average: Perceptions and Expectations of Divorce at the Time of Marriage,* 17 Law & Behavior 439 (1993).

21. Carl E. Schneider, *Bioethics in the Language of the Law,* 24 HCR 16 (Jul/Aug 1994). I do not mean law never matters. There are, for example, economic studies "that find that individuals—specifically, automobile drivers—do respond to legal rules. . . . [L]iability insurance premiums affect the decision to drive, . . . the number of automobile deaths has risen as a result of the no-fault movement . . . [, and] safety-belt requirements increase the number of pedestrian deaths because people who feel safer drive faster." Richard A. Posner, *Can Lawyers Solve the Problems of the Tort System?,* 73 California L Rev 747, 749–50 (1985). As this suggests, the difference the law makes is not always the difference it intends.

22. Linda L. Emanuel, *Structured Deliberation to Improve Decisionmaking for the Seriously Ill,* 25 HCR, Special Supp S14 (Nov/Dec 1995).

23. Joel M. Zinberg, *Decisions for the Dying: An Empirical Study of Physicians' Responses to Advance Directives,* 13 Vermont L Rev 445, 472 (1989). Use of advance directives may have increased since this study. However, their impact is checked by the fact that "the most important determinants of treatment decisions for incompetent patients are the physician–family consensus as to the proposed treatment and the physician's perception of potential civil or criminal liability." Idem at 476.

24. Arthur L. Caplan, *Can Autonomy be Saved?,* in *If I Were a Rich Man Could I Buy a Pancreas? and Other Essays on the Ethics of Health Care* 261 (Indiana U Press, 1992).

25. Idem.

26. Russell S. Kramer, et al, *Effect of New York State's Do-Not-Resuscitate Legislation on In-Hospital Cardiopulmonary Resuscitation Practice,* 88 American J Medicine 108, 109–10 (1990).

27. Robert Zussman, *Reflections on Fieldwork in a Medical Setting: Medicine, Medical Ethics, and the Sociological Voice,* paper presented at the Conference on the Sociology of Medical Ethics, Ann Arbor, Michigan, Sept 15–17, 1995.

28. Arthur L. Caplan, *Can Autonomy be Saved?,* in *If I Were a Rich Man Could I Buy a Pancreas? and Other Essays on the Ethics of Health Care* 262–63 (Indiana U Press, 1992).

29. Idem at 265.

30. Barry R. Furrow, et al, *Health Law: Cases, Materials and Problems* 187 (West, 2d ed, 1991).

31. Paul S. Appelbaum, Charles W. Lidz, & Alan Meisel, *Informed Consent: Legal Theory and Clinical Practice* 46 (Oxford U Press, 1987).

32. Jay Katz, *Informed Consent—A Fairy Tale,* 39 U Pittsburgh L Rev 137, 139 (1977).

33. Appelbaum, et al, *Informed Consent* at 202 (cited in note 31).

34. Paul C. Weiler, *Medical Malpractice On Trial* 13 (Harvard U Press, 1991).

35. Howard Brody, *Stories of Sickness* x (Yale U Press, 1987). On stories in medicine, see Kathryn Hunter, *Doctors' Stories: The Narrative Structure of Medical Knowledge* (Princeton U Press, 1991).

36. For an extended description of the distance between bioethics and the social sciences, see Renée C. Fox, *The Evolution of American Bioethics: A Sociological Perspective,* in George Weisz, ed, *Social Science Perspectives on Medical Ethics* 185 (U Pennsylvania Press, 1990).

37. See Charles E. Lindblom & David K. Cohen, *Usable Knowledge: Social Science and Social Problem Solving* (Yale U Press, 1979).

38. Pearl Katz, *How Surgeons Make Decisions*, in Robert A. Hahn & Atwood D. Gaines, eds, *Physicians of Western Medicine* 157 (Reidel, 1985).

39. For an example of such a result, see Debra L. Roter & Judith A. Hall, *Studies of Doctor–Patient Interaction*, 10 Annual Rev of Public Health 163 (1989). See Alan Meisel & Loren H. Roth, *Toward an Informed Discussion of Informed Consent: A Review and Critique of the Empirical Studies*, 25 Arizona L Rev 265 (1983), for a thorough demonstration of the problems with empirical research in many kinds of bioethical problems.

40. Recent monographic examples include, but are not limited to, Charles L. Bosk, *All God's Mistakes: Genetic Counseling in a Pediatric Hospital* (U Chicago Press, 1992); Robert Zussman, *Intensive Care: Medical Ethics and the Medical Profession* (U Chicago Press, 1992); Renée Anspach, *Deciding Who Lives: Fateful Choices in the Intensive Care Nursery* (U California Press, 1993). Anspach and Zussman provide instructive apologias for the usefulness of social science in bioethics; Bosk presents somewhat more guarded reflections on the same topic. Janis concludes that "a substantial number of studies can now be drawn upon to provide promising leads for explaining health-related behavior and for developing practical applications . . . ." Irving L. Janis, *The Patient as Decision Maker*, in W. Doyle Gentry, ed, *Handbook of Behavioral Medicine* 326, 343 (Guilford, 1984). Baruch Brody, *Quality of Scholarship in Bioethics*, 15 J Medicine & Philosophy 161 (1990), and Robert A. Pearlman, Steven H. Miles, & Robert M. Arnold, *Contributions of Empirical Research To Medical Ethics*, 14 Theoretical Medicine 197 (1993), show how empirical studies have promoted discussion of some specific ethical issues. For an informative discussion of the relative contributions of "epidemiological" surveys and sociological field work, see Robert Zussman, *Reflections on Fieldwork in a Medical Setting: Medicine, Medical Ethics, and the Sociological Voice,* paper presented at the Conference on the Sociology of Medical Ethics, Ann Arbor, Michigan, Sept 15–17, 1995. More broadly, see Renée C. Fox, *The Evolution of American Bioethics: A Sociological Perspective,* in George Weisz, ed, *Social Science Perspectives on Medical Ethics* 206 (U Pennsylvania Press, 1990).

41. An important exception is Renée Anspach, *Deciding Who Lives: Fateful Choices in the Intensive Care Nursery* (U California Press, 1993). But it deals with decisions about infants, not the adults with whom I am concerned. Another important exception is Robert Zussman, *Intensive Care: Medical Ethics and the Medical Profession* (U Chicago Press, 1992). However, many of the patients in Zussman's study were too ill to participate in the medical decisions made about them.

42. On the memoirs of patients as a window into the experience of illness, see Anne Hunsaker Hawkins, *Reconstructing Illness: Studies in Pathography* (Purdue U Press, 1993); Lucy Bregman & Sara Thiermann, *First Person Mortal: Personal Narratives of Illness, Dying and Grief* (Paragon, 1995); Arthur W. Frank, *The Wounded Storyteller: Body, Illness, and Ethics* (U Chicago Press, 1995); Faith McLellan, *From Book to Byte: Narratives of Physical Illness,* 8 Medical Humanities Rev 9 (1994). These memoirs have burgeoned into a small literary subgenre: Hawkins lists 153 of them, despite her efforts she did not find them all, and they are still emerging rapid-fire.

43. For example, Simone de Beauvoir, *A Very Easy Death* (Pantheon, 1965); Joseph Heller & Speed Vogel, *No Laughing Matter* (G.P. Putnam, 1986); Madeleine L' Engle, *Two-Part Invention: The Story of a Marriage* (Harper & Row, 1988); May Sarton, *After the Stroke: A Journal* (Norton, 1988); John Updike, *At War with My Skin,* in *Self-Consciousness: Memoirs* (Fawcett Crest, 1989); Christy Brown, *My Left Foot* (Minerva,

1990); Philip Roth, *Patrimony: A True Story* (Simon & Schuster, 1991); Anatole Broyard, *Intoxicated by My Illness: And Other Writings on Life and Death* (Fawcett Columbine, 1992); Donald Hall, *Life Work* (Beacon Press, 1993); Reynolds Price, *A Whole New Life* (Atheneum, 1994); Paul West, *A Stroke of Genius: Illness and Self-Discovery* (Viking, 1995); Wilfrid Sheed, *In Love with Daylight: A Memoir of Recovery* (Simon & Schuster, 1995); William Styron, *A Case of the Great Pox,* The New Yorker 62 (Sept 18, 1995); Kenzaburo Oe, *A Healing Family* (Kodansha, 1996).

44. Eric Hodgins, *Episode: Report on the Accident Inside My Skull* (Atheneum, 1964); Stewart Alsop, *Stay of Execution: A Sort of Memoir* (Lippincott, 1973); Michael Halberstam & Stephan Lesher, *A Coronary Event* (Popular Library, 1976); Norman Cousins, *Anatomy of an Illness as Perceived by the Patient: Reflections on Healing and Regeneration* (Bantam, 1979); Cornelius & Kathryn Morgan Ryan, *A Private Battle* (Simon & Schuster, 1979); Marvin Barrett, *Spare Days* (Morrow, 1988); Molly Haskell, *Love and Other Infectious Diseases: A Memoir* (Citadel, 1990); Barbara Creaturo, *Courage: The Testimony of a Cancer Patient* (Pantheon, 1991); Andrew H. Malcolm, *Someday* (Harper Perennial, 1991); Betty Rollin, *First You Cry* (HarperPaperback, 1993); Tim Brookes, *Catching My Breath: An Asthmatic Explores His Illness* (Times Books, 1994); Gayle Feldman, *You Don't Have to Be Your Mother* (Norton, 1994); Ellen Burstein MacFarlane with Patricia Burstein, *Legwork: An Inspiring Journey Through a Chronic Illness* (Charles Scribner, 1994); Jimmy Breslin, *I Want to Thank My Brain for Remembering Me: A Memoir* (Little, Brown, 1996); Michael Korda, *Man to Man: Surviving Prostate Cancer* (Random House, 1996); Jean-Dominique Bauby, *The Diving Bell and the Butterfly* (Knopf, 1997).

45. Ernest A. Hirsch, *Starting Over* (Christopher Publishing House, 1977); Robert V. Hine, *Second Sight* (U California Press, 1983); Gerda Lerner, *A Death of One's Own* (U Wisconsin Press, 1985); Esther Goshen-Gottstein, *Recalled to Life: The Story of a Coma* (Yale U Press, 1988); Ilza Veith, *Can You Hear the Clapping of One Hand? Learning to Live with a Stroke* (U California Press, 1988); John M. Hull, *Touching the Rock: An Experience of Blindness* (Vintage, 1990); Max Lerner, *Wrestling With the Angel: A Memoir of My Triumph Over Disease* (Touchstone, 1990); Robert F. Murphy, *The Body Silent* (Norton, 1990); Arthur W. Frank, *At the Will of the Body: Reflections on Illness* (Houghton Mifflin, 1991); Evelyn Shirk, *After the Stroke: Coping With America's Third Leading Cause of Death* (Prometheus, 1991); Max Apple, *Roommates: My Grandfather's Story* (Warner Books, 1994); William Martin, *My Prostate and Me: Dealing With Prostate Cancer* (Cadell & Davies, 1994); Gillian Rose, *Love's Work: A Reckoning With Life* (Schocken, 1995); Louise DeSalvo, *Breathless: An Asthma Journal* (Beacon Press, 1997).

46. Max Pinner & Benjamin F. Miller, *When Doctors Are Patients* (Norton, 1952); William A. Nolen, *Surgeon Under the Knife* (Dell, 1976); Anthony J. Sattilaro, *Recalled by Life* (Avon, 1982); Fitzhugh Mullan, *Vital Signs: A Young Doctor's Struggle With Cancer* (Farrar, Straus, Giroux, 1983); Oliver Sacks, *A Leg to Stand On* (HarperCollins, 1984); Harvey Mandell & Howard Spiro, eds, *When Doctors Get Sick* (Plenum Medical, 1987); Edward E. Rosenbaum, *The Doctor* (Ballantine Books, 1988); Siegfried J. Kra, *The Three-Legged Stallion and Other Tales From a Doctor's Notebook* (Fawcett Crest, 1989); Arnold R. Beisser, *Flying Without Wings: Personal Reflections on Being Disabled* (Doubleday, 1989); G. Edward Rozar & David B. Biebel, *Laughing in the Face of AIDS: A Surgeon's Personal Battle* (Baker, 1992); Richard Selzer, *Raising the Dead* (Whittle Books, 1993); Robert Pensack & Dwight Williams, *Raising Lazarus* (G.P. Putnam, 1994); Jody Heymann, *Equal Partners: A Physician's Call for a New Spirit of Medicine* (Little, Brown, 1995).

47. For example, Jill Ireland, *Life Wish* (Jove, 1987); Gilda Radner, *It's Always Something* (Avon, 1989); Evan Handler, *Time on Fire: My Comedy of Terrors* (Little, Brown, 1996); Ben Watt, *Patient: The True Story of a Rare Illness* (Grove Press, 1996); Barbara Barrie, *Second Act: Life After Colostomy and Other Adventures* (Scribner, 1997).

48. Sandi Cooper, for instance, was a special-education teacher who left that job to become the mother of four children and who lived in a "modest, middle-class home." *Parkinson's: A Personal Story of Acceptance* 13 (Branden, 1992). Several other housewives of apparently quite middle-class resources have described their experiences, including Mary Cooper Greene, *Living With a Broken String* (no publisher, 1987); Eileen Radziunas, *Lupus: My Search for a Diagnosis* (Hunter House, 1989); Pat Brack, *Moms Don't Get Sick* (Melius, 1990). Louie Nassaney, *I Am Not a Victim: One Man's Triumph Over Fear and Aids* (Hay House, 1990), tells of a young man of limited means and education. William F. Sayers, *Don't Die on My Shift* (Major Books, 1977), is the story of a man with polio whose circumstances were so desperate that his mother won an episode of *Queen for a Day*. Regina Woods was another polio patient with little money. She relates her story in *Tales From Inside the Iron Lung: And How I Got Out of It* (U Pennsylvania Press, 1994). Marjorie McVicker Sutcliffe, *Grandma Cherry's Spoon: A Story of Tuberculosis* (Geronima, 1991), is a memoir about a truly impoverished rural family.

49. I say "a few" instead of "one" because people acquire end-stage renal disease (ESRD) in several ways, often because of another disease. Many ESRD patients have diabetes, many have high blood pressure, many have had specifically nephrological illnesses, and some have suffered kidney failure for yet other reasons. In addition, ESRD may be treated either with dialysis or a transplant, so ESRD patients have experienced more various medical experiences than many other patients.

Chapter 1

1. Thomas S. Kuhn, *The Structure of Scientific Revolutions* 23 (U Chicago Press, 1970). It is hard for a late–twentieth-century academic to think about the development of a field of scholarship without adverting to Kuhn's magisterial work. Perhaps it applies better to scientific scholarship than to other kinds. Perhaps it applies awkwardly to a field as deeply theoretical and as frankly practical as bioethics. Perhaps it does not even describe all scientific work. But it has enormous resonance, and it will prove a useful point of embarkation. For a recent survey of Kuhn's work, see Paul Hoyningen-Huene, *Reconstructing Scientific Revolutions: Thomas S. Kuhn's Philosophy of Science* (U Chicago Press, 1993).

2. On the origins of bioethics, see David J. Rothman, *Strangers at the Bedside: A History of How Law and Bioethics Transformed Medical Decision Making* (Basic Books, 1991).

3. Renée C. Fox, *The Evolution of American Bioethics: A Sociological Perspective,* in George Weisz, ed, *Social Science Perspectives on Medical Ethics* 206 (U Pennsylvania Press, 1990).

4. See Daniel Wikler, *What Has Bioethics to Offer Health Policy?,* 69 Milbank Quarterly 233 (1991).

5. For example, Beauchamp and Childress labor to show there is more to bioethics than autonomy. Tom L. Beauchamp & James F. Childress, *Principles of Biomedical Ethics* (Oxford U Press, 3d ed, 1987).

6. Carl E. Schneider, *Moral Discourse and the Transformation of American Family Law,* 83 Michigan L Rev 1803, 1846 (1985).

7. See, e.g., Philip Rieff, *The Triumph of the Therapeutic: Uses of Faith After Freud* (U Chicago Press, 1966); Philip Rieff, *Freud: The Mind of the Moralist* (U Chicago Press, 1979).

8. Troyen A. Brennan, *Just Doctoring: Medical Ethics in the Liberal State* 76 (U California Press, 1991).

9. See, e.g., Arthur L. Caplan, *Can Autonomy be Saved?*, in *If I Were a Rich Man Could I Buy a Pancreas? and Other Essays on the Ethics of Health Care* 257 (Indiana U Press, 1992).

10. Idem at 259. In this same colorful vein: "[T]he 'new' medical ethics . . . views physician paternalism as a sin on a par with matricide and child abuse." Howard Brody, *The Healer's Power* 15 (Yale U Press, 1992).

11. See, for example, the various editions of Tom L. Beauchamp & James F. Childress, *Principles of Biomedical Ethics* (Oxford U Press).

12. Renée C. Fox, *The Evolution of American Bioethics: A Sociological Perspective,* in George Weisz, ed, *Social Science Perspectives on Medical Ethics* 206–07 (U Pennsylvania Press, 1990).

13. AMA, *Current Opinions of the Judicial Council of the AMA—1982* § 8.07 (AMA, 1982), quoted in Brennan, *Just Doctoring* at 66 (cited in note 8).

14. Robert Zussman, *Intensive Care: Medical Ethics and the Medical Profession* 85 (U Chicago Press, 1992).

15. Idem at 81.

16. Eric J. Cassell, *The Changing Concept of the Ideal Physician,* 115 Daedalus 185, 199 (Spring 1986).

17. Bebe Lavin, et al, *Change in Student Physicians' Views on Authority Relationships With Patients*, 28 J Health & Social Behavior 258, 263 (1987).

18. Norio Higuchi, *The Patient's Right to Know of a Cancer Diagnosis: A Comparison of Japanese Paternalism and American Self-Determination,* 31 Washburn L J 455, 456 (1992). These changes are reported in Dennis H. Novack, et al, *Changes in Physicians' Attitudes Toward Telling the Cancer Patient,* 241 JAMA 897 (1979).

19. Brennan, *Just Doctoring* at 120 (cited in note 8).

20. Debra L. Roter & Judith A. Hall, *Studies of Doctor–Patient Interaction,* 10 Annual Rev Public Health 163, 178 (1989).

21. Arthur L. Caplan, *Can Autonomy be Saved?*, in *If I Were a Rich Man Could I Buy a Pancreas? and Other Essays on the Ethics of Health Care* 261 (Indiana U Press, 1992). To like effect, see, e.g., Brennan, *Just Doctoring* at 66 (cited in note 8). For a less sanguine evaluation of changes in attitudes toward patient autonomy in decisions to terminate treatment, see David Orentlicher, *The Illusion of Patient Choice in End-of-Life Decisions,* 267 JAMA 2101 (1992).

22. Benjamin N. Cardozo, *The Nature of the Judicial Process* 168 (Yale U Press, 1921). Cardozo was referring to judges.

23. Zussman, *Intensive Care* at 87 (cited in note 14). Or, as Bosk puts it, "The dark side of patient autonomy was patient abandonment." Charles L. Bosk, *All God's Mistakes: Genetic Counseling in a Pediatric Hospital* 158 (U Chicago Press, 1992). Burt explains, "The physician who is now instructed to obey the 'informed consent' of his patient, no matter how harmful he feels that action to be for the patient, is not only permitted but positively enjoined to separate himself from his patient, to respect his patient's 'autonomy' by suppressing his own identifications, his self-confusions, with that patient." Robert A. Burt, *The Limits of Law in Regulating Health Care Decisions,* 7 HCR 29, 32 (Dec 1977). This is a danger Katz fair-mindedly acknowledges. Jay Katz, *The Silent World of Doctor and Pa-*

tient 163 (Free Press, 1984). The tendency may well be increased by doctors' fretful views about their risks of legal liability for giving medical advice. For a bracing and intelligent comment on this problem and the hospital attorney's role in it, see Alan Weisbard, *Defensive Law: A New Perspective on Informed Consent,* 146 Archives of Internal Medicine 860 (1986).

24. Paul S. Appelbaum & Loren H. Roth, *Patients Who Refuse Treatment in Medical Hospitals,* 250 JAMA 1296, 1301 (1983).

25. Tim Brookes, *Catching My Breath: An Asthmatic Explores His Illness* 280 (Times Books, 1994).

26. Kenneth A. Shapiro, *Dying and Living: One Man's Life with Cancer* 7 (U Texas Press, 1985).

27. *Natanson v. Kline,* 350 P2d 1093, 1104 (Kan, 1960).

28. For a pointed history of that doctrine, see Jay Katz, *The Silent World of Doctor and Patient* 41–84 (Free Press, 1984). For a particularly well-informed and complex view of that history, see Martin S. Pernick, *The Patient's Role in Medical Decisionmaking: A Social History of Informed Consent in Medical Therapy,* in President's Commission for the Study of Ethical Problems in Medicine and Biomedical and Behavioral Research, *Making Health Care Decisions: The Ethical and Legal Implications of Informed Consent in the Patient–Practitioner Relationship,* Volume Three: Appendices (U S Gov't Printing Office, 1982).

29. 42 USC §§ 1395cc(f), 1396a(w). In addition, of course, many public and private health-care providers have written rules (governing DNR orders, for example) and established programs (ethics committees, for instance) intended at least partly to protect patients' autonomy.

30. 497 US 261 (1990). For sound views of these constitutional issues, see Yale Kamisar, *When Is There a Constitutional "Right to Die"? When Is There No Constitutional "Right to Live"?,* 25 Georgia L Rev 1203 (1991); John Robertson, Cruzan *and the Constitutional Status of Nontreatment Decisions for Incompetent Patients,* 25 Georgia L Rev 1139 (1991). I analyze *Cruzan* in Cruzan *and the Constitutionalization of American Life,* 17 J Medicine & Philosophy 589 (1992).

31. 117 S Ct 2258 (1997).

32. Idem at 2269.

33. I do not mean that the law has failed to recognize some important reasons patient autonomy must be limited. For a helpful and refreshing argument that "autonomy does not seem to be as dominant a value as rhetoric would suggest," see Roger B. Dworkin, *Medical Law and Ethics in the Post-Autonomy Age,* Indiana L J 727, 728 (1993).

34. Ezekiel J. Emanuel & Linda L. Emanuel, *Four Models of the Physician–Patient Relationship,* 267 JAMA 2221, 2223 (1992) (emphasis in original) (quoting the President's Commission for the Study of Ethical Problems in Medicine and Biomedical and Behavioral Research, *Making Health Care Decisions* (U S Gov't Printing Office, 1982)).

35. Lachlan Forrow, Steven A. Wartman, & Dan Brock, *Science, Ethics, and the Making of Clinical Decisions,* 259 JAMA 3161, 3166 (1988).

36. Dan W. Brock, *The Ideal of Shared Decision Making Between Physicians and Patients,* 1 Kennedy Institute of Ethics J 28, 28 (1991). Brock's own views on the subject are well worth reading. For similar descriptions of how medical decisions ought to be made, see, e.g., Richard Sherlock, *Reasonable Men and Sick Human Beings,* 80 American J Medicine 2, 2 (1986).

37. Instead of precision, readers of bioethical writing must often settle for such uninformative terms as "shared," or "collaborative," or "participatory." The Emanuels have

made a step in the right direction by proposing ideal types of medical decisions. Emanuel & Emanuel, 267 JAMA 2221 (cited in note 34). They identify a "paternalistic" model in which doctors decide what is best, subject to patients' assent; an "informative" model in which doctors present information to patients and patients decide; an "interpretive" model in which doctors help patients discover what they want and how best to get it; and a "deliberative" model in which doctors "help the patient determine and choose the health-related values that can be realized in the clinical situation." Idem at 2222. The Emanuels conclude there has been a "shift toward the informative model." Idem at 2223. For another set of ideal types, see James F. Childress, *Metaphors and Models of Medical Relationships,* in Louis W. Hodges, ed, 8 Social Responsibility: Journalism, Law, Medicine 47 (1982).

38. Mark Siegler & Peter A. Singer, *Clinical Ethics,* in William N. Kelley, ed, *Textbook of Internal Medicine* 4 (Lippincott, 2d ed, 1992).

39. Tom L. Beauchamp & James F. Childress, *Principles of Biomedical Ethics* 76 (Oxford U Press, 3d ed, 1989) (emphases in original).

40. For an imposing list of articles to this effect, see Marjorie Maguire Shultz, *From Informed Consent to Patient Choice,* 95 Yale L J 219, 226 n. 30 (1985).

41. *Canterbury v. Spence,* 464 F2d 772, 781 (DC Cir, 1972).

42. Idem at 780.

43. Idem at 784.

44. Idem at 781.

45. Jay Katz, *The Silent World of Doctor and Patient* 99 (Free Press, 1984).

46. Jay Katz, *Informed Consent—A Fairy Tale? Law's Vision,* 39 U Pittsburgh L Rev 137 (1977). Echoing Katz, Brennan writes that "doctors have consistently sought to maximize their own paternalistic prerogatives. The notion of informed consent thus remains a fairy tale." Troyen A. Brennan, *Silent Decisions: Limits of Consent and the Terminally Ill Patient,* 16 Law, Medicine & Health Care 204, 204 (1988).

47. Paul S. Appelbaum, Charles W. Lidz, & Alan Meisel, *Informed Consent: Legal Theory and Clinical Practice* 130 (Oxford U Press, 1987).

48. Marjorie M. Shultz, *From Informed Consent to Patient Choice: A New Protected Interest,* 95 Yale L J 219 (1985). For other criticisms of informed consent, see, e.g., Alan Meisel, *A "Dignitary Tort" as a Bridge Between the Idea of Informed Consent and the Law of Informed Consent,* 16 Law, Medicine & Health Care 210 (1988); Howard Brody, *Transparency: Informed Consent in Primary Care,* 19 HCR 5 (Sept/Oct 1989); Cathy J. Jones, *Autonomy and Informed Consent in Medical Decisionmaking: Toward a New Self-Fulfilling Prophecy,* 47 Washington & Lee L Rev 379 (1990); Howard Brody, *The Healer's Power* 83–119 (Yale U Press, 1992).

49. Susan M. Wolf, *Ethics Committees and Due Process: Nesting Rights in a Community of Caring,* 50 Maryland L Rev 798, 824 (1991).

50. Idem at 857.

51. Idem at 855.

52. For a critical examination of the centrality of rights thinking in American politics, law, and life, see Mary Ann Glendon, *Rights Talk: The Impoverishment of Political Discourse* (Free Press, 1991). For an argument stressing that centrality but arguing that alternatives yearn to break through, see Robert N. Bellah, et al, *Habits of the Heart: Individualism and Commitment in American Life* (U California Press, 1985). On rights thinking at the intersection of bioethics and law, see Carl E. Schneider, *Rights Discourse and Neonatal Euthanasia,* 76 California L Rev 151 (1988); and Carl E. Schneider, *Cruzan and the Constitutionalization of American Life,* 17 J Medicine & Philosophy 589 (1992). On the

role of rights in medical decisions, see Robert Zussman, *Intensive Care: Medical Ethics and the Medical Profession* 81–97 (Chicago U Press, 1992). The emphasis on the distinctively American quality of the autonomy paradigm is not accidental. There are few countries in the world where autonomy has so influenced thinking about the authority of the patient. There are many countries—even highly industrialized countries—where a strikingly different paradigm presides. Japan is a conspicuous example. There, for instance, a substantial number of doctors continue to conceal some fatal diagnoses from patients. See Robert B. Leflar, *Informed Consent and Patients' Rights in Japan,* 33 Houston L Rev 1 (1995).

53. Dan Brock, *Informed Consent,* in *Life and Death: Philosophical Essays in Biomedical Ethics* 33 (Cambridge U Press, 1993).

54. Idem at 34.

55. William James, *The Varieties of Religious Experience: A Study in Human Nature* 186 (Modern Library, 1994).

56. Tom L. Beauchamp & James F. Childress, *Principles of Biomedical Ethics* 105 (Oxford U Press, 3d ed, 1989).

57. Dan Brock, *Informed Consent,* in *Life and Death: Philosophical Essays in Biomedical Ethics* 33 (Cambridge U Press, 1993). It is not clear how Beauchamp and Childress understand the obligation of physicians faced with patients reluctant to make medical decisions. They say, for instance, that the autonomy principle "engenders a positive or affirmative obligation of respectful treatment in disclosing information and fostering autonomous decision making," Beauchamp & Childress, *Principles of Biomedical Ethics* at 73 (cited in note 56), but they leave tantalizingly unspecified what "fostering autonomous decision making" might mean.

58. President's Commission for the Study of Ethical Problems in Medicine and Biomedical and Behavioral Research, *Making Health Care Decisions: The Ethical and Legal Implications of Informed Consent in the Patient–Practitioner Relationship,* Volume One: Report 46 (U S Gov't Printing Office, 1982).

59. E Haavi Morreim, *Balancing Act: The New Medical Ethics of Medicine's New Economics* 139 (Georgetown U Press, 1995) (footnote omitted).

60. Idem at 141.

61. Idem.

62. Idem at 140.

63. Idem.

64. Idem at 146.

65. Idem at 134.

66. Idem at 136–37.

67. Jay Katz, *The Silent World of Doctor and Patient* 122 (Free Press, 1984).

68. Idem.

69. Idem.

70. Idem at 123.

71. Idem at 125.

72. Idem at 141.

73. Idem at 137.

74. See, e.g., idem at 154–55. But, of course, "Dostoyevsky's Grand Inquisitor predicted that patients may not wish to assume the responsibilities engendered by that 'terrible gift of freedom.'" Idem at 164.

75. Idem at 200.

76. Idem.

77. Idem at 154.

78. Idem at 207.

79. William G. Bartholome, *A Revolution in Understanding: How Ethics Has Transformed Health Care Decision Making,* 18 Quality Rev Bulletin 6, 10 (1992). (By this point, the patient may be so repelled by the "provider's" patronizing and self-satisfied manner that no further "dialogue" between them will ever be necessary.)

80. Cathy J. Jones, *Autonomy and Informed Consent in Medical Decisionmaking: Toward a New Self-Fulfilling Prophecy,* 47 Washington & Lee L Rev 379, 421 (1990).

81. Idem at 429.

82. Robert M. Veatch, *Abandoning Informed Consent,* 25 HCR 5, 9 (Mar/Apr 1995).

83. Idem at 11.

84. Idem at 10.

85. Idem at 11.

86. *Changing Medical Organization and the Erosion of Trust,* 74 Milbank Quarterly 171, 178 (1996).

87. Eliot Freidson, *Professional Dominance: The Social Structure of Medical Care* 236 (Atherton, 1970).

88. Mark A. Chesler & Barbara K. Chesney, *Cancer and Self-Help: Bridging the Troubled Waters of Childhood Illness* 229 (U Wisconsin Press, 1995) (footnote omitted).

89. This makes this doctor sound more peremptory than he is. While explaining why he sometimes did not tell patients everything right away, he said,

> As I am talking about this I am thinking about a kind of scenario where I know it is going to happen. I am not ready to talk about it yet. I was doing labs of today's clinic and this young woman who I have seen three or four times since September . . . . [Sigh.] The renal function on this visit today is half what it was at the last visit in early January, and I was disappointed when I saw the labs. You know something? Today, right now, I don't want to talk to her about it. I need to chew it and sit on it for a couple of days, because I am pissed off and I am discouraged by it.

One of the reasons this doctor's patients overwhelmingly like him is they think he cares about them. This passage indicates why they might think so.

90. Timothy E. Quill & Howard Brody, *Physician Recommendations and Patient Autonomy: Finding a Balance Between Physician Power and Patient Choice,* 125 Annals of Internal Medicine 763, 763 (1996).

91. Idem at 764.

92. Idem (footnotes omitted).

93. *Foreword,* in Claire Sylvia with William Novak, *A Change of Heart: A Memoir* xii (Little, Brown, 1997).

94. For a social scientist's analysis of genetic counseling and that ethos, see Charles L. Bosk, *All God's Mistakes: Genetic Counseling in a Pediatric Hospital* (U Chicago Press, 1992). Psychiatry, of course, is another medical field where nondirectiveness has flourished.

95. Eleanor Gordon Applebaum & Stephen K. Firestein, *The Need for Time to Work Through an Agonizing Decision: Werdnig-Hoffmann Disease,* in Eleanor Gordon Applebaum & Stephen K. Firestein, eds, *A Genetic Counseling Casebook* 210 (Free Press, 1983).

96. Donald R. Cohodes, *Through the Looking Glass: Decision Making and Chemotherapy,* 14 Health Affairs 203, 208 (1995).

97. James C. Wade, *The Patient/Physician Relationship: One Doctor's View,* 14 Health Affairs 209, 209 (1995).

98. Regina Woods, *Tales from Inside the Iron Lung: And How I Got Out of It* 31 (U Pennsylvania Press, 1994).

99. Lucy Bregman & Sara Thiermann, *First Person Mortal: Personal Narratives of Dying, Death, and Grief* 81 (Paragon House, 1995).

100. Susan Wolf Sternberg, *A Year of Miracles: A Healing Journey From Cancer to Wholeness* 5 (Star Mountain Press, 1995).

101. *Taking on Prostate Cancer,* Fortune 55, 72 (May 13, 1996). This article was the cover story in this issue of *Fortune.* The teaser on the cover read: "When Intel's CEO got the chilling diagnosis, he didn't just follow doctor's orders. Neither should you."

102. Idem at 60.

103. *Man to Man: Surviving Prostate Cancer* 253 (Random House, 1996).

104. Idem at 66.

105. Idem at 214.

106. Idem at 213. For a picture of support groups as agents for encouraging parents of ill children to "express their needs, reassert active control over their lives, and play active roles in the care of their children," see Mark A. Chesler & Barbara K. Chesney, *Cancer and Self-Help: Bridging the Troubled Waters of Childhood Illness* 106 (U Wisconsin Press, 1995).

107. Michael Korda, *Man to Man: Surviving Prostrate Cancer* 222 (Random House, 1996).

108. Troyen A. Brennan, *Just Doctoring: Medical Ethics in the Liberal State* 90 (U California Press, 1991).

109. See pages 15–16.

110. Barbara Creaturo, *Courage: The Testimony of A Cancer Patient* viii (Pantheon, 1991).

111. Brennan, *Just Doctoring* at 91 (cited in note 108).

112. That reminder is powerfully put in Jay Katz, *The Silent World of Doctor and Patient* (Free Press, 1984), and David J. Rothman, *Strangers at the Bedside: A History of How Law and Bioethics Transformed Medical Decision Making* (Basic Books, 1991). For one repellent story that exemplifies what made the bad old days bad, see Cornelius & Kathryn Morgan Ryan, *A Private Battle* 83–89 (Simon & Schuster, 1979).

113. Musa Mayer, *Examining Myself: One Woman's Story of Breast Cancer Treatment and Recovery* 53 (Faber & Faber, 1993).

114. George R. Melton & Wil Garcia, *Beyond AIDS: A Journey Into Healing* 40 (Brotherhood Press, 1988).

115. Gregory White Smith & Steven Naifeh, *Making Miracles Happen* 18 (Little, Brown, 1997).

116. Robert M. Kaplan, *Health-Related Quality of Life in Patient Decision Making,* 47 J Social Issues 69, 70 (1991).

117. Tim Brookes, *Catching My Breath: An Asthmatic Explores His Illness* 283 (Times Books, 1994).

118. See, e.g., Sheldon Greenfield, Sherrie Kaplan, & John E. Ware, *Expanding Patient Involvement in Care: Effects on Patient Outcomes,* 102 Annals of Internal Medicine 520 (1985); Sheldon Greenfield, et al, *Patients' Participation in Medical Care: Effects on Blood Sugar Control and Quality of Life in Diabetes,* 3 J General Internal Medicine 448 (1988).

119. Lachlan Forrow, Steven A. Wartman, & Dan W. Brock, *Science, Ethics, and the Making of Clinical Decisions,* 259 JAMA 3161, 3166 (1988).

On noncompliance, see L. Stockwell Morris & R.M. Schulz, *Patient Compliance—An Overview,* 17 J Clinical Pharmacy & Therapeutics 283 (1992). The extent of noncompliance is commonly thought to be vast, so that "[n]oncompliance may be the most significant problem facing medical practice today." Stephen A. Eraker, John P. Kirscht, & Marshall H. Becker, *Understanding and Improving Patient Compliance,* 100 Annals of Internal Medicine 258, 258 (1984). Morris and Schulz estimate that half the patients in long-term therapy are noncompliant.

120. Max Lerner, *Wrestling With the Angel: A Memoir of My Triumph Over Illness* 69 (Simon & Schuster, 1990)121. Anne Hunsaker Hawkins, *Reconstructing Illness: Studies in Pathography* 65 (Purdue U Press, 1993). "Pathography" is Hawkins' term for patients' memoirs.

122. Joyce Slayton Mitchell, *Winning the Chemo Battle* 203 (Norton, 1988). For a more critical look at this argument, see Chapter 5.

123. Tom L. Beauchamp & James F. Childress, *Principles of Biomedical Ethics* 68 (Oxford U Press, 3d ed, 1989).

124. Robert M. Kaplan, *Health-Related Quality of Life in Patient Decision Making,* 47 J Social Issues 69, 70 (1991).

125. Joseph Schneider & Peter Conrad, *Having Epilepsy: The Experience and Control of Illness* (Temple U Press, 1983).

126. Brookes, *Catching My Breath* at 280 (cited in note 117).

127. "Physicians who say the patient 'has a low pain threshold' have probably not had the same disorder that is causing 'the low pain threshold' patient to howl with agony at the passage of his ureteral stone." Harvey Mandell & Howard Spiro, *Preface*, in Harvey Mandell & Howard Spiro, eds, *When Doctors Get Sick* xi (Plenum Medical, 1988).

128. Jody Heymann, *Equal Partners: A Physician's Call for a New Spirit of Medicine,* 3–4 (Little, Brown, 1995).

129. For an instance, see Sue Fisher, *In the Patient's Best Interest: Women and the Politics of Medical Decisions* (Rutgers U Press, 1986). I develop this point in Chapter 6.

130. Idem. at 7.

131. See, of course, Jay Katz, *The Silent World of Doctor and Patient* (Free Press, 1984).

132. Fisher, *In the Patient's Best Interest* at 188 n. 3 (cited in note 129).

133. Idem at 161, quoting Mary Daly, *Gyn/Ecology* 109 (Beacon Press, 1978).

134. Idem at 162.

135. *Tales from Inside the Iron Lung: And How I Got Out of It* 31 (U of Pennsylvania Press, 1994).

136. Idem.

137. Charles Taylor, *Multiculturalism and "The Politics of Recognition"* 30 (Harvard U Press, 1992).

138. Idem at 29.

139. Charles Taylor, *The Ethics of Authenticity* 26 (Harvard U Press, 1992).

140. Lawrence M. Friedman, *The Republic of Choice: Law, Authority, and Culture* 2 (Harvard U Press, 1990).

141. Taylor, *The Ethics of Authenticity* at 27 (cited in note 139).

142. Rachelle Breslow, *Who Said So?: How Our Thoughts and Beliefs Affect Our Physiology* 57 (Celestial Arts, 1991) (emphasis in original).

143. Robert N. Bellah, et al, *Habits of the Heart: Individualism and Commitment in American Life* 15 (U California Press, 1985). See also Carl E. Schneider, *Marriage, Morals, and the Law: No-Fault Divorce and Moral Discourse,* Utah L Rev 503 (1994).

144. George Kateb, *Democratic Individuality and the Meaning of Rights,* in Nancy L. Rosenblum, ed, *Liberalism and the Moral Life* 198 (Harvard U Press, 1991).

145. Bellah, et al, *Habits of the Heart* at 82 (cited in note 143).

146. Kenneth A. Shapiro, *Dying and Living: One Man's Life With Cancer* 7 (U Texas Press, 1985).

147. Ezekiel J. Emanuel & Linda L. Emanuel, *Four Models of the Physician–Patient Relationship,* 267 JAMA 2221, 2225 (1992) (footnotes omitted).

148. William James, *The Varieties of Religious Experience: A Study in Human Nature* 341 (Modern Library, 1994).

149. Isaiah Berlin, *Two Concepts of Liberty,* in *Four Essays on Liberty* 131 (Oxford U Press, 1969).

150. Gertrude Himmelfarb, *On Looking Into the Abyss: Untimely Thoughts on Culture and Society* 79 (Vintage, 1995).

151. John Stuart Mill, *On Liberty,* in *The Philosophy of John Stuart Mill: Ethical, Political, and Religious* 252 (Modern Library, 1961).

152. Idem at 254.

153. Idem at 255.

154. Anne Hunsaker Hawkins, *Reconstructing Illness: Studies in Pathography* 129 (Purdue U Press, 1993).

155. Alexis de Tocqueville, 2 *Democracy in America* 4 (Vintage, 1957).

156. Idem at 107.

157. Ralph Waldo Emerson, *Self-Reliance,* in *The Selected Writings of Ralph Waldo Emerson* 146 (Modern Library, 1992).

158. Peter Clecak, *America's Quest for the Ideal Self: Dissent and Fulfillment in the 60s and 70s* 10 (Oxford U Press, 1983).

159. Robert N. Bellah, et al, *Habits of the Heart: Individualism and Commitment in American Life* 23 (U California Press, 1985).

160. Gail Sheehy, *Passages: Predictable Crises of Adult Life* 364 (Bantam, 1977), quoted idem at 79.

161. Carl E. Schneider, *Moral Discourse and the Transformation of American Family Law,* 83 Michigan L Rev 1803, 1847 (1985). For a somewhat skeptical view of the life of psychologic man in America today, see idem at 1845–1851. For a vibrantly jaundiced one, see Philip Rieff, *The Triumph of the Therapeutic* (U Chicago Press, 1987).

162. Clecak, *America's Quest for the Ideal Self* at 11 (cited in note 158).

163. Claudine Herzlich & Janine Pierret, *From Self-help to the Duty to Be Healthy,* in *Illness and Self in Society* 210 (Johns Hopkins U Press, 1987).

164. Idem at 212.

165. Idem at 215.

166. Idem at 230 (footnote omitted).

167. Ellen C. Annandale, *Dimensions of Patient Control in a Free-Standing Birth Center,* 25 Social Science Medicine 1235, 1246 (1987).

168. For an indignant review of these developments, see Robert Crawford, *You Are Dangerous to Your Health: The Ideology and Politics of Victim Blaming,* 7 International J Health Policy 663 (1977). See also Barry Glassner, *Fitness and the Postmodern Self,* 30 J Health & Social Behavior 180 (1989), and David Wagner, *The New Temperance: The American Obsession With Sin and Vice* (Westview, 1997). I sometimes think that, in our therapeutic society, health is one of the few remaining areas in which we may indulge in the pleasures of moralism. Russian children used to be urged to turn in their parents when they disserved the Party; today, American children must "intervene" when their parents jog too little, eat too much, or smoke at all.

169. Paul Reed, *The Q Journal: A Treatment Diary* 38 (Celestial Arts, 1991).

170. See Carl E. Schneider, *Brothers and Strangers: Moral Discourse and Mutual Incomprehension,* paper presented to the International Society of Family Law, Durban, South Africa, July 30, 1997.

171. Charles Taylor, *The Ethics of Authenticity* 18 (Harvard U Press, 1992).

172. Anne Hunsaker Hawkins, *Reconstructing Illness: Studies in Pathography* 129 (Purdue U Press, 1993).

173. Idem at 76–77.

174. Arnold R. Beisser, *Flying Without Wings* 42 (Doubleday, 1989).

175. Tim Brookes, *Catching My Breath: An Asthmatic Explores His Illness* 276–77 (Times Books, 1994) (emphasis in original).

176. Mary Alice Geier, *Cancer: What's It Doing in My Life?* 114 (Hope Publishing, 1985) (emphasis in original).

177. Max Lerner, *Wrestling With the Angel: A Memoir of My Triumph Over Illness* 45 (Simon & Schuster, 1990).

178. Idem at 105. Nevertheless Lerner thought it *hubris* "to substitute my judgment" for that of specialists and said "the province of autonomy I sought was more modest, quite simply to inform myself—by every available means—to play whatever role came to me, because it was my life and my death." Idem at 69.

179. Suzy Szasz, *Living With It: Why You Don't Have to Be Healthy to Be Happy* 10 (Prometheus, 1991).

180. Michael Korda, *Man to Man: Surviving Prostate Cancer* 66 (Random House, 1996) (emphasis in original).

181. Renée C. Fox, *Medical Morality Is Not Bioethics*, in *Essays in Medical Sociology* 663 (Transaction Books, 1988).

182. Lawrence J. Schneiderman, et al, *Do Physicians' Own Preferences for Life-Sustaining Treatment Influence Their Perceptions of Patients' Preferences?,* 4 J Clinical Ethics 28 (1993).

183. See Carl E. Schneider, *The Mystery of Doctors' Attitudes Toward Malpractice Law,* Address to University of Michigan Law School Alumni, New York State Bar Association Meeting, 1995. For example, doctors overestimate the annual rate of suits for malpractice by a factor of three, overestimate the risk of suit from an incident of negligence by a factor of almost five, and overestimate the risk of suit from an adverse event by a factor of eleven. Paul C. Weiler, et al, *A Measure of Malpractice: Medical Injury, Malpractice Litigation, and Patient Compensation* 124 (Harvard U Press, 1993). For evidence of the sensitivity of at least some physicians to criticism generally, see Grace Budrys, *When Doctors Join Unions* (Cornell U Press, 1997). For an examination of doctors' misperceptions of the law, see Marshall B. Kapp & Bernard Lo, *Legal Perceptions and Medical Decision Making,* 64 Milbank Quarterly 163 (Supp 2, 1986).

184. Timothy E. Quill & Howard Brody, *Physician Recommendations and Patient Autonomy: Finding a Balance Between Physician Power and Patient Choice,* 125 Annals of Internal Medicine 763, 764 (1996). One patient says: "In some ways the medical profession has rushed to meet patients' demand for more control. . . . Surely the compliance of so many doctors stemmed more from their relative helplessness in the face of cancer, their inability to predict the results of their own interventions, than from any new-found respect for their patients." Juliet Wittman, *Breast Cancer Journal: A Century of Petals* 22 (Fulcrum, 1993).

185. A. Peter Lundin, *Chronic Renal Failure and Hemodialysis,* in Harvey Mandell & Howard Spiro, eds, *When Doctors Get Sick* 366–67 (Plenum Medical, 1988).

186. Thomas S. Kuhn, *The Structure of Scientific Revolutions* 52 (U Chicago Press, 1970).

187. Prominent criticisms include Daniel Callahan, *Contemporary Biomedical Ethics,* 302 NEJM 1228 (1980); Daniel Callahan, *Autonomy: A Moral Good, Not a Moral Obsession,* 14 HCR 40 (Oct 1984); Willard Gaylin, *Introduction: Autonomy, Paternalism, and Community,* 14 HCR 5 (Oct 1984); Robert M. Veatch, *Autonomy's Temporary Triumph,* 14 HCR 38 (Oct 1984); Edmund D. Pellegrino & David C. Thomasma, *For the Patient's Good: The Restoration of Beneficence in Health Care* (Oxford U Press, 1988). I express some of my own discomforts in Carl E. Schneider, *Rights Discourse and Neonatal Euthanasia,* 76 California L Rev 151 (1988).

188. For a survey, see Susan M. Wolf, *Shifting Paradigms in Bioethics and Health Law: The Rise of a New Pragmatism,* 20 American J Law & Medicine 395 (1994).

189. Thomas S. Kuhn, *The Structure of Scientific Revolutions* 91 (U Chicago Press, 1970).

190. See, e.g., Analee E. Beisecker, *Aging and the Desire for Information and Input in Medical Decisions: Patient Consumerism in Medical Encounters,* 28 Gerontologist 330 (1988).

191. If I seem overemphatic, it is because the autonomy paradigm in bioethics is so exalted that any failure of complete allegiance is taken by the devout as a complete renunciation of it. See, e.g., Wolf, *Shifting Paradigms,* 20 American J Law & Medicine at 411 (cited in note 188), which announces that "there are renewed challenges now to the very notion of patients' rights in the face of clinical realities" and cites two of the articles from which this book grows as (the only) evidence of this perfidy.

192. Gerald Dworkin, *The Theory and Practice of Autonomy* 32 (Cambridge U Press, 1988).

Chapter 2

1. Jay Katz, *The Silent World of Doctor and Patient* 228 (Free Press, 1984). In the tendentious way Katz phrases this "prevalent assertion" it is indeed dubious. Who does not doubt patients want to trust their doctors "blindly"?

2. President's Commission for the Study of Ethical Problems in Medicine and Biomedical and Behavioral Research, *Making Health Care Decisions: The Ethical and Legal Implications of Informed Consent in the Patient–Practitioner Relationship,* Volume One: Report 17 (U S Gov't Printing Office, 1982). For a more exact description of these data, see text at notes 41–43. The President's Commission is now widely taken to have said "that the vast majority of respondents to its survey wanted information and participation in medical decisions." Marjorie Maguire Shultz, *From Informed Consent to Patient Choice: A New Protected Interest,* 95 Yale L Rev 219, 222 n. 10 (1985).

3. Jack Ende, et al, *Measuring Patients' Desire for Autonomy: Decision Making and Information-Seeking Preferences Among Medical Patients,* 4 J General Internal Medicine 23 (1989). "Upper respiratory tract illness (URI) represented mild disease; hypertension (HBP), moderate disease; and myocardial infarction (MI), severe or most threatening disease." Idem at 23.

4. Idem at 25. These results were confirmed in a study of the membership of an HMO. Suzanne C. Thompson, Jennifer Pitts, & Lenore Schwankovsky, *Preferences for Involvement in Medical Decision Making: Situational and Demographic Influences,* 22 Patient Education & Counseling 133 (1993).

5. Ende, et al, 4 J General Internal Medicine at 26–27 (cited in note 3).

6. Idem at 26.

7. William M. Strull, Bernard Lo, & Gerald Charles, *Do Patients Want to Participate in Medical Decision Making?*, 252 JAMA 2990 (1984).

8. Idem at 2991. The clinicians "reported giving these amounts of information in only 38% of cases."

9. Idem at 2991.

10. Idem at 2992.

11. Idem.

12. Idem.

13. Idem at 2993.

14. Robert F. Nease, Jr., & W. Blair Brooks, *Patient Desire for Information and Decision Making in Health Care Decisions: The Autonomy Preference Index and the Health Opinion Survey,* 10 J General Internal Medicine 593, 594 (1995).

15. Idem at 594 (emphasis in original).

16. Idem (emphasis in original).

17. Idem at 596.

18. Idem.

19. Ilan B. Vertinsky, et al, *Measuring Consumer Desire for Participation in Clinical Decision Making,* 9 Health Services Research 121 (1974).

20. Idem at 128. This factor comprised statements like, "Ask the doctor to give him all the information he has, and then the patient decides what to do." Idem.

21. Idem at 133. Avoidance was the researchers' summarizing term for those "items indicating propensity to delegate the decision function completely (A3, 'Just follow the doctor's orders and go home')." Idem at 128.

22. Ruth R. Faden, et al, *Disclosure of Information to Patients in Medical Care,* 19 Medical Care 718 (1981).

23. What makes the study particularly interesting was that 93% of the neurologists interviewed believed the doctor should make the choices. However, here, as in a number of other efforts, the usefulness of the study's results is diminished because its respondents were forced to choose between only two options. Once again, too, the study reported widespread interest in information about available medications and their risks. However, the information least wanted was about "drug-related mortality."

24. Idem at 720.

25. Analee E. Beisecker, *Aging and the Desire for Information and Input in Medical Decisions: Patient Consumerism in Medical Encounters,* 28 Gerontologist 330, 330 (1988).

26. Idem.

27. Jennifer S. Mark & Howard Spiro, *Informed Consent For Colonoscopy,* 150 Archives of Internal Medicine 777, 777–78 (1990).

28. Idem at 778.

29. Charles W. Lidz, et al, *Barriers to Informed Consent,* 99 Annals of Internal Medicine 539 (1983). One more impressionistic study of informed consent reported that the researcher's "period of observation bore out, that in many cases patients do request or allow physicians to make decisions for them." Cathy J. Jones, *Autonomy and Informed Consent in Medical Decisionmaking: Toward a New Self-Fulfilling Prophecy,* 47 Washington & Lee L Rev 379, 419–20 (1990).

30. Lidz, et al, 99 Annals of Internal Medicine at 540 (cited in note 29).

31. Idem at 541.

32. Suzanne M. Miller, David S. Brody, & Jeffrey Summerton, *Styles of Coping With*

Threat: Implications for Health, 54 J Personality & Social Psychology 142, 146 (1988). They found that 48.1% of the former personality type ("high monitors") and 71.4% of the latter ("low monitors") "preferred that treatment decisions be made jointly by themselves and their physicians." Idem.

33. Lesley F. Degner & Jeffrey A. Sloan, *Decision Making During Serious Illness: What Role Do Patients Really Want to Play?,* 45 J Clinical Epidemiology 941 (1992).

34. Idem at 945–46.

35. Idem at 946. Once again, age was the best (though not a strong) predictor of a desire to participate in decisions. Interestingly, "[t]he clinical hypothesis that patients who are more ill prefer less control in cancer treatment decision making was not supported. Neither symptom distress levels nor stage of disease were related to patients' role preferences." Idem at 947.

36. H.J. Sutherland, et al, *Cancer Patients: Their Desire for Information and Participation in Treatment Decisions,* 82 J Royal Society of Medicine 260 (1989).

37. Idem at 262.

38. Barrie R. Cassileth, et al, *Information and Participation Preferences Among Cancer Patients,* 92 Annals of Internal Medicine 832, 832–834 (1980). Once again, information was more valued than control: The parallel assents to the statement "I want as *much* information as possible, good and bad" were 96%, 79%, and 80%.

39. Health Services Research Group, *Studying Patients' Preferences in Health Care Decision Making,* 147 Canadian Medical Association J 859, 862 (1992).

40. For criticisms of this feature of the Cassileth study, see Lesley F. Degner & Jeffrey A. Sloan, *Decision Making During Serious Illness: What Role Do Patients Really Want to Play?,* 45 J Clinical Epidemiology 941, 948 (1992); Jack Ende, et al, *Measuring Patient's Desire for Autonomy: Decision Making and Information-Seeking Preferences Among Medical Patients,* 4 J General Internal Medicine 23, 27 (1989). Other studies have used the same two questions about decision-making employed in the Cassileth study and have yielded relatively high desires to make decisions, although still with substantial numbers preferring to avoid decisions. Marc D. Silverstein, et al, *Amyotrophic Lateral Sclerosis and Life-Sustaining Therapy: Patients' Desires for Information, Participation in Decision Making, and Life-Sustaining Therapy,* 66 Mayo Clinic Proceedings 906, 908 (1991), for instance, reported that 70% of their respondents wanted to participate in medical decisions. Similarly, Christina G. Blanchard, et al, *Information and Decision-Making Preferences of Hospitalized Adult Cancer Patients,* 27 Social Science Medicine 1139, 1143 (1988), found that "almost one-third (30.5%) [of the cancer patients they interviewed] stated that they preferred to leave decisions about their medical care and treatment up to their physician."

41. Louis Harris & Associates, *Views of Informed Consent and Decisionmaking: Parallel Surveys of Physicians and the Public,* in President's Commission for the Study of Ethical Problems in Medicine and Biomedical and Behavioral Research, *Making Health Care Decisions: The Ethical and Legal Implications of Informed Consent in the Patient–Practitioner Relationship,* Volume Two: Appendices *Empirical Studies of Informed Consent* 17 (U S Gov't Printing Office, 1982).

42. Idem at 209. (Once again, the sicker the respondents, the less likely they were to want to make decisions.)

43. Jack Ende, et al, *Measuring Patients' Desire for Autonomy: Decision Making and Information-Seeking Preferences among Medical Patients,* 4 J General Internal Medicine 23, 27 (1989). For a persuasive effort to demonstrate that all the studies showing a higher desire for participation do not conflict with the conclusions of those studies showing a lower desire, see idem at 27–28.

44. Louis Harris & Associates, *Views of Informed Consent and Decisionmaking* at 17 (cited in note 41); Jack Ende, et al, *Measuring Patient's Desire for Autonomy: Decision Making and Information-Seeking Preferences among Medical Patients,* 4 J General Internal Medicine 23, 26–27 (1989); H.J. Sutherland, et al, *Cancer Patients: Their Desire for Information and Participation in Treatment Decisions,* 82 J Royal Society Medicine 260 (1989). Similarly, another study found that patients "who preferred leaving decisions to the physician had a lower performance status, i.e., in bed more than half of the day or totally bed-ridden, than those who preferred to participate in decisions . . . ." Christina G. Blanchard, et al, *Information and Decision-Making Preferences of Hospitalized Adult Cancer Patients,* 27 Social Science Medicine 1139, 1142 (1988). And it is suggestive that older people, who are likelier than younger people to be seriously ill or to have experienced serious illness, are also likelier to wish to delegate decisions. See, e.g., Cassileth, et al, 92 Annals of Internal Medicine 832 (cited in note 38). It is also suggestive that people with histories of serious illness were particularly unlikely to be anxious that their advance directives be strictly followed. But cf. Lesley F. Degner & Jeffrey A. Sloan, *Decision Making During Serious Illness: What Role Do Patients Really Want to Play?,* 45 J Clinical Epidemiology 941, 947 (1992), which found that symptom-distress levels were not related to patients' preferences about decisions.

45. *In re Quinlan,* 355 A2d 647 (NJ, 1976).

46. *Cruzan v. Director,* Missouri Department of Health, 497 US 261 (1990).

47. For instance, Caplan concludes that no more than 10% of the population has an advance directive. Arthur L. Caplan, *Can Autonomy be Saved?,* in *If I Were a Rich Man Could I Buy a Pancreas? and Other Essays on the Ethics of Health Care* 261 (Indiana U Press, 1992). Even those presumptively most in need of advance directives prepare them with surprising infrequency. Thus one study found that, while half of the thirty-nine nursing-home patients questioned had thought about end-of-life decisions, only six had actually signed advance directives. Eric L. Diamond, et al, *Decision-Making Ability and Advance Directive Preferences in Nursing Home Patients and Their Proxies,* 29 Gerontologist 622 (1989). One random survey of outpatients found that only 11% had discussed cardiopulmonary resuscitation with their doctors, while 67% had thought of doing so. (Forty-four percent had discussed the issue with someone else.) Mark H. Ebell, et al, *The Do-Not-Resuscitate Order: Outpatient Experience and Decision-Making,* 31 J Family Practice 630 (1990). Another study reports that only 9% of its respondents had discussed surrogate decision-makers with their doctors and that only 6% had discussed life-sustaining treatment. Bernard Lo, Gary A. McLeod, & Glenn Saika, *Patient Attitudes to Discussing Life-Sustaining Treatment,* 146 Archives of Internal Medicine 1613 (1986). For a review of studies suggesting that people rarely discuss termination of treatment with either their families or their doctors, see Ezekiel J. Emanuel & Linda L. Emanuel, *Proxy Decision Making for Incompetent Patients,* 267 JAMA 2067, 2068–69 (1992).

48. Arthur L. Caplan, *Can Autonomy be Saved?,* in *If I Were a Rich Man Could I Buy a Pancreas? and Other Essays on the Ethics of Health Care* 263 (Indiana U Press, 1992). For a thoughtful defense of people who decline to write advance directives, see Joanne Lynn, *Why I Don't Have a Living Will,* 19 Law, Medicine, & Health Care 101 (1991).

49. Ashwini Sehgal, et al, *How Strictly Do Dialysis Patients Want Their Advance Directives Followed?,* 267 JAMA 59, 60 (1992).

50. Idem at 61. "Sixty percent of subjects with prior written directives wanted advance directives followed strictly in our scenarios. By contrast, 33% of subjects without prior written directives wanted advance directives followed strictly . . . ." Idem. People with histories of other serious illness (cancer or stroke) were particularly unlikely to want their

advance directives strictly followed. Idem. For reflections on this problem, see Dan W. Brock, *Trumping Advance Directives,* 21 HCR 55 (Sept/Oct 1991).

51. Ruth R. Faden, et al, *Disclosure of Information to Patients in Medical Care,* 19 Medical Care 718, 732 (1981). Similarly, "the empirical and anecdotal studies of patients who refuse treatment almost never portray the process of obtaining informed consent as playing a causative role." Paul S. Appelbaum, Charles W. Lidz, & Alan Meisel, *Informed Consent: Legal Theory and Clinical Practice* 202 (Oxford U Press, 1987).

52. Paul S. Appelbaum & Loren Roth, *Patients Who Refuse Treatment in Medical Hospitals,* 250 JAMA 1296 (1983). The Harris Report observes that 79% of all those surveyed reported they had never refused treatment a doctor recommended. The report does not reveal what kind of treatment the other 21% refused or why. Louis Harris & Associates, *Making Health Care Decisions: Appendix B* at 184 (cited in note 41).

53. "Even when patients refuse recommended treatment, they do so usually not for elaborate reasons of religious or moral principle but most often because they have lost the trust essential for care, i.e., they do not believe the physician or the staff cares for them and they can no longer entrust their care to these persons . . . ." Richard Sherlock, *Reasonable Men and Sick Human Beings,* 80 American J Medicine 2 (1986). Perhaps the widespread phenomenon of patient "noncompliance" represents a kind of passive resistance to doctors making medical decisions. I suspect, however, it represents a good deal more as well.

54. Of course, there are good reasons not to expect massive patient refusals. Informed consent often comes late in the process of making decisions, doctors can frame information to make the recommended choice relatively attractive, and so on. But the virtual absence of patient refusals is too impressive to be accounted for just in terms of the defects of informed consent.

55. Marlynn L. May & Daniel B. Stengel, *Who Sues Their Doctors? How Patients Handle Medical Grievances,* 24 Law & Society Rev 105, 116 (1990). Their results "tentatively suggest that patients are not affected by many of the procedural niceties of these efforts [to improve communication between doctor and patient]: involving the patient as partner, informing the patient about care, not rushing the patient's visit, and taking personal care about the patient's medical problem." Idem at 118.

56. Katz (disapprovingly) quotes Richard Selzer in a hyperbolic version of such comments: "When I try to call the patient in on a consultation and say, 'Which alternative would you prefer?' *invariably* the patient says, 'What do you mean, which alternative? I want you to tell me what to do. You're the doctor.'" Jay Katz, *The Silent World of Doctor and Patient* 126 (Free Press, 1984) (quoting F. Middleton, *Profile: Richard Selzer,* 1 New Haven Magazine 37 (July 1983)) (emphasis in original).

57. See, e.g., William M. Strull, Bernard Lo, & Gerald Charles, *Do Patients Want to Participate in Medical Decision Making?,* 252 JAMA 2990, 2992 (1984).

58. Cornelius & Kathryn Morgan Ryan, *A Private Battle* (Simon & Schuster, 1979).

59. His story is described in his wife's memoir: Martha Weinman Lear, *Heartsounds* (Simon & Schuster, 1980). She herself, however, exclaims at one point to one of her husband's doctors, "Damn, don't give me options. Give me guidance." Idem at 291.

60. Gayle Feldman, *You Don't Have to Be Your Mother* 22 (Norton, 1994).

61. William Martin, *My Prostate and Me: Dealing with Prostate Cancer* (Cadell & Davies, 1994).

62. Lest this seem too strange to be true, I provide a citation—idem at 54—and quote one sentence of the passage I am referring to: "By noon, I was totally engrossed in trying to unravel the riddles of prostate cancer, sometimes almost to the point of forgetting just

why I had developed such a keen interest in the subject." Another victim of prostate cancer—the president and CEO of Intel—said the more he read medical articles, "the clearer they got, just as had been the case when I was studying silicon device physics 30 years ago. That added a strange element of enjoyment to a process that was, overall, very scary." Andy Grove, *Taking on Prostate Cancer,* Fortune 55, 60 (May 13, 1996).

63. To name just some of many: Bernice Kavinoky, *Voyage and Return* (Norton, 1966); Fitzhugh Mullan, *Vital Signs: A Young Doctor's Struggle with Cancer* (Farrar, Straus, Giroux, 1983); Sue Baier & Mary Zimmeth Schomaker, *Bed Number Ten* (CRC Press, 1985); Oliver Sacks, *A Leg to Stand On* (HarperCollins, 1987); Madeleine L'Engle, *Two-Part Invention: The Story of a Marriage* (Harper & Row, 1988); Betty Garton Ulrich, *Rooted in the Sky: A Faith to Cope With Cancer* (Judson, 1989); Barbara D. Webster, *All of a Piece: A Life With Multiple Sclerosis* (Johns Hopkins U Press, 1989); Molly Haskell, *Love and Other Infectious Diseases: A Memoir* (Citadel, 1990); Robert F. Murphy, *The Body Silent* (Norton, 1990); Philip Roth, *Patrimony: A True Story* (Simon & Schuster, 1991); Anatole Broyard, *Intoxicated by My Illness, And Other Writings on Life and Death* (Fawcett Columbine, 1992); G. Edward Rozar & David B. Biebel, *Laughing in the Face of AIDS: A Surgeon's Personal Battle* (Baker, 1992).

64. Mary Cooper Greene, *Living With a Broken String* (no publisher, 1987).

65. Sue Baier & Mary Zimmeth Schomaker, *Bed Number Ten* no page number (CRC Press, 1985).

66. Idem.

67. William D. Sharpe, *Meniere's Disease,* in Harvey Mandell & Howard Spiro, eds, *When Doctors Get Sick* 62 (Plenum Medical, 1988).

68. Joyce L. Dunlop, *Prosthetic Hips,* in Harvey Mandell & Howard Spiro, eds, *When Doctors Get Sick* 80 (Plenum Medical, 1988).

69. Laura Chester, *Lupus Novice: Toward Self-Healing* 73 (Station Hill Press, 1987).

70. Idem at 76.

71. Such an olio of methods is common: "In reading these pathographies, one is struck partly by the bizarreness of the combinations of treatment: also by the ease with which health care is treated as a commodity and pursued as such. Orthodox medicine is but one of several 'brands' available." Anne Hunsaker Hawkins, *Reconstructing Illness: Studies in Pathography* 147–48 (Purdue U Press, 1993). "Several" hardly captures the cavalcade of alternative remedies people not only try but passionately endorse. For an astonishing list of the remedies pressed on one sick man, see Floyd Skloot, *The Night-Side: Chronic Fatigue Syndrome and the Illness Experience* 105–18 (Troy Line Press, 1996). On the relationship between conventional and alternative medicine in black culture, see Loudell F. Snow, *Walkin' Over Medicine* (Westview, 1993).

72. Victor G. Cicirelli, *Family Caregiving: Autonomous and Paternalistic Decision Making* 111 (Sage, 1992). Another 20% "felt they should discuss the decisions with their daughters but make their own decisions." Idem at 112. (The mothers "had sufficient cognitive abilities to comprehend and respond to a wide variety of questions." Idem at 113. They were generally not seriously ill or frail, and they had enough initiative to volunteer for the study.) Cicirelli also reports that elderly parents were significantly more willing than the children who cared for them to countenance paternalistic decisions. Cicirelli hypothesizes "that elderly care receivers were more concerned with issues about the health and safety of the older people in the vignettes presented to them than with any considerations of autonomy." Idem at 108–9.

73. Dallas M. High, *Standards for Surrogate Decision Making: What the Elderly Want,* 17 J Long-Term Administration 8 (1989). The study asked patients whether they

wanted surrogates to make the decision they would have made or the decision that was best for them. The patients split evenly.

74. Leslie J. Blackhall, et al, *Ethnicity and Attitudes Toward Patient Autonomy,* 274 JAMA 820 (1995). On the role of families in medical decisions, see Richard Sherlock & C. Mary Dingus, *Families and the Gravely Ill: Roles, Rules, and Rights* (Greenwood, 1988); John Hardwig, *What About the Family?,* 20 HCR 5 (Mar/Apr 1990); Symposium, *Ethics, Bioethics, and Family Law,* 1992 Utah L Rev 735; Jeffrey Blustein, *The Family in Medical Decisionmaking,* 23 HCR 6 (May/June 1993); Hilde Lindemann Nelson & James Lindemann Nelson, *The Patient in the Family: An Ethics of Medicine and Families* (Routledge, 1995). For an extended description of how one father and son handled the father's medical problems, see Philip Roth, *Patrimony: A True Story* (Simon & Schuster, 1991).

Chapter 3

1. For a passionate statement of this position, see Jay Katz, *The Silent World of Doctor and Patient* (Free Press, 1984). For a more matter-of-fact one, see David S. Brody, *The Patient's Role in Clinical Decision-Making,* 93 Annals of Internal Medicine 718, 719 (1980), which can imagine no other reason that patients might delegate decisions than that physicians have traditionally controlled decisions and that patients "may be comforted by the belief that their physician is all-knowing and all-powerful" and "may not want to be responsible for decisions that may ultimately lead to unfavorable outcomes." For a sympathetic though ultimately critical statement of the old tradition, see Albert R. Jonsen, *The New Medicine and the Old Ethics* 80–102 (Harvard U Press, 1990). For an effective attack on it, see Allen Buchanan, *Medical Paternalism,* 7 Philosophy & Public Affairs 370 (1978). On the role of professions generally, see Andrew Abbott, *The System of Professions: An Essay on the Division of Expert Labor* (U Chicago Press, 1988), and Elliott A. Krause, *Death of the Guilds: Professions, States, and the Advance of Capitalism, 1930 to the Present* (Yale U Press, 1996).

2. *A Leg to Stand On* 158 (HarperCollins, 1984).

3. Irving L. Janis & Leon Mann, *Decision Making: A Psychological Analysis of Conflict, Choice, and Commitment* 6 (Free Press, 1977).

4. Idem at 15.

5. Donald A. Redelmeier, Paul Rozin, & Daniel Kahneman, *Understanding Patients' Decisions: Cognitive and Emotional Perspectives,* 270 JAMA 72, 72 (1993).

6. Marvin S. Cohen, *Three Paradigms for Viewing Decision Biases,* in Gary A. Klein, et al, eds, *Decision Making in Action: Models and Methods* 46 (Ablex Publishers, 1993).

7. Irving L. Janis, *The Patient as Decision Maker,* in W. Doyle Gentry, ed, *Handbook of Behavioral Medicine* 326, 358 (Guilford, 1984).

8. Janis & Mann, *Decision Making* at 16 (cited in note 3). On the sadly numerous defects of human reasoning, see Richard Nisbett & Lee Ross, *Human Inference: Strategies and Shortcomings of Social Judgment* (Prentice-Hall, 1980); Daniel Kahneman, Paul Slovic, & Amos Tversky, *Judgment Under Uncertainty: Heuristics and Biases* (Cambridge U Press, 1982); Amitai Etzioni, *The Moral Dimension: Toward a New Economics* (Free Press, 1988). For discussion of how those defects affect medical decisions, see Janis, *The Patient as Decision Maker* (cited in note 7); Jon F. Merz & Baruch Fischhoff, *Informed Consent Does Not Mean Rational Consent: Cognitive Limitations on Decision-Making,* 11 J Legal Medicine 321 (1990); Donald A. Redelmeier, Paul Rozin, & Daniel

Kahneman, *Understanding Patients' Decisions: Cognitive and Emotional Perspectives,* 270 JAMA 72 (1993).

9. Lee Roy Beach & Raanan Lipshitz, *Why Classical Decision Theory is an Inappropriate Standard for Evaluating and Aiding Most Human Decision Making,* in Gary A. Klein, et al, eds, *Decision Making in Action: Models and Methods* 28 (Ablex Publishers, 1993). "Studies of the psychological and physiological concomitants of decision making have found that there are increases in anxiety symptoms, sleeplessness, and psychosomatic symptoms, as well as marked changes in heart rate, finger pulse amplitude, and galvanic skin response, when a person is required to make a difficult choice . . . ." Janis, *The Patient as Decision Maker* at 335 (cited in note 7).

10. "The overall conclusion of the investigators is that patients are not active in seeking information and doctors are not active in giving it. Our own empirical investigations are in agreement with these findings, as is the bulk of the literature on patient 'compliance.'" Alan Meisel & Loren H. Roth, *Toward an Informed Discussion of Informed Consent: A Review and Critique of the Empirical Studies,* 25 Arizona L Rev 265, 274–75 (1983) (footnotes omitted).

11. Edward E. Rosenblum, *The Doctor* 52 (Ballantine, 1988).

12. Idem at 115.

13. On the impediments to securing information from patients, see Irving Kenneth Zola, *Structural Constraints in the Doctor–Patient Relationship: The Case of Non-Compliance,* in Leon Eisenberg & Arthur Kleinman, eds, *The Relevance of Social Science for Medicine* 245 (D. Reidel, 1981).

14. Virginia Woolf, *On Being Ill,* in *The Moment and Other Essays* 15–16 (Hogarth, 1952). As one journalist found, "In trying to describe—or even to think about—what goes on in the body, the politics of the body, we exhaust the simple vocabularies almost immediately (*hurts here . . . numb . . . sharp . . . dull ache . . . sore*) and must invent images and metaphors. These images take on a life of their own, a reality . . . ." Lance Morrow, *Heart: A Memoir* 114 (Warner, 1995). And a poet: "The house of the body in pain is furnished with inexact metaphors that resist tidy medical labeling, and with approximate descriptions of extreme states. You find yourself at a loss, with language running dry just when needed most—that is, when explaining an internal teeming microcosm to the medical world, the physical therapy world, *and* to the macrocosmic world of relationship to others in general." Suzanne E. Berger, *Horizontal Woman: The Story of a Body in Exile* 49 (Houghton Mifflin, 1996).

15. Ian Stevenson, *Observations on Illness from the Inside (Bronchiectasis),* in Max Pinner & Benjamin F. Miller, eds, *When Doctors Are Patients* 223–24 (Norton, 1952).

16. Louise DeSalvo, *Breathless: An Asthma Journal* 25 (Beacon Press, 1997).

17. Giorgio Pressburger, *The Law of White Spaces* 137 (Vintage, 1994).

18. Arnold R. Beisser, *Flying Without Wings* 18 (Doubleday, 1989).

19. Suzanne E. Berger, *Horizontal Woman: The Story of a Body in Exile* 49 (Houghton Mifflin, 1996).

20. Charles L. Bosk, *Occupational Rituals in Patient Management,* 303 NEJM 71, 72 (1980). On the centrality of uncertainty in medical training and practice, see Charles L. Bosk, *Forgive and Remember: Managing Medical Failure* (U Chicago Press, 1979); Joseph W. Schneider & Peter Conrad, *Having Epilepsy: The Experience and Control of Illness* 60 (Temple U Press, 1983); Jay Katz, *The Silent World of Doctor and Patient* 165–206 (Free Press, 1984); Renée C. Fox, *Training for Uncertainty,* in *Essays in Medical Sociology* 25 (Transaction Books, 1988); Renée C. Fox, *The Evolution of Medical Uncertainty* at 533 in idem; Robert Zussman, *Intensive Care: Medical Ethics and the Medical*

Profession 116–22 (U Chicago Press, 1992). On uncertainty in the work of one internist, see Robert A. Hahn, *Sickness and Healing: An Anthropological Perspective* 173–208 (Yale U Press, 1995). On the social nature of medical uncertainty, see Zussman, *Intensive Care* at 116–22 (cited in this note).

21. Jay Katz, *The Silent World of Doctor and Patient* 166 (Free Press, 1984).

22. Eric J. Cassell, *The Changing Concept of the Ideal Physician,* Daedalus 185, 186 (Spring 1986).

23. Idem at 191.

24. Renée C. Fox, *Experiment Perilous: Physicians and Patients Facing the Unknown* 238 (U Pennsylvania Press, 1974) (quoting Walsh McDermott, *A Consideration of the Present Ethics of Clinical Investigation*).

25. George Eliot, *Middlemarch* 93 (Penguin Books, 1994).

26. H. A. Waldron & L. Vickerstaff, *Intimations of Quality. Ante-Mortem and Post-Mortem Diagnoses* (Nuffield Provincial Hospitals Trust, 1977), quoted in Thomas McKeown, *The Role of Medicine: Dream, Mirage, or Nemesis* 32 (Princeton U Press, 1979).

27. For a fine explanation of why professional diagnoses are complex and arduous, see Andrew Abbott, *The System of Professions: An Essay on the Division of Expert Labor* 40–44 (U Chicago Press, 1988).

28. Donald R. Cohodes, *Through the Looking Glass: Decision Making and Chemotherapy,* 14 Health Affairs 203, 206 (1995). Cohodes was the director of federal systems for the Blue Cross and Blue Shield Association and a member of the editorial board of the journal *Health Affairs.*

29. On how hard put physicians must be to find language for describing magnitudes of risk, see Peter H. Schuck, *Rethinking Informed Consent,* 103 Yale L J 899, 948–49 (1994). Yet less sanguine is Claire O. Leonard, Gary A. Chase, & Barton Childs, *Genetic Counseling: A Consumer's View,* 287 NEJM 433, 438 (1972), which suggests that a failure to understand probability is an important barrier to the success of genetic counseling and cites psychological studies indicating "that probability comprehension is a developmental trait and there are differences in the degree to which individuals achieve competence."

30. Edward E. Rosenbaum, *The Doctor* 119 (Ballantine, 1988).

31. Renée C. Fox, *The Human Condition of Health Professionals*, in *Essays in Medical Sociology* 576 (Transaction Books, 1988).

32. "Only statistics seem able to handle the high degree of variability and the complex pattern of correlated data. With so many variables, practically nothing comes clear and distinct; there are thousands of combinations possible. So calculating the odds of this and that, given such and such, seems the only way to have a reasonable basis for decision." K.D. Clouser, *Approaching the Logic of Diagnosis,* in K. Schaffner, ed, *Logic of Discovery and Diagnosis in Medicine* (U California Press, 1985), quoted in Marc Berg, *Rationalizing Medical Work: Decision-Support Techniques and Medical Practices* 30 (MIT Press, 1997).

33. The insistent difficulty of these decisions is suggested by the greatly complex attempt to work out in "greatly simplified form" the expected values of two treatment options in Norman F. Boyd, et al, *Whose Utilities for Decision Analysis?,* 10 Medical Decision Making 58 (1990). Robert Zussman argues that even discussions about withdrawing treatment are often not "either/or" decisions, but rather a series of discrete decisions about whether to attempt one treatment among many. Robert Zussman, *Intensive Care: Medical Ethics and the Medical Profession* 139–60 (U Chicago Press, 1992).

34. Edward E. Rosenbaum, *The Doctor* 154 (Ballantine, 1988).

35. Laura Evans, *The Climb of My Life: A Miraculous Journey From the Edge of Death to the Victory of a Lifetime* 134 (HarperSanFrancisco, 1996).

36. *My Breast: One Woman's Cancer Story* 158 (Addison-Wesley, 1992).

37. Idem.

38. Idem at 109.

39. Evelyn Shirk, *After the Stroke: Coping With America's Third Leading Cause of Death* 75 (Prometheus Books, 1991).

40. Marc Berg, *Rationalizing Medical Work: Decision-Support Techniques and Medical Practices* 55 (MIT Press, 1997).

41. Ben Watt, *Patient: The True Story of a Rare Illness* 32 (Grove Press, 1996).

42. *Love's Work: A Reckoning with Life* 102–3 (Schocken, 1995).

43. Eric Hodgins, *Episode: Report on the Accident Inside My Skull* 15–16 (Atheneum, 1964) (emphasis in original).

44. Ernest A. Hirsch, *Starting Over* 50 (Christopher Publishing House, 1977).

45. Tim Brookes, *Catching My Breath: An Asthmatic Explores His Illness* 72 (Times Books, 1994).

46. Rosalind MacPhee, *Picasso's Woman: A Breast Cancer Story* 41 (Kodansha, 1996).

47. Idem at 47.

48. Fanny Gaynes, *How am I Gonna Find a Man if I'm Dead?* 57–58 (Morgin Press, 1994).

49. William Martin, *My Prostate and Me: Dealing With Prostate Cancer* 103 (Cadell & Davies, 1994).

50. Joyce Wadler, *My Breast: One Woman's Cancer Story* 39 (Addison-Wesley, 1992).

51. Tim Brookes, *Catching My Breath: An Asthmatic Explores His Illness* 140 (Times Books, 1994).

52. Agnes de Mille, *Reprieve: A Memoir* 135–36 (Doubleday, 1981).

53. Thomas S. Kuhn, *The Structure of Scientific Revolutions* 44 n. 1 (U Chicago Press, 1970). See also Donald A. Schon, *The Reflective Practitioner: How Professionals Think in Action* (Basic Books, 1983).

53a. Gary Klein, *Sources of Power: How People Make Decisions* 17 (MIT Press, 1998).

53b. Raanan Lipshitz, *Converging Themes in the Study of Decision Making in Realistic Settings,* in Gary A. Klein, et al, eds, *Decision Making in Action: Models and Methods* 124 (Ablex Publishers, 1993).

53c. Klein, *Sources of Power* at 280 (cited in note 53a).

54. *Courage: The Testimony of a Cancer Patient* (Pantheon, 1991).

55. Intensive Care at 112 (cited in note 33). On cultural and individual differences that complicate discussions of symptoms like pain, see Arthur Kleinman, *The Illness Narratives: Suffering, Healing, and the Human Condition* 1–30 (Basic Books, 1988). On cultural differences, see, e.g., M. Azorowski, *Cultural Components in Response to Pain,* 8 J Social Issues 16 (1952); Ronald C. Kessler, et al, *Social Psychology and Health,* in Karen Cook, Gary Fine, & James S. House, eds, *Sociological Perspectives on Social Psychology* 558 (Allyn & Bacon, 1995). On differences between the ways doctors and patients understand illness, see S. Kay Toombs, *The Meaning of Illness: A Phenomenological Account of the Different Perspectives of Physician and Patient* (Kluwer Academic, 1992).

56. Donna McFarlane, *Division of Surgery* 61 (Women's Press, 1994).

57. Kessler, et al, *Social Psychology and Health* at 548 (cited in note 55); M. Zborowski, *Cultural Components in Response to Pain,* 8 J Social Issues 16 (1952); Irving

Kenneth Zola, *Culture and Symptoms—An Analysis of Patients' Presenting Complaints,* 31 American Sociological Rev 615 (1966).

58. Francesca Morosani Thompson, *Going for the Cure* 131 (International Myeloma Foundation, 1989).

59. Michael P. Kelly, *Colitis* 68 (Routledge, 1992). For a litany of doubts about "the cognitive and psychological capacity of the nondisabled to form meaningful judgments about various health states," see Ellen Smith Pryor, *The Tort Law Debate, Efficiency, and the Kingdom of the Ill: A Critique of the Insurance Theory of Causation,* 79 Virginia L Rev 91, 114 (1993).

60. For a sophisticated statement of this point, see Dan W. Brock, *The Ideal of Shared Decision Making Between Physicians and Patients,* 1 Kennedy Institute of Ethics J 28 (1991).

61. *The Illusion of Patient Choice in End-of-Life Decisions,* 267 JAMA 2101, 2102 (1992), citing T. R. Malloy, et al, *How Interventions Are Described Affects Patients' Decisions About Life Sustaining Treatment,* in *Program of the American Geriatric Society/ American Federation for Aging Research Annual Scientific Meeting.* Abstract A2 (1991). To like effect is Barbara J. McNeil, et al, *On the Elicitation of Preferences for Alternative Therapies,* 306 NEJM 1259 (1982). This problem is helpfully discussed in Amos Tversky & Daniel Kahneman, *Rational Choice and the Framing of Decisions,* in Karen Schweers Cook & Margaret Levi, *The Limits of Rationality* 60 (U Chicago Press, 1990). When the inconsistency of their response is explained to people, many say both that they wish to be consistent and that they wish to adhere to their inconsistent preferences. Idem at 70.

62. Renée R. Anspach, *Deciding Who Lives: Fateful Choices in the Intensive-Care Nursery* 101 (U California Press, 1993).

63. Thus Max Lerner discovered "something I didn't know at the start: that in a serious illness the news comes in installments, and the second may make the initial news look pale. The first installment told me I 'had a problem,' as my internist put it, as gently as he could. The second told me how much time I had left." *Wrestling With the Angel: A Memoir of My Triumph Over Illness* 24 (Simon & Schuster, 1990).

64. Paulette Bates Alden, *Crossing the Moon: A Journey Through Infertility* 264 (Hungry Mind Press, 1996).

65. *In Love with Daylight: A Memoir of Recovery* 177 (Simon & Schuster, 1995).

66. Specialization means new illnesses require new doctors, and hospital stays have shortened, so doctors and patients have less time to become acquainted. John F. Steiner, et al, *Changing Patterns of Disease on an Inpatient Medical Service: 1961–62 to 1981–82,* 83 American J Medicine 331, 334 (1987).

67. For an argument that patients have, personally and vicariously, had experience with the uncertainty of medical practice and with medical error and that they are familiar with medical "controversies, contradictions, and even reversals," see Stephen A. Eraker, John P. Kirscht, & Marshall H. Becker, *Understanding and Improving Patient Compliance,* 100 Annals of Internal Medicine 258, 259 (1984).

68. Francesca Morosani Thompson, *Going for the Cure* 141 (International Myeloma Foundation, 1989).

69. Joseph W. Schneider & Peter Conrad, *Having Epilepsy: The Experience and Control of Illness* 172 (Temple U Press, 1983).

70. Claire O. Leonard, Gary A. Chase, & Barton Childs, *Genetic Counseling: A Consumer's View,* 287 NEJM 433, 437–38 (1972).

71. Joel Solkoff, *Learning to Live Again: My Triumph Over Cancer* 39–40 (Holt, Rinehart, & Winston, 1983). In Schneider and Conrad's experience, this "'research' activ-

ity produced results that were not always accurate . . . ." *Having Epilepsy* at 210 (cited in note 69). Nor do patients keep clearly in mind who said what so they can assign each datum the weight it deserves. In my interviews, for instance, I virtually never find patients who remember the source of what they have learned about their illness.

72. Amitai Etzioni, *The Moral Dimension: Toward A New Economics* 117 (Free Press, 1988). "The number of crucially relevant categories [in making decisions] usually far exceeds 7 ± 2, the limits of man's capacity for processing information in immediate memory . . . ." Irving L. Janis & Leon Mann, *Decision Making: A Psychological Analysis of Conflict, Choice, and Commitment* 22 (Free Press, 1977).

73. Barbara J. McNeil, et al, *On the Elicitation of Preferences for Alternative Therapies,* 306 NEJM 1259, 1262 (1982): "The finding that radiation therapy was less attractive when the treatments were identified indicates that people relied more on preexisting beliefs regarding the treatments than on the statistical data presented to them."

74. Paul Slovic, Baruch Fischhoff, & Sarah Lichtenstein, *Facts Versus Fears: Understanding Perceived Risk,* in Daniel Kahneman, Paul Slovic, & Amos Tversky, eds, *Judgment Under Uncertainty: Heuristics and Biases* 467–68 (Cambridge U Press, 1982). These unrepresentative reports help lead to wildly inaccurate (but nevertheless confident) estimates of various kinds of risk. See idem.

75. See, e.g., Lesley Fallowfield with Andrew Clark, *Breast Cancer* 17–26 (Routledge, 1991).

76. Joseph Heller & Speed Vogel, *No Laughing Matter* 90 (Putnam, 1986).

77. Tim Brookes, *Catching My Breath: An Asthmatic Explores His Illness* 72 (Times Books, 1994).

78. Gayle Feldman, *You Don't Have to Be Your Mother* 37 (Norton, 1994).

79. Lee Modjeska, *Keeper of the Night: A Portrait of Life in the Shadow of Death* 18–19 (LuraMedia, 1995).

80. Idem at 93–94.

81. As one of Cornelius Ryan's doctors commented to Mrs. Ryan,

"In the course of a long conversation having to do with explaining the nature of the disease process and the treatment options that are open to the patient, there are often many misconceptions. This seems to be particularly true when a patient has taken an avowed interest in finding out as much as possible about his disease. . . . This often generates preconceived notions which become increasingly difficult for the patient to deal with."

Cornelius & Kathryn Morgan Ryan, *A Private Battle* 178 n.* (Simon & Schuster, 1979).

82. *Sources of Power: How People Make Decisions* 280 (MIT Press, 1998). See Ellen J. Langer, *The Illusion of Control,* 32 J Personality & Social Psychology 311 (1975), for the evidence that people overestimate their control over events.

83. James C. Wade, *The Patient/Physician Relationship: One Doctor's View,* 14 Health Affairs 209, 211 (1995).

84. Idem at 211–12.

84a. *Sources of Power* at 104–05 (cited in note 82).

85. Tim Brookes, *Catching My Breath: An Asthmatic Explores His Illness* 277 (Times Books, 1994).

86. Ben Watt, *Patient: The True Story of a Rare Illness* 82 (Grove Press, 1996).

87. May Sarton, *After the Stroke: A Journal* 37 (Norton, 1988).

88. Max Lerner, *Wrestling With the Angel: A Memoir of My Triumph Over Illness* 32 (Simon & Schuster, 1990).

89. For a disturbingly vivid description of this problem, see Robert Jon Pensack & Dwight Arnan Williams, *Raising Lazarus* (G.P. Putnam, 1994).

90. Floyd Skloot, *The Night-Side: Chronic Fatigue Syndrome and the Illness Experience* 121 (Story Line Press, 1996).

91. Sally Wagner, *How Do You Kiss a Blind Girl?* 5 (Charles C. Thomas, 1986).

92. Brookes, *Catching My Breath* at 33 (cited in note 85).

93. Lesley Fallowfield with Andrew Clark, *Breast Cancer* 38 (Routledge, 1992).

94. Musa Mayer, *Examining Myself: One Woman's Story of Breast Cancer Treatment and Recovery* 12 (Faber & Faber, 1993).

95. Philip Roth, *Patrimony: A True Story* 143 (Simon & Schuster, 1991). For a review of evidence that a wish to terminate treatment is often occasioned by treatable depression, see Yale Kamisar, *Are Laws Against Assisted Suicide Unconstitutional?*, 23 HCR 32 (May/June 1993).

96. Robert Pensack & Dwight Williams, *Raising Lazarus* 122–23 (G. P. Putnam, 1994).

97. Evan Handler, *Time on Fire: My Comedy of Terrors* 205 (Little, Brown, 1996).

98. Rosalind MacPhee, *Picasso's Woman: A Breast Cancer Story* 56 (Kodansha, 1996).

99. Juliet Wittman, *Breast Cancer Journal: A Century of Petals* 280 (Fulcrum, 1993).

100. Troyen A. Brennan, *Just Doctoring: Medical Ethics in the Liberal State* 77 (U California Press, 1991).

101. Bradford H. Gray, *The Profit Motive and Patient Care: The Changing Accountability of Doctors and Hospitals* 218–19 (Harvard U Press, 1991).

102. See Arnold S. Relman, *The New Medical–Industrial Complex,* 303 NEJM 963 (1980).

103. On the bureaucratization of medical care, see Eviatar Zerubavel, *Patterns of Time in Hospital Life: A Sociological Perspective* (U Chicago Press, 1979); Paul Starr, *The Social Transformation of American Medicine* (Basic Books, 1982); Anselm Strauss, et al, *Social Organization of Medical Work* (U Chicago Press, 1985); Victor R. Fuchs, *The Health Economy* (Harvard U Press, 1986); Eli Ginzberg, *The Medical Triangle: Physicians, Politicians, and the Public* (Harvard U Press, 1990); Gray, *The Profit Motive and Patient Care* (cited in note 101); Robert Zussman, *Intensive Care: Medical Ethics and the Medical Profession* (U Chicago Press, 1992). I discuss bureaucratization in Chapter 6.

104. Eliot Freidson, *Doctoring Together: A Study of Professional Social Control* 10 (U Chicago Press, 1975).

105. Renée R. Anspach, *Deciding Who Lives: Fateful Choices in the Intensive-Care Nursery* 117 (U California Press, 1993).

106. See Joel E. Frader, *Difficulties in Providing Intensive Care,* 64 Pediatrics 10, 14 (1979).

107. Carolyn Wiener, et al, *Patient Power: Complex Issues Need Complex Answers,* 11 Social Policy 30, 34 (1980).

108. Charles L. Bosk, *Occupational Rituals in Patient Management,* 303 NEJM 71, 72 (1980).

109. For an impressive statement of how different professional tasks produce different perspectives, see Renée R. Anspach, *Prognostic Conflict in Life-and-Death Decisions: The Organization as an Ecology of Knowledge,* 28 J Health & Social Behavior 215 (1987), and Renée R. Anspach, *Deciding Who Lives: Fateful Choices in the Intensive Care Nursery* (U California Press, 1993).

110. On utilization management, see Gray, *The Profit Motive and Patient Care* at 274–320 (cited in note 101).

111. "[P]eople generally neither make a single choice nor plan a set of choices; they continue to ask advice and seek help from a wide variety of lay, professional, and semi-

professional others until the situation is resolved or options are exhausted." Bernice A. Pescosolido, *Beyond Rational Choice: The Social Dynamics of How People Seek Help,* 97 American J Sociology 1096, 1113 (1992).

112. On this problem, see Anspach, *Deciding Who Lives* at 110–23 (cited in note 109). On the way the structure of the hospital influences medical decisions, see Zussman, *Intensive Care* at 116–22 (cited in note 103). On shifts and rotations, see Eviatar Zerubavel, *Patterns of Time in Hospital Life: A Sociological Perspective* (U Chicago Press, 1979).

113. Daniel F. Chambliss, *Beyond Caring: Hospitals, Nurses, and the Social Organization of Ethics* 65 (U Chicago Press, 1996).

114. Carol A. Heimer, *Your Baby's Fine, Just Fine: Certification Procedures, Meetings, and the Supply of Information in Neonatal Intensive Care Units,* in James F. Short, Jr., & Lee Clarke, eds, *Organizations, Uncertainties, and Risk* 180 (Westview, 1992).

115. Idem at 181–82.

116. Idem at 180.

117. Fred Davis, *Passage Through Crisis: Polio Victims and Their Families* 65–66 (Transaction Books, 1991).

118. Chambliss, *Beyond Caring* at 177 (cited in note 113).

119. H. T. Wright, *The Matthew Tree* 12 (Pantheon, 1975). In addition, the "organizational complexity of group practices can be a barrier to client utilization of services because people are unused to dealing with bureaucracies for their medical care." Edward J. Speedling, *Heart Attack: The Family Response at Home and in the Hospital* 128 (Tavistock, 1982).

120. Joie Harrison McGrail, *Fighting Back: One Woman's Struggle Against Cancer* 79 (Harper & Row, 1978).

121. Sue Baier & Mary Zimmeth Schomaker, *Bed Number Ten* 141 (CRC Press, 1986). One illuminating study, for instance, reports that, in the cardiology unit studied, five or more doctors were "not infrequently" making decisions about a single patient. Charles W. Lidz, Alan Meisel, & Mark Munetz, *Chronic Disease: The Sick Role and Informed Consent,* 9 Culture, Medicine & Psychiatry 8 (1985).

122. Gillian Rose, *Love's Work: A Reckoning with Life* 101 (Schocken, 1995).

123. Judith Alexander Brice, *Ulcerative Colitis and Avascular Necrosis of Hips,* in Harvey Mandell and Howard Spiro, eds, *When Doctors Get Sick* 182 (Plenum Medical, 1988) (emphasis in original).

124. Abraham Verghese, *My Own Country: A Doctor's Story* 266 (Vintage, 1995). Group meetings, sometimes quite large ones, certainly occur. But they are expensive, time-consuming, and hard to convene, and they thus cannot be called too often. Meetings to provide patients information compete with meetings for other organizational purposes, including internal communication.

125. On this point and how to adapt informed-consent law to it, see Paul S. Appelbaum, Charles W. Lidz, & Alan Meisel, *Informed Consent: Legal Theory and Clinical Practice* (Oxford U Press, 1987).

126. Roberta G. Simmons, Susan Klein Marine, & Richard L. Simmons, *Gift of Life: The Effect of Organ Transplantation on Individual, Family, and Societal Dynamics* 260 (Transaction Books, 1987).

127. On the merits of such a decisional approach, particularly for medical decisions, see Amitai Etzioni, *The Moral Dimension: Toward a New Economics* 128–35 (Free Press, 1988).

128. Dan W. Brock, *The Ideal of Shared Decision Making Between Physicians and Patients,* 1 Kennedy Institute of Ethics J 28, 28 (1991).

129. Or as some commentators seem to believe. For example, Shultz remarks confidently that patients "are capable, indeed uniquely so, of balancing ultimate costs and benefits of care decisions." Marjorie Maguire Shultz, *From Informed Consent to Patient Choice: A New Protected Interest,* 95 Yale L J 219, 281 (1985).

130. Lee Clarke, *Context Dependency and Risk Decision Making,* in James F. Short, Jr., & Lee Clarke, eds, *Organizations, Uncertainties, and Risk* 28 (Westview, 1992).

131. Max Lerner, *Wrestling With the Angel: A Memoir of My Triumph Over Illness* 40 (Simon & Schuster, 1990).

132. Idem at 42.

133. For a moving expression of this discovery, see Vicki Williams, *The Horror Is Worth It,* Newsweek 14 (Oct 9, 1989). Or take the case of Elizabeth Bouvia. *Bouvia v. Superior Court,* 225 Cal Rptr 297 (Cal App 2 Dist 1986). Bouvia was a twenty-eight-year-old quadriplegic. She was capable and intelligent. But her arms and legs were useless. She suffered from cruel and crippling arthritis. She could do nothing for herself. She asked to be denied food so that she might die. She fought a bitter and determined battle for death through the courts. Eventually, they granted her wish. But when they did, she changed her mind and chose to live. Hers is a common experience—that until people are confronted with the final reality of their own case, they do not know how they would react. If Elizabeth Bouvia was uncertain after so much time, thought, and struggle whether she wanted to live, how easy will patients with fewer resources find it to reach settled views on these perplexing problems?

134. Amitai Etzioni, *The Moral Dimension: Toward a New Economics* 147 (Free Press, 1988).

134a. Judith Orasanu & Terry Connolly, *The Reinvention of Decision Making,* in Gary A. Klein, et al, eds, *Decision Making in Action: Models and Methods* 18 (Ablex Publishers, 1993). For the argument that "it is impossible to free ourselves from inconsistency," see Gary Klein, *Sources of Power: How People Make Decisions* 264–67 (MIT Press, 1998).

135. Howard S. Becker, *Notes on the Concept of Commitment,* 66 American J Sociology 32, 38 (1960).

136. Lee Clarke, *Context Dependency and Risk Decision Making,* in James F. Short, Jr., & Lee Clarke, eds, *Organizations, Uncertainties, and Risk* 30 (Westview, 1992).

137. Idem at n.4.

138. Wilfrid Sheed, *In Love With Daylight: A Memoir of Recovery* 21 (Simon & Schuster, 1995).

139. Arthur W. Frank, *The Wounded Storyteller: Body, Illness, and Ethics* 1 (U Chicago Press, 1995).

140. Idem at 54–55.

141. J. J. Christensen-Szalanski, *Discount Functions and the Measurement of Patients' Values: Women's Values During Childbirth,* 4 Medical Decision Making 47 (1984).

141a. R. H. Shmerling, et al, *Discussing Cardiopulmonary Resuscitation: A Study of Elderly Outpatients,* 3 J General Internal Medicine 317 (1988).

142. Maria A. Everhart & Robert A. Pearlman, *Stability of Patient Preferences Regarding Life-Sustaining Treatments,* 97 Chest 159, 162 (1990).

142a. Linda L. Emanuel, et al, *Advance Directives: Stability of Patients' Treatment Choices,* 154 Archives of Internal Medicine 209 (1994).

142b. Marion Danis, et al, *Stability of Choices About Life-Sustaining Treatments,* 120 Annals of Internal Medicine 567, 572 (1994).

143. Idem at 568–69.

144. Marc D. Silverstein, et al, *Amyotrophic Lateral Sclerosis and Life-Sustaining*

Therapy: Patients' Desires for Information, Participation in Decision Making, and Life-Sustaining Therapy, 66 Mayo Clinic Proceedings 907, 912 (1991).

145. Hugh L. Dwyer, *Malignant Fibrous Histiocytoma and Limb Amputation,* in Harvey Mandell & Howard Spiro, eds, *When Doctors Get Sick* 65 (Plenum Medical, 1988).

146. Ernest A. Hirsch, *Starting Over* 36 (Christopher Publishing House, 1977).

147. Idem at 146.

148. Idem at 142.

149. Idem at 149.

150. Jerome Groopman, *The Last Deal,* The New Yorker 62, 67 (Sept 8, 1997).

151. Idem at 74.

152. Idem at 62.

153. Robert Pensack & Dwight Williams, *Raising Lazarus* 226–27 (G. P. Putnam, 1994).

154. Wilfrid Sheed, *In Love With Daylight: A Memoir of Recovery* 45 (Simon & Schuster, 1995).

155. Amitai Etzioni, *The Moral Dimension: Toward a New Economics* 103 (Free Press, 1988).

156. Roberta G. Simmons, Susan Klein Marine, & Richard L. Simmons, *Gift of Life: The Effect of Organ Transplantation on Individual, Family, and Societal Dynamics* 258 (Transaction Books, 1987).

157. Lee Modjeska, *Keeper of the Night: A Portrait of Life in the Shadow of Death* 27 (LuraMedia, 1995).

158. Betty Rollin, *First, You Cry* 51–52 (HarperPaperback, 1993).

159. Allison B. Seckler, et al, *Substituted Judgment: How Accurate Are Proxy Predictions?,* 115 Annals of Internal Medicine 92, 92–93 (1991). Their own data showed that "although the concordance of family members' predictions achieved statistical significance, the kappas . . . did not achieve even the moderate strength of agreement . . . that should be required of surrogates making life and death decisions . . . ." Idem at 95. To like effect, see R. R. Uhlmann, et al, *Physicians' and Spouses' Predictions of Elderly Patients' Resuscitation Preferences,* 43 J Gerontological Medicine 115 (1988); Joseph G. Ouslander, et al, *Health Care Decisions Among Elderly Long-Term Care Residents and Their Potential Proxies,* 149 Archives of Internal Medicine 1367 (1989); Tom Tomlinson, et al, *An Empirical Study of Proxy Consent for Elderly Persons,* 30 Gerontologist 54 (1990). A useful survey of such studies is Ezekiel J. Emanuel & Linda L. Emanuel, *Proxy Decision Making for Incompetent Patients,* 267 JAMA 2067, 2068 (1992).

160. For a statement of this point through a detailed examination of one patient's case, see Stuart J. Eisendrath & Albert R. Jonsen, *The Living Will: Help or Hindrance?,* 249 JAMA 2054 (1983). For a perceptive analysis of the reasons for these difficulties, see Patricia D. White, *Appointing a Proxy Under the Best of Circumstances,* Utah L Rev 849 (1992). Because of the reasons I have surveyed I am puzzled by the confidence of some bioethicists that a "good values baseline" can be assembled and used to guide decisions. Compare Arthur L. Caplan, *Can Autonomy be Saved?,* in *If I Were a Rich Man Could I Buy a Pancreas? and Other Essays on the Ethics of Health Care* 256 (Indiana U Press, 1992).

161. Louie Nassaney with Glenn Kolb, *I Am Not a Victim: One Man's Triumph Over Fear & AIDS* 29 (Hay House, 1990).

162. Paulette Bates Alden, *Crossing the Moon: A Journey Through Infertility* 168 (Hungry Mind Press, 1996).

163. Guido Calabresi & Philip Bobbitt, *Tragic Choices* 18–19 (Norton, 1978).

164. Eileen Radziunas, *Lupus: My Search for a Diagnosis* 65 (Hunter House, 1989).

165. See Talcott Parsons, *The Social System,* ch. 10 (Free Press, 1951); Talcott Parsons, *Illness and the Role of the Physician: A Sociological Perspective,* 27 American J Orthopsychiatry 452 (1951). By citing Parsons, I am not adopting all his views. Rather, I am acknowledging his work in directing attention to what it means to be sick. A good introduction to Parsons on medicine is Renée C. Fox, *Medical Evolution,* in *Essays in Medical Sociology* (Transaction Books, 2d ed, 1988). For an application, see Renée C. Fox, *Experiment Perilous: Physicians and Patients Facing the Unknown,* ch. 4 (U Pennsylvania Press, 1974). For an extended examination of Parsons' place in medical sociology, see Uta Gerhardt, *Ideas About Illness: An Intellectual and Political History of Medical Sociology* 1–71 (NYU Press, 1989). For critical reviews of the literature on the sick role, see Andrew C. Twaddle, *Health Decisions and Sick Role Variations: An Exploration,* 10 J Health & Social Behavior 105 (1969); Alexander Segall, *The Sick Role Concept: Understanding Illness Behavior,* 17 J Health & Social Behavior 163 (1976); and Sol Levine & Martin A. Kozloff, *The Sick Role: Assessment and Overview,* 4 Annual Rev Sociology 317 (1978). For a wider array of sick roles, see Howard Brody, *Stories of Sickness* (Yale U Press, 1987). On the sick role in postmodern times, see Arthur W. Frank, *The Wounded Storyteller: Body, Illness, and Ethics* (U Chicago Press, 1995).

166. Oliver Sacks, *A Leg to Stand On* 164 (HarperCollins, 1984).

167. Merritt B. Low, *Poliomyelitis with Residual Paralysis,* in Max Pinner & Benjamin F. Miller, eds, *When Doctors Are Patients* 77 (Norton, 1952).

168. Reynolds Price, *A Whole New Life* 112 (Atheneum, 1994).

169. The curse of fatigue unto exhaustion pervades patients' memoirs. For a particularly draining instance, see Eileen Radziunas, *Lupus: My Search for a Diagnosis* (Hunter, House 1989).

170. Kenneth H. Cohn, *Chemotherapy From an Insider's Perspective,* Lancet 1006, 1007 (May 1, 1982).

171. Mary Alice Geier, *Cancer: What's It Doing in My Life?* 12 (Hope Publishing House, 1985).

172. Claudine Herzlich & Janine Pierret, *From Self-help to the Duty to Be Healthy,* in *Illness and Self in Society* 214 (Johns Hopkins U Press, 1987).

173. Fitzhugh Mullan, *Vital Signs: A Young Doctor's Struggle With Cancer* 42 (Farrar, Straus, Giroux, 1983).

174. Michael P. Kelly, *Colitis* 70 (Routledge, 1992).

175. James L. Johnson, *Coming Back* 120 (Springhouse Publishing, 1979).

176. Joie Harrison McGrail, *Fighting Back: One Woman's Struggle Against Cancer* 28 (Harper & Row, 1978).

177. Eileen Radziunas, *Lupus: My Search for a Diagnosis* 64 (Hunter House, 1989).

178. Kenneth H. Cohn, *Chemotherapy From an Insider's Perspective,* Lancet 1006, 1008 (May 1, 1982).

179. Agnes de Mille, *Reprieve: A Memoir* 46 (Doubleday, 1981). De Mille did not hand things over exclusively to her doctor quite as much as this passage suggests. Like many patients, she also relied on her husband, who consulted regularly with her doctors.

180. William James, *The Varieties of Religious Experience: A Study in Human Nature* 158 (Modern Library, 1994).

181. May Sarton, *After the Stroke: A Journal* 44 (Norton, 1988).

182. De Mille, *Reprieve* at 61–62 (cited in note 179).

183. Robert E. Kravetz, *Bleeding Ulcer,* in Harvey Mandell & Howard Spiro, eds, *When Doctors Get Sick* 433 (Plenum Medical, 1988).

184. Pat Brack, *Moms Don't Get Sick* 11 (Melius, 1990).

185. Jay Katz, *The Silent World of Doctor and Patient* 100 (Free Press, 1984).

186. Oliver Sacks, *A Leg to Stand On* 167 (HarperCollins, 1989) (emphasis in original).

187. Roberta G. Simmons, Susan Klein Marine, & Richard L. Simmons, *Gift of Life* 270–71 (Transaction Books, 1987).

188. Robert F. Murphy, *The Body Silent* 51–52 (Norton, 1990).

189. Lesley F. Degner & Jeffrey A. Sloan, *Decision Making During Serious Illness: What Role Do Patients Really Want to Play?*, 45 J Clinical Epidemiology 941, 949 (1992). Sherlock suggests sick people "want, often desperately, to *entrust* themselves and their care to the physician, believing that his or her judgment about how to care for them is better than theirs, and caring little for the formalities of consent or the ideal of shared decision-making." Richard Sherlock, *Reasonable Men and Sick Human Beings,* 80 American J Medicine 2, 3 (1986).

190. Simmons, Marine, & Simmons, *Gift of Life* at 271 (cited in note 187).

191. William Martin, *My Prostate and Me: Dealing With Prostate Cancer* 54 (Cadell & Davies, 1994).

192. Wilfrid Sheed, *In Love With Daylight: A Memoir of Recovery* 9 (Simon & Schuster, 1995). Sheed "couldn't read a whole book about health matters without alternately flinching and falling asleep . . . ." Idem at 12. Of course, he eventually wrote such a book (and a fine and funny book it is). But like many patients' memoirs, it is more about being sick than about making decisions.

193. Philip & Joyce Bedsworth, *Fight the Good Fight* 96 (Herald Press, 1991).

194. On the distress of uncertainty, see Renée C. Fox, *Experiment Perilous: Physicians and Patients Facing the Unknown* 127–30 (U Pennsylvania Press, 1974); David C. Stewart & Thomas J. Sullivan, *Illness Behavior and the Sick Role in Chronic Disease: The Case of Multiple Sclerosis,* 16 Social Science Medicine 1307 (1982); Charles Waddell, *The Process of Neutralization and the Uncertainties of Cystic Fibrosis,* 4 Sociology of Health & Illness 210 (1982); Joseph W. Schneider & Peter Conrad, *Having Epilepsy: The Experience and Control of Illness* 53–76, 207–11 (Temple U Press, 1983); Peter Conrad, *The Experience of Illness: Recent and New Directions,* in Julius A. Roth & Peter Conrad, eds, *Research in the Sociology of Health Care: The Experience and Management of Chronic Illness* 7–9 (1987); S. Kay Toombs, *The Meaning of Illness: A Phenomenological Account of the Different Perspectives of Physician and Patient* 97 (Kluwer Academic, 1992).

195. "[S]eeking a doctor's help is a relatively infrequent response to symptoms. . . . Delay is the statistical norm. Fear and anxiety the psychological ones." Irving Kenneth Zola, *Structural Constraints in the Doctor–Patient Relationship: The Case of Non-Compliance,* in Leon Eisenberg & Arthur Kleinman, eds, *The Relevance of Social Science for Medicine* 244 (D. Reidel, 1981).

196. Patients repeatedly testify in memoirs that many of their friends disappeared when they fell ill.

197. See Stewart Alsop, *Stay of Execution: A Sort of Memoir* (Lippincott, 1973), for one patient's gradual decision to limit the information he received about his condition.

198. Lance Morrow, *Heart: A Memoir* 121 (Warner Books, 1995).

199. Joseph Heller & Speed Vogel, *No Laughing Matter* 7–8 (Putnam, 1986).

200. Mary Winfrey Trautman, *The Absence of the Dead Is Their Way of Appearing* 10 (Cleis Press, 1984).

201. Ernest A. Hirsch, *Starting Over* 13–14 (Christopher Publishing House, 1977).

202. Reynolds Price, *A Whole New Life* viii (Atheneum, 1994). And thus Jimmy Breslin on his reactions to reading about proposed brain surgery: "Pliers in my head. I put that

book down and that was the end of that reading. I knew in there somewhere was a description of how they get through the skull to work on the brain. They would break into my head like it was a store. I didn't want to read a line about that." *I Want to Thank My Brain for Remembering Me: A Memoir* 69 (Little, Brown, 1996).

203. Molly Haskell, *Love and Other Infectious Diseases: A Memoir* 115 (Citadel, 1990).

204. Janet Lee James, *One Particular Harbor* 9–10 (Nobel Press, 1993).

205. James L. Johnson, *Coming Back* 12 (Springhouse Publishing, 1979).

206. Natalie Davis Spingarn, *Hanging in There* 21 (Stein & Day, 1982).

207. Richard E. Thompson, *Benign Giant Cell Tumor of Sacrum,* in Harvey Mandell & Howard Spiro, eds, *When Doctors Get Sick* 338 (Plenum Medical, 1988).

208. Edward E. Rosenbaum, *The Doctor* 137 (Ballantine, 1988).

209. Fitzhugh Mullan, *Vital Signs: A Young Doctor's Struggle With Cancer* 104 (Farrar, Straus, Giroux, 1983).

210. Robert L. Seaver, *Myocardial Infarction,* in Harvey Mandell & Howard Spiro, eds, *When Doctors Get Sick* 36–37 (Plenum Medical, 1988).

211. Michael P. Kelly, *Colitis* 54 (Routledge, 1992).

212. Idem at 55.

213. Idem.

214. Gerda Lerner, *A Death of One's Own* 145 (U Wisconsin Press, 1985).

215. On some of the causes, see Elaine J. Sobo, *Choosing Unsafe Sex: AIDS-Risk Denial Among Disadvantaged Women* (U Pennsylvania Press, 1995).

216. William James, *The Varieties of Religious Experience: A Study in Human Nature* 101 (Modern Library, 1994).

217. Paul Monette, *Borrowed Time: An Aids Memoir* 83 (Avon, 1988).

218. Robert F. Murphy, *The Body Silent* 24–25 (Norton, 1990).

219. Idem at 26.

220. Idem at 29. Alsop reacted similarly to some grim news: "The background music, the music of fear, blared high again for a moment. But I put John's [the doctor's] remark out of my mind—an essential art for one in fear of death—and the background music became almost inaudible again." Stewart Alsop, *Stay of Execution: A Sort of Memoir* 116 (Lippincott, 1973).

221. Abraham Myerson, *Vascular Disease,* in Max Pinner & Benjamin F. Miller, eds, *When Doctors Are Patients* 200 (Norton, 1952).

222. Arthur Kleinman, *The Illness Narratives: Suffering, Healing, and the Human Condition* 48 (Basic, 1988). For further praise of this technique (under the label of "suppression") see George E. Vaillant, *Adaptation to Life: How the Best and the Brightest Came of Age* 105–26 (Little, Brown, 1977). On the frequency of this response, see Suzanne M. Miller & Charles E. Mangan, *Interacting Effects of Information and Coping Style in Adapting to Gynecologic Stress: Should the Doctor Tell All?,* 45 J Personality & Social Psychology 223, 223 (1983).

223. Michael P. Kelly, *Colitis* 112 (Routledge, 1992).

224. Miller & Mangan, 45 J Personality & Social Psychology at 224 (cited in note 222). "To integrate this otherwise conflicting range of evidence requires attention to individual differences in preference for information or distraction . . . ." Idem.

225. Idem at 223.

226. Hacib Aoun & Glen Arm, *From the Eye of the Storm, With the Eyes of a Physician,* 116 Annals of Internal Medicine 335, 337 (1992).

227. Natalie Davis Spingarn, *Hanging in There* 11–12 (Stein & Day, 1982).

228. Idem at 56.

229. Idem at 106 (emphases in original).

230. Idem at 56.

231. Franz J. Ingelfinger, *Arrogance,* 303 NEJM 1507, 1510 (1980). Another doctor writes, "I had to be quite desperate and afraid before I was willing to give up control of my body, my future, myself. That decision was very difficult. When I finally felt bad enough, I had to say to my doctors, 'Okay, I give up. Do with me what you will.'" He had then "made the decision to put myself in their hands, to relinquish the need to control my case and myself. I had become a patient and was enormously relieved." Maurice Fox, *Coronary Artery Disease and Coronary After Bypass Graft,* in Harvey Mandell & Howard Spiro, eds, *When Doctors Get Sick* 5 (Plenum Medical, 1988).

232. Harvey Mandell & Howard Spiro, eds, *Epilogue,* in *When Doctors Get Sick* 455–56 (Plenum Medical, 1988).

233. Henrietta Aladjem, *The Sun Is My Enemy: One Woman's Victory Over a Mysterious and Dreaded Disease* 142 (Prentice-Hall, 1972).

234. Paulette Bates Alden, *Crossing the Moon: A Journey Through Infertility* 162 (Hungry Mind Press, 1996).

235. Ellen C. Annandale, *Dimensions of Patient Control in a Free-Standing Birth Center,* 25 Social Science Medicine 1235, 1244 (1987).

236. Wilfrid Sheed, *In Love With Daylight: A Memoir of Recovery* 160 (Simon & Schuster, 1995).

237. William James, *The Varieties of Religious Experience: A Study in Human Nature* 7 (Modern Library, 1994).

238. David A. Tate, *Health, Hope, and Healing* (M. Evans, 1989).

239. One author and patient who impressively explores the moral aspects of illness is Arthur W. Frank. See particularly *The Wounded Storyteller: Body, Illness, and Ethics* (U Chicago Press, 1995).

240. Wilfrid Sheed, *In Love With Daylight: A Memoir of Recovery* 227 (Simon & Schuster, 1995).

241. Idem.

242. Idem at 16.

243. Thomas C. Schelling, *The Intimate Contest for Self-Command,* in *Choice and Consequence: Perspectives of an Errant Economist* 57 (Harvard U Press, 1984).

244. Idem at 78. For an ingenious list of ways we order the world to frustrate our preferences, see Thomas C. Schelling, *Self-Command in Practice, in Policy, and in a Theory of Rational Choice,* 74 American Economic Rev 1 (1984). For example: "My back book prescribes exercises that are to be done faithfully every day. I am certain that some of them need to be done only two or three times a week. But the author knows that 'two or three times a week' is not a schedule conducive to self-discipline." Idem at 7 n. 5.

245. William J. Donoghue, *Medical Language as Symptom: Doctor Talk in Teaching Hospitals,* 30 Perspectives in Biology & Medicine 81, 83 (1986). For a strikingly similar analysis from a patient, see Evan Handler, *Time on Fire: My Comedy of Terrors* 193–94 (Little, Brown, 1996). For a less severe but still critical view, see Franz J. Ingelfinger, *Arrogance,* 303 NEJM 1507, 1510–11 (1980). For a less severe analyses of the often jocular language of medical people, see, e.g., Daniel F. Chambliss, *Beyond Caring: Hospitals, Nurses, and the Social Organization of Ethics* 45–49 (U Chicago Press, 1996); Renée C. Fox, *Experiment Perilous* 76–82 (U Pennsylvania Press, 1974). (For a diverting description of the often-parallel black humor of patients, see idem at 170–77.)

246. Rosemary Breslin, *Not Exactly What I Had in Mind: An Incurable Love Story* 194 (Villard, 1997).

247. Joseph Heller & Speed Vogel, *No Laughing Matter* 116 (Putnam, 1986).

248. David E. Hein, *Crohn's Disease,* in Harvey Mandell & Howard Spiro, eds, *When Doctors Get Sick* 251 (Plenum Medical, 1988).

249. Idem at 249.

250. Idem at 254.

251. These terms do not define themselves, but I believe there is a rough social consensus about what they mean in many cases.

252. Gretel Ehrlich, *A Match to the Heart* 88 (Pantheon, 1994).

253. Carolyn Wiener, et al, *Patient Power: Complex Issues Need Complex Answers,* 11 Social Policy 30, 35 (1980) (emphasis in original).

254. Daniel Defoe, *The Life and Strange Surprising Adventures of Robinson Crusoe* 37 (Harmondsworth, 1985).

255. Augustine, *Confessions* Book VIII.

256. One measure of the patient's challenge in both categories comes in studies of noncompliance. Compliance with short-term medications is apparently higher than with long-term ones, Sandra Berman Bernstein, *Breaking the Vicious Cycle of Noncompliance,* 19 Nursing 74, 75 (1989), and "patients who have chronic illnesses with few or no symptoms" are particularly likely to have troubles with compliance, William S. Bond & Daniel A. Hussar, *Detection Methods and Strategies for Improving Medication Compliance,* 48 American J Hospital Pharmacists 1978, 1979 (1991).

257. Anselm Strauss, et al, *Social Organization of Medical Work* 1–2 (U Chicago Press, 1985).

258. Leo G. Reeder, *The Patient-Client as a Consumer: Some Observations on the Changing Professional-Client Relationship,* 13 J Health & Social Behavior 406, 407 (1972).

259. Lachlan Forrow, Steven A. Wartman, & Dan W. Brock, *Science, Ethics, and the Making of Clinical Decisions,* 259 JAMA 3161, 3164 (1988).

260. Arthur Kleinman, *The Illness Narratives: Suffering, Healing, and the Human Condition* 32–39 (Basic Books, 1988).

261. Idem at 38.

262. Idem. For further examples, see Terrence F. Ackerman, *Why Doctors Should Intervene,* 12 HCR 14 (Aug 1982); Anselm Strauss, et al, *Social Organization of Medical Work* 15–19 (U Chicago Press, 1985). Caplan, to take another example, suggests that suddenly impaired patients may be competent but so debilitated that people rehabilitating them "take, and ought to take, a more directive and tacitly paternalistic approach to those in their care than would be found ethically acceptable" ordinarily. Arthur L. Caplan, *Informed Consent and Provider/Patient Relationships in Rehabilitation Medicine,* in *If I Were a Rich Man Could I Buy a Pancreas? and Other Essays on the Ethics of Health Care* 248 (Indiana U Press, 1992). He argues patients who are "depressed, disoriented, or demoralized by the severity of their impairments" might "need to be motivated or encouraged, rather than merely having their options presented in a disinterested or neutral manner." Idem at 249. The question—raised by the case of Alice Alcott—is whether to limit this principle to the recently and severely impaired.

263. These patients were not alone in skepticism about full disclosure: "Lankton *et al.* found that patients who were given a detailed disclosure of risks of anesthesia stated that they would not like to have complete disclosure if they were to have surgery again. One-fourth indicated that they had been frightened by the disclosure, and three of the sixteen

frightened patients indicated that they had asked to have disclosure stopped while it was in progress." Alan Meisel & Loren H. Roth, *Toward an Informed Discussion of Informed Consent: A Review and Critique of the Empirical Studies,* 25 Arizona L Rev 265, 279 (1983) (footnotes omitted). Such reactions must of course be understood against the background of evidence that patients generally want information.

264. James L. Johnson, *Coming Back* 117 (Springhouse Publishing, 1979).

265. Michael P. Kelly, *Colitis* 56 (Routledge, 1992).

266. Arnold R. Beisser, *Flying Without Wings* 135 (Doubleday, 1989).

267. *In Love With Daylight: A Memoir of Recovery* 13 (Simon & Schuster, 1995).

268. Idem at 14.

269. Idem at 14–15.

270. Norman F. Boyd, et al, *Whose Utilities for Decision Analysis?,* 10 Medical Decision Making 58 (1990).

271. *Love's Work: A Reckoning With Life* 96 (Schocken, 1995).

272. Boyd, et al, 10 Medical Decision Making at 58 (cited in note 270).

273. Irving L. Janis, *The Patient as Decision Maker,* in W. Doyle Gentry, ed, *Handbook of Behavioral Medicine* 333 (Guilford, 1984).

274. Carl H. Fellner & John R. Marshall, *Kidney Donors—The Myth of Informed Consent,* 126 American J Psychiatry 1245, 1247 (1970). Five donors hoped they would not be selected, but decided well before receiving their full dose of informed consent they would donate if they qualified. Donors were given a face-saving way to withdraw (the transplant team would tell the family the potential donor was unsuitable), but none took it.

275. Idem at 1250. On the other hand, see the (ambiguously reported) study of kidney recipients in which "[f]ifty percent of the patients indicated that there had been a distinct period when they had deliberated about their decision. For 34%, the decision had been made gradually, but for 16% there was no period of mulling over—the decision had been made immediately." J. John Wagener & Shelley E. Taylor, *What Else Could I Have Done? Patients' Responses to Failed Treatment Decisions,* 5 Health Psychology 481, 487 (1986).

276. Roberta G. Simmons, Susan Klein Marine, & Richard L. Simmons, *Gift of Life: The Effect of Organ Transplantation on Individual, Family, and Societal Dynamics* (Transaction Books, 1987).

277. Idem at 241 (emphasis in original).

278. Idem at 255 (emphasis in original).

279. Idem at 283.

280. Idem.

281. Idem at 260 (emphasis in original).

282. Idem at 265 (emphasis in original).

283. Idem.

284. Idem at 264.

285. Idem.

286. Idem at 268.

287. Idem at 269.

288. Penny F. Pierce, *Deciding on Breast Cancer Treatment: A Description of Decision Behavior,* 42 Nursing Research 20, 23 (1993).

289. Idem. This is not, of course, an argument against providing patients with information, since it will often be unclear in advance which information a patient will find dispositive.

290. Richard Nisbett & Lee Ross, *Human Inference: Strategies and Shortcomings of Social Judgment* 41–42 (Prentice-Hall, 1980).

291. This may seem an improbably trivial basis for such a decision, but some people really hate needles. One cancer patient whose story I followed believed, as her husband reported at the beginning of her illness, "that if she has to do chemotherapy that involves IVs, she would regard the prospect of facing repeated IVs as less attractive than death, and might just refuse treatment that most would regard as not all that terrible." Eventually, she found she needed anti-anxiety drugs and hypnotherapy to make IVs even barely tolerable. While she could "go through the actual procedure," the "fear and apprehension the night before and the morning of" the procedure were acute. And even when she needed to take a blood thinner for pulmonary emboli, she chose what she understood to be "the riskier alternative" of taking pills rather than an IV. This patient fought through these fears with strength, determination, courage, and the sympathy and imaginative help of her husband.

292. Similarly, when Frank talks "to people about to begin chemotherapy, a common reaction is for fears of immediate side-effects, particularly hair loss, to be more of a topic than fears of the treatment not working." Arthur W. Frank, *The Wounded Storyteller: Body, Illness, and Ethics* 44 (U Chicago Press, 1995).

293. Musa Mayer, *Examining Myself: One Woman's Story of Breast Cancer Treatment and Recovery* 26 (Faber & Faber, 1993).

294. *Change of Heart* 86 (Sayre, 1973).

295. *Limbo* 10 (Chandler & Sharpe, 1979).

296. *A Whole New Life* 133–34 (Atheneum, 1994).

297. *Cancer: What's It Doing in My Life?* 18 (Hope Publishing House, 1985).

298. For a description of them and their reasons, see Chapter 4.

299. Louie Nassaney with Glenn Kolb, *I Am Not a Victim: One Man's Triumph Over Fear & AIDS* 29 (Hay House, 1990).

300. Idem at 86.

301. Kenneth A. Shapiro, *Dying and Living: One Man's Life With Cancer* 170 (U Texas Press, 1985).

302. Betty Johnson, *Change of Heart* 77 (Sayre, 1973).

303. Anatole Broyard, *Intoxicated By My Illness: And Other Writings on Life and Death* 39–40 (Fawcett Columbine, 1992).

304. Rachelle Breslow, *Who Said So?: How Our Thoughts and Beliefs Affect Our Physiology* 15 (Celestial Arts, 1991).

305. Idem at 23.

306. Idem at 98.

307. Idem.

308. Idem at 99.

309. Susan Wolf Sternberg, *A Year of Miracles: A Healing Journey From Cancer to Wholeness* 151 (Star Mountain Press, 1995).

310. Idem at 68. Sternberg is quoting a professor of pharmacology whose guidance she valued.

311. Michael Korda, *Man to Man: Surviving Prostate Cancer* 101 (Random House, 1996).

312. Evan Handler, *Time on Fire: My Comedy of Terrors* 141–42 (Little, Brown, 1996).

313. *My Prostate and Me: Dealing With Prostate Cancer* 114 (Cadell & Davies, 1994).

314. Irving L. Janis & Leon Mann, *Decision Making: A Psychological Analysis of Conflict, Choice, and Commitment* 230 (Free Press, 1977).

315. T.P. Hackett & N.H. Cassem, *Psychological Management of the Myocardial Infarction Patient*, 1 J Human Stress 25, 27 (1975).

316. Richard P. Brickner, *My Second Twenty Years: An Unexpected Life* 197 (Basic Books, 1976).

317. Janis & Mann, *Decision Making* at 230 (cited in note 314).

318. See R.K. Goldsen, P.T. Gerhardt, & V. Handy, *Some Factors Related to Patient Delay in Seeking Diagnosis for Cancer Symptoms*, 10 Cancer 1 (1957); B. Kutner, H.B. Makover, & A. Oppenheim, *Delay in the Diagnosis and Treatment of Cancer: A Critical Analysis of the Literature*, 7 J Chronic Diseases 95 (1958); Raymond Rink, *Delay Behavior in Breast Cancer Screening*, in J.W. Cullen, B.H. Fox, & R.N. Isom, eds, *Cancer: The Behavioral Dimensions* 23 (Raven Press, 1976).

319. Harvey Mandell & Howard Spiro, eds, *When Doctors Get Sick* (Plenum Medical, 1987). Similarly, Hahn observes of his study of memoirs by doctors who became patients that some of them "manifest the denial and delay commonly reported of nonphysician patients." Robert A. Hahn, *Sickness and Healing: An Anthropological Perspective* 257 (Yale U Press, 1995).

320. Tim Brookes, *Catching My Breath: An Asthmatic Explores His Illness* 39 (Times Books, 1994).

321. Edward E. Rosenbaum, *The Doctor* 52 (Ballantine, 1988).

322. Reynolds Price, *A Whole New Life* 11 (Atheneum, 1994) (emphasis in original).

323. Tom L. Beauchamp & James F. Childress, *Principles of Biomedical Ethics* 76 (Oxford U Press, 3d ed, 1989) (emphases in original).

324. Canterbury v. Spence, 464 F2d 772, 781 (DC Cir, 1972).

325. Thomas Mann, *The Magic Mountain* 33 (Vintage International, 1992).

326. For accounts of how people choose careers and spouses, see Janis & Mann, *Decision Making* at 35 (cited in note 314).

327. "I have never been anywhere but sick. In a sense sickness is a place, more instructive than a long trip to Europe, and it's always a place where there's no company, where nobody can follow." Flannery O'Connor, *The Habit of Being* 163 (Noonday Press, 1995).

328. Lachlan Forrow, Steven A. Wartman, & Dan W. Brock, *Science, Ethics, and the Making of Clinical Decisions: Implications for Risk Factor Intervention*, 259 JAMA 3161, 3165 (1988) (footnotes omitted).

329. Amitai Etzioni, *The Moral Dimension: Toward a New Economics* 121 (Free Press, 1988).

330. Barbara J. McNeil, et al, *On the Elicitation of Preferences for Alternative Therapies*, 306 NEJM 1259, 1262 (1982).

331. See, e.g., David M. Eddy, *Probabilistic Reasoning in Clinical Medicine: Problems and Opportunities*, in Daniel Kahneman, Paul Slovic, & Amos Tversky, eds, *Judgment Under Uncertainty: Heuristics and Biases* 249 (Cambridge U Press, 1982).

332. Jonathan Borak & Suzanne Veilleux, *Errors of Intuitive Logic Among Physicians*, 16 Social Science Medicine 1939, 1942 (1982).

333. Richard Nisbett & Lee Ross, *Human Inference: Strategies and Shortcomings of Social Judgment* 286–94 (Prentice-Hall, 1980).

334. Forrow, et al, 259 JAMA at 3165 (cited in note 328). For a vivid demonstration of the extent to which medical practices vary from place to place, see John E. Wennberg, et al, *Are Hospital Services Rationed in New Haven or Over-Utilised in Boston?*, Lancet 1185 (May 23, 1987). To like effect, see Mark R. Chassin, et al, *Variations in*

the Use of Medical and Surgical Services by the Medicare Population, 314 NEJM 285 (1986). On variation from country to country, see Lynn Payer, *Medicine and Culture: Varieties of Treatment in the United States, England, West Germany and France* (H. Holt, 1988).

335. Bradford H. Gray, *The Profit Motive and Patient Care: The Changing Accountability of Doctors and Hospitals* 252 (Harvard U Press, 1991) (emphasis in original).

336. Idem at 253.

337. David J. Rothman, *Strangers at the Bedside: A History of How Law and Bioethics Transformed Medical Decision Making* (Basic Books, 1991).

338. Pearl Katz, *How Surgeons Make Decisions,* in Robert A. Hahn & Atwood D. Gaines, eds, *Physicians of Western Medicine* 166 (D. Reidel, 1985).

339. Idem.

340. Idem at 172.

341. Idem at 160.

342. Gray, *The Profit Motive and Patient Care* at 188 (cited in note 335).

343. Idem at 255.

344. Idem. See Marc A. Rodwin, *Medicine, Money, and Morals: Physicians' Conflicts of Interest* (Oxford U Press, 1993).

345. See E. Haavi Morreim, *Balancing Act: The New Medical Ethics of Medicine's New Economics* (Georgetown U Press, 1995).

346. G. Edward Rozar & David B. Biebel, *Laughing in the Face of AIDS: A Surgeon's Personal Battle* 81 (Baker, 1992).

347. See note 159.

348. See, e.g., Robert A. Hahn, *Sickness and Healing: An Anthropological Perspective* 173–208 (Yale U Press, 1995).

349. Idem at 190.

350. Idem at 189.

351. Irving L. Janis & Leon Mann, *Decision Making: A Psychological Analysis of Conflict, Choice, and Commitment* 50 (Free Press, 1977).

352. "When the case involves me, or my family, my judgment is not to be trusted. As has been said, so many times, 'The doctor who takes care of himself has a fool for a patient.'" William A. Nolen, *Surgeon Under the Knife* 88 (Dell, 1976).

353. *Sources of Power: How People Make Decisions* 31 (MIT Press, 1998) (emphasis in original).

354. Idem at 24 (emphasis in original).

355. Raanan Lipshitz, *Converging Themes in the Study of Decision Making in Realistic Settings,* in Gary A. Klein, ed, *Decision Making in Action: Models and Methods* 137 (Ablex Publishers, 1993).

356. Arthur S. Elstein, Lee S. Schulman, & Sarah A. Sprafka, *Medical Problem Solving: A Ten-Year Retrospective,* 13 Evaluation & the Health Professions 5, 13 (1990).

357. Klein, *Sources of Power* at 103 (cited in note 353).

358. Idem at 263.

359. Marvin S. Cohen, *The Naturalistic Basis of Decision Biases,* in Gary A. Klein, ed, *Decision Making in Action: Models and Methods* 59 (Ablex Publishers, 1993).

360. Judith Orasanu & Terry Connolly, *The Reinvention of Decision Making,* in Gary A. Klein, ed, *Decision Making in Action: Models and Methods* 11 (Ablex Publishers, 1993).

361. Klein, *Sources of Power* at 52 (cited in note 353).

362. Idem at 152.

363. Orasanu & Connolly, *The Reinvention of Decision Making* at 18 (cited in note 360).

364. Klein, *Sources of Power* at 280 (cited in note 353).

365. Orasanu & Connolly, *The Reinvention of Decision Making* at 18 (cited in note 360).

366. Klein, *Sources of Power* at 272 (cited in note 353). Similarly Orasanu & Connolly argue that studies of reasoning "cast little light on the performance of the expert operating in his or her regular environment with normal decision aids, time sequences, cue sets, and so on." *The Reinvention of Decision Making* at 15 (cited in note 360). And Christensen-Szalanski "cites the example of an impressive cluster of biases discovered in medical diagnosis, whose opportunities for occurrence turned out to be 'embarrassingly small' and whose effects on treatment choices when they did occur were found to be negligible." Marvin S. Cohen, *The Naturalistic Basis of Decision Biases,* in Gary A. Klein, ed, *Decision Making in Action: Models and Methods* 54 (Ablex Publishers, 1993).

367. On "collective rationality," see Amitai Etzioni, *The Moral Dimension: Toward a New Economics* 185–98 (Free Press, 1988).

368. Donald A. Redelmeier, Paul Rozin, & Daniel Kahneman, *Understanding Patients' Decisions: Cognitive and Emotional Perspectives,* 270 JAMA 72, 73 (1993).

369. See Charles Bosk, *Forgive and Remember: Managing Medical Failure* (U Chicago Press, 1979).

370. Eric J. Cassell, *The Healer's Art* 143 (MIT Press, 1985).

371. Orasanu & Connolly, *The Reinvention of Decision Making* at 19 (cited in note 360)

372. Lee Roy Beach & Raanan Lipshitz, *Why Classical Decision Theory is an Inappropriate Standard for Evaluating and Aiding Most Human Decision Making,* in Gary A. Klein, et al, eds, *Decision Making in Action: Models and Methods* 25 (Ablex Publishers, 1993).

373. Klein, *Sources of Power* at 123 (cited in note 353).

Chapter 4

1. In like manner, an editorial in the New England Journal of Medicine (written before some but not all the studies I have reviewed) concluded confidently that "[r]ecent surveys have shown that most people, whether well or seriously ill, wish to be informed of their condition and to participate in medical decisions." Marcia Angell, *Respecting the Autonomy of Competent Patients,* 310 NEJM 1115 (1984).

1a. Suzanne C. Thompson, *Will It Hurt Less If I Can Control It? A Complex Answer to a Simple Question,* 90 Psychological Bulletin 89, 95 (1981).

2. Stewart Alsop, *Stay of Execution: A Sort of Memoir* 84 (Lippincott, 1973).

3. Idem at 173.

4. Musa Mayer, *Examining Myself: One Woman's Story of Breast Cancer Treatment and Recovery* 28 (Faber & Faber, 1993).

5. Cornelius & Kathryn Morgan Ryan, *A Private Battle* (Simon & Schuster, 1979).

6. Edward E. Rosenbaum, *The Doctor* 121 (Ballantine, 1988).

7. Anatole Broyard, *Toward a Literature of Illness,* in *Intoxicated by My Illness: And Other Writings on Life and Death* 19–20 (Fawcett Columbine, 1992).

8. Roberta G. Simmons, Susan Klein Marine, & Richard L. Simmons, *Gift of Life: The Effect of Organ Transplantation on Individual, Family, and Societal Dynamics* 359 (Transaction Books, 1987).

9. *In Love with Daylight: A Memoir of Recovery* 17 (Simon & Schuster, 1995).

10. Joseph W. Schneider & Peter Conrad, *Having Epilepsy: The Experience and Control of Illness* 177 (Temple U Press, 1983). For a similar reaction, see Barbara D. Webster, *All of a Piece: A Life With Multiple Sclerosis* 23–35 (Johns Hopkins U Press, 1989).

11. Molly Haskell, *Love and Other Infectious Diseases: A Memoir* 179 (Citadel, 1990).

12. See Renée C. Fox, *Experiment Perilous: Physicians and Patients Facing the Unknown* 127–30 (U Pennsylvania Press, 1974); Joseph W. Schneider & Peter Conrad, *Having Epilepsy: The Experience and Control of Illness* 53–76 (Temple U Press, 1983); Barbara D. Webster, *All of a Piece: A Life with Multiple Sclerosis* 39–40, 86–97 (Johns Hopkins U Press, 1989).

13. Fox, *Experiment Perilous* at 165 (cited in note 12).

14. Idem.

15. Schneider & Conrad, *Having Epilepsy* at 168 (cited in note 10).

16. Webster comments, "It took me almost a year before I relaxed and stopped seeing impending disaster in every new sensation and symptom. It took time to learn the new parameters of normality." Webster, *All of a Piece* at 37 (cited in note 10). She also valued learning that "some very strange things that had happened to me" were simply symptoms of her disease: "Explanation even in retrospect is very comforting." Idem.

17. Schneider & Conrad, *Having Epilepsy* at 178 (cited in note 10). Webster, *All of a Piece* (cited in note 10), reports many of the same reasons for her anxiety for information about her disease. She particularly wanted information that would help her with her feelings about her disease and with the reactions of other people. Webster also provides a reminder that even copious information may not always work. Idem at 39.

18. Jeannie Morton, *Personal View,* 295 British Medical J 1482 (1987).

19. Donna McFarlane, *Division of Surgery* 17–18 (Women's Press, 1994).

20. Henry D. Weaver, *Confronting the Big C: A Family Faces Cancer* 47–48 (Herald Press, 1984).

21. Schneider & Conrad, *Having Epilepsy* at 178 (cited in note 10).

22. Haskell, *Love and Other Infectious Diseases* at 29 (cited in note 11).

23. See M. Davis, *Variations in Patients' Compliance With Doctors' Advice: An Empirical Analysis of Patterns of Communication,* 58 American J Public Health 274 (1969); M. Davis, *Variation in Patients' Compliance with Doctors' Orders: Medical Practice and Doctor–Patient Interaction,* 2 Psychiatry in Medicine 31 (1971); B. Freeman, et al, *Gaps in Doctor Patient Communication,* 5 Pediatric Research 298 (1971); W. Stiles, et al, *Dimensions of Patient and Physician Roles in Medical Screening Interviews,* 13A Social Science Medicine 335 (1979); W. Stiles, et al, *Interaction Exchange Structure and Patient Satisfaction with Medical Interviews,* 17 Medical Care 667 (1979).

24. Debra L. Roter & Judith A. Hall, *Studies of Doctor–Patient Interaction,* 10 Annual Rev Public Health 163, 174 (1989).

25. Idem at 175.

26. See Charles W. Lidz, et al, *Barriers to Informed Consent,* 99 Annals of Internal Medicine 539 (1983).

27. Patients may need less information for this purpose than for "informed consent," since they may only want to veto plans of treatment that are particularly flagrant or menacing.

28. One illustration of the awkwardness of law's language is its inability to handle these considerations fully yet delicately. Informed consent is commonly justified in terms of patients' needs to make their own decisions, while it might find an equally persuasive rationale in the other reasons patients want information. And doctors might respond to the

law more willingly if its justification were expressed more convincingly. On the other hand, expanding the doctrine's rationale might produce uncertainty about the scope of the duty to disclose and an unrewarding expansion of the cause of action.

29. Jerry M. Burger, *Negative Reactions to Increases in Perceived Personal Control,* 56 J Personality & Social Psychology 246, 246 (1989). See also Suzanne C. Thompson, Paul R. Cheek, & Melody A. Graham, *The Other Side of Perceived Control: Disadvantages and Negative Effects,* in Shirlynn Spacapan & Stuart Oskamp, eds, *The Social Psychology of Health: The Claremont Symposium on Applied Social Psychology* 85 (Sage, 1987), which concludes, "Many studies have found that individuals can benefit from perceptions of control over aversive events." I have drawn gratefully on these two helpful summaries of the literature on control.

30. Eric J. Cassell, *The Healer's Art* 44 (Lippincott, 1976).

31. David S. Brody, *The Patient's Role in Clinical Decision-Making,* 93 Annals of Internal Medicine 718, 720 (1980). Even writers who are cautious about the autonomy paradigm write that the chronically ill "must strive to prevent the illness from overwhelming their sense of efficacy and the control they, like all of us, wish to exercise over their lives and activities." Bruce Jennings, Daniel Callahan, & Arthur L. Caplan, *Ethical Challenges of Chronic Illness,* HCR, Special Supp 11 (Feb/March 1988).

32. Michael Korda, *Man to Man: Surviving Prostate Cancer* 215 (Random House, 1996) (emphases in original).

32a. Gregory White Smith & Steven Naifeh, *Making Miracles Happen* 18 (Little, Brown, 1997).

33. *Moving Violations: War Zones, Wheelchairs, and Declarations of Independence* 79 (Hyperion, 1995).

34. Pat Brack, *Moms Don't Get Sick* 46 (Melius, 1990).

35. Jerry M. Burger, *Negative Reactions to Increases in Perceived Personal Control,* 56 J Personality & Social Psychology 246, 246 (1989).

36. Judith Rodin, *Aging and Health: Effects of the Sense of Control,* 233 Science 1271, 1271 (1986).

37. *It's Always Something* 183 (Avon, 1990).

38. Kenneth A. Shapiro, *Dying and Living: One Man's Life With Cancer* 126 (U Texas Press, 1985).

39. Jerry M. Burger & Harris M. Cooper, *The Desirability of Control,* 3 Motivation & Emotion 381, 382 (1979).

40. Thompson, et al, *The Other Side of Perceived Control* at 89 (cited in note 29).

41. Idem at 73–74.

42. Idem at 74.

43. Idem.

44. Idem at 75. For a case in which (Howard Brody suggests) a physician–patient who should have known better sought too much control, see Howard Brody, *Stories of Sickness* 137–42 (Yale U Press, 1987). The same story is told in different terms by the patient's widow. Martha W. Lear, *Heartsounds* (Simon & Schuster, 1980).

45. Apparently "individuals will not be motivated to have or exercise control if sufficient information to evaluate the alternatives effectively is not available." Thompson, et al, *The Other Side of Perceived Control* at 73 (cited in note 29).

46. Idem at 79. So great can be the wish to escape blame—one's own and others'—that where "failure is anticipated, subjects will often choose a condition that increases their chances of failure, but that has the advantage of avoiding the costs of self-responsibility." Idem.

47. Jerry M. Burger, *Negative Reactions to Increases in Perceived Personal Control,* 56 J Personality & Social Psychology 246 (1989).

48. Irving L. Janis, *The Patient as Decision Maker,* in W. Doyle Gentry, ed, *Handbook of Behavioral Medicine* 326, 326 (Guilford, 1984).

49. Ellen C. Annandale, *Dimensions of Patient Control in a Free-Standing Birth Center,* 25 Social Science Medicine 1235, 1245 (1987).

50. Thompson et al, *The Other Side of Perceived Control* at 87 (cited in note 29).

51. Idem at 71–72.

52. Idem at 85–86.

53. Jerry M. Burger, *Negative Reactions to Increases in Perceived Personal Control,* 56 J Personality & Social Psychology 246, 254 (1989).

54. David S. Krantz, Andrew Baum, & Margaret v. Wideman, *Assessment of Preferences for Self-Treatment and Information in Health Care,* 39 J Personality & Social Psychology 977, 987 (1980).

55. Ellen J. Langer, *The Illusion of Control,* 32 J Personality & Social Psychology 311 (1975). Langer reports many people believe the world is basically just, so that people get what they earn, and she reports experiments which suggest that people often believe they can affect chance events like lotteries. See Melvin J. Lerner, *The Belief in a Just World: A Fundamental Delusion* (Plenum Press, 1980)

56. Ullabeth Sätterlund Larsson, et al, *Patient Involvement in Decision-making in Surgical and Orthopaedic Practice,* 6 Scandinavian J Caring Sciences 87, 91 (1992).

57. *The Illusion of Control* (cited in note 55).

58. Thompson et al, *The Other Side of Perceived Control* at 80–81 (cited in note 29).

59. The other was "not caring enough to make the effort." Idem at 83–84. For a review of the literature on reluctance to make decisions when abler people are available, see Jerry M. Burger, *Negative Reactions to Increases in Perceived Personal Control,* 56 J Personality & Social Psychology 246, 250–51 (1989).

60. "[P]eople want information as a resource for managing illness . . . ." Julius A. Roth & Peter Conrad, *Research in the Sociology of Health Care: The Experience and Management of Chronic Illness* 14 (JAI Press, 1987).

61. Michael P. Kelly, *Colitis* 46–48 (Routledge, 1992).

62. See, e.g., Louise DeSalvo, *Breathless: An Asthma Journal* (Beacon Press, 1997).

63. Louise Scott, *Ulcerative Colitis,* in Harvey Mandell & Howard Spiro, eds, *When Doctors Get Sick* 198–99 (Plenum Medical, 1988).

64. Robert Pensack & Dwight Williams, *Raising Lazarus* 99–100 (Putnam, 1994).

65. Janet Lee James, *One Particular Harbor* 189 (Nobel Press, 1993).

66. On the importance to sick people of such mundane things, see Renée C. Fox, *Experiment Perilous: Physicians and Patients Facing the Unknown* 116–18 (U Pennsylvania Press, 1974). On how they seek mastery over them, see idem at 143–47 and Michael P. Kelly, *Colitis* (Routledge, 1992).

67. Alexis de Tocqueville, 2 *Democracy in America* 338 (Vintage, 1957).

68. Herbert M. Howe, *Do Not Go Gentle* 91 (Norton, 1981).

69. Joyce Slayton Mitchell, *Winning the Chemo Battle* 203 (Norton, 1988).

70. Michael Korda, *Man to Man: Surviving Prostate Cancer* 87 (Random House, 1996).

71. *A Match to the Heart* 57 (Pantheon, 1994).

72. Gerda Lerner, *A Death of One's Own* 60 (U Wisconsin Press, 1985).

73. Marvin Barrett, *Spare Days* 13 (Morrow, 1988).

74. Ben Watt, *Patient: The True Story of a Rare Illness* 113 (Grove Press, 1996).

75. Howard Brody, *Stories of Sickness* 116–17 (Yale U Press, 1987). On the "power of powerlessness," see, e.g., John M. Hull, *Touching the Rock: An Experience of Blindness* 106 (Vintage, 1990).

76. William James, *The Varieties of Religious Experience: A Study in Human Nature* 101–2 (Modern Library, 1994).

77. Arnold R. Beisser, *Flying Without Wings* 112–13 (Doubleday, 1989).

78. George R. Melton & Wil Garcia, *Beyond AIDS: A Journey Into Healing* 45 (Brotherhood Press, 1988).

79. James, *The Varieties of Religious Experience* at 108 (cited in note 76).

80. Idem at 109.

81. Norman Cousins, *Anatomy of an Illness as Perceived by the Patient: Reflections on Healing and Regeneration* 45 (Bantam, 1979).

82. Idem at 44.

83. Joie Harrison McGrail, *Fighting Back: One Woman's Struggle Against Cancer* 51 (Harper & Row, 1978). For a summary of the evidence about some of these ideas, see Christopher Peterson & Lisa M. Bossio, *Health and Optimism* (Free Press, 1991). For an intriguing study of a similar attitude among the Navajo, see Joseph A. Carrese & Lorna A. Rhodes, *Western Bioethics on the Navajo Reservation: Benefit or Harm?*, 274 JAMA 826 (1996).

84. Evan Handler, *Time on Fire: My Comedy of Terrors* 55 (Little, Brown, 1996).

85. Laura Evans, *The Climb of My Life: A Miraculous Journey From the Edge of Death to the Victory of a Lifetime* 136–37 (HarperSanFrancisco, 1996).

86. Handler, *Time on Fire* at 31 (cited in note 84).

87. James, *The Varieties of Religious Experience* at 117 (cited in note 76).

88. See, as two among the host, McGrail, *Fighting Back* (cited in note 83); Gilda Radner, *It's Always Something* (Avon, 1989). A doctor of this persuasion (in a macrobiotic vein) is Anthony J. Sattilaro, *Recalled by Life* (Avon, 1982).

89. For example, Laura Chester, *Lupus Novice: Toward Self-Healing* (Station Hill Press, 1987).

90. Jill Ireland, *Life Wish* 1 (Jove, 1987).

91. Idem at 81.

92. Idem at 212.

93. Idem at 77.

94. Idem at 39.

95. Idem at 185.

96. Renée C. Fox, *Experiment Perilous: Physicians and Patients Facing the Unknown* 132 (U Pennsylvania Press, 1974).

97. Arnold R. Beisser, *Flying Without Wings* 107 (Doubleday, 1989).

98. Fox, *Experiment Perilous* at 177–79 (cited in note 96). The mighty locus classicus of the attempt to understand illness in religious terms is John Donne, *Devotions Upon Emergent Occasions* (U Michigan Press, 1959). Modern illness memoirs with a religious perspective include James L. Johnson, *Coming Back* (Springhouse Publishing, 1979); Mary Alice Geier, *Cancer: What's It Doing in My Life?* (Hope Publishing House, 1985); Mary Cooper Greene, *Living With a Broken String* (no publisher, 1987); Marvin Barrett, *Spare Days* (Morrow, 1988); Madeleine L'Engle, *Two-Part Invention: The Story of a Marriage* (Harper & Row, 1988); Betty Garton Ulrich, *Rooted in the Sky: A Faith to Cope With Cancer* (Judson Press, 1989); Becky Lynn Wecksler & Michael Wecksler, *In God's Hand: One Woman's Experience With Breast Cancer* (Herald Press, 1989); John M. Hull, *Touching the Rock: An Experience of Blindness* (Vintage, 1990); Philip & Joyce Bedsworth,

Fight the Good Fight (Herald Press, 1991); and G. Edward Rozar & David B. Biebel, *Laughing in the Face of AIDS: A Surgeon's Personal Battle* (Baker Book House, 1992). It is hardly surprising religion is central in the lives of citizens of the most devout industrialized society. Theodore Caplow, et al, *All Faithful People: Change and Continuity in Middletown's Religion* 26–27 (U Minnesota Press, 1983). As Tocqueville remarked, "It must never be forgotten that religion gave birth to Anglo-American society. In the United States, religion is therefore mingled with all the habits of the nation . . . ." Alexis de Tocqueville, 2 *Democracy in America* 6 (Vintage, 1957).

99. Terry A. Cronan, et al, *Prevalence of the Use of Unconventional Remedies for Arthritis in a Metropolitan Community,* 32 Arthritis & Rheumatism 1604 (1989).

100. Rozar & Biebel, *Laughing in the Face of AIDS* at 77 (cited in note 98).

101. Fox, *Experiment Perilous* at 133 (cited in note 96). For an informative contrast between religious and secular attempts to assert control through explanation, see Anne Hawkins, *Two Pathographies: A Study in Illness and Literature,* 9 J Medicine & Philosophy 231 (1984).

102. McGrail, *Fighting Back* at 35 (cited in note 83).

103. Fitzhugh Mullan, *Vital Signs: A Young Doctor's Struggle With Cancer* 43 (Farrar, Straus, Giroux, 1983).

104. Kathy Charmaz, *Good Days, Bad Days: The Self in Chronic Illness and Time* 15 (Rutgers U Press, 1991).

105. Idem.

106. Anne Hunsaker Hawkins, *Reconstructing Illness: Studies in Pathography* (Purdue U Press, 1993).

107. Arthur W. Frank, *The Wounded Storyteller: Body, Illness, and Ethics* 115 (U Chicago Press, 1995).

108. Reynolds Price, *A Whole New Life* 184 (Atheneum, 1994) (emphasis in original).

109. Hawkins, *Reconstructing Illness* at 24 (cited in note 106).

110. *Moving Violations: War Zones, Wheelchairs, and Declarations of Independence* 79 (Hyperion, 1995).

111. This paragraph owes much to Arthur W. Frank's perceptive and moving *The Wounded Storyteller: Body, Illness, and Ethics* (U Chicago Press, 1995).

112. Paul Reed, *The Q Journal: A Treatment Diary* 13 (Celestial Arts, 1991).

113. Anatole Broyard, *Toward a Literature of Illness,* in *Intoxicated by My Illness: And Other Writings on Life and Death* 19 (Fawcett Columbine, 1992).

114. *The Habit of Being* 57 (Noonday Press, 1995).

115. Henry D. Weaver, *Confronting the Big C: A Family Faces Cancer* 76 (Herald Press, 1984).

116. Joanna Baumer Permut, *Embracing the Wolf* 165 (Cherokee Publishing, 1989).

117. Patricia Hingle, *A Coming of Roses* 37 (Home Plates of Ascension, 1988).

118. G. Edward Rozar & David B. Biebel, *Laughing in the Face of AIDS: A Surgeon's Personal Battle* 78 (Baker Book House, 1992) (emphasis in original).

119. Sandi Gordon, *Parkinson's: A Personal Story of Acceptance* 67 (Branden, 1992).

120. Betty Johnson & Constance Collier, *Change of Heart* 131 (Sayre, 1973).

121. Idem.

122. Anthony J. Sattilaro with Tom Monte, *Recalled by Life* 207 (Avon, 1982).

123. Barry L. Zaret, *Trauma,* in Harvey Mandell & Howard Spiro, eds, *When Doctors Get Sick* 410 (Plenum Medical, 1988).

124. Hawkins, *Reconstructing Illness* at 43 (cited in note 106).

125. Hadley L. Conn, Jr., *Renal Carcinoma,* in Harvey Mandell & Howard Spiro, eds, *When Doctors Get Sick* 355 (Plenum Medical, 1988).

126. Lesley Fallowfield with Andrew Clark, *Breast Cancer* 73 (Routledge, 1992).

127. Robert L. Yocum, *My Adventure With Lupus: Living With a Chronic Illness* 42–43 (Griffin, 1995).

128. Linda R. Bell, *The Red Butterfly: Lupus Patients Can Survive* 51 (Branden, 1983).

129. Kenneth H. Cohn, *Chemotherapy From an Insider's Perspective,* Lancet 1006, 1008 (May 1, 1982).

130. Abraham Verghese, *My Own Country: A Doctor's Story* 413 (Vintage, 1995).

130a. Suzanne C. Thompson, *Will It Hurt Less If I Can Control It? A Complex Answer to a Simple Question,* 90 Psychological Bulletin 89, 98 (1981). Interestingly, Thompson reports that having behavioral control over an unpleasant event does not seem to make it less painful, although it can lessen anxiety about it and increase tolerance for it. However, she says, "Cognitive control appears to have uniformly positive effects on the experience of an aversive event. Knowing that one has a cognitive strategy lessens anticipatory anxiety, reduces the impact of the stimulus, and improves the postevent effects." Idem at 95.

131. William James, *The Varieties of Religious Experience: A Study in Human Nature* 158 (Modern Library, 1994).

132. Eileen Radziunas, *Lupus: My Search for a Diagnosis* xiii (Hunter House, 1989).

133. Arthur W. Frank, *The Wounded Storyteller: Body, Illness, and Ethics* 126 (U Chicago Press, 1995).

134. Howard Brody, *Transparency: Informed Consent in Primary Care,* 19 HCR 5, 5 (Sept/Oct 1989). Similarly, "the examples and paradigms discussed in most of the bioethics literature are drawn almost exclusively from the content of either emergency or acute medical care." Arthur L. Caplan, *Informed Consent and Provider/Patient Relationships in Rehabilitation Medicine,* in *If I Were a Rich Man Could I Buy a Pancreas? and Other Essays on the Ethics of Health Care* 241 (Indiana U Press, 1992). To like effect is Lachlan Forrow, Steven A. Wortman, & Dan Brock, *Science, Ethics, and the Making of Clinical Decisions,* 259 JAMA 3161, 3164 (1988). On the difference between making medical decisions in tertiary- and primary-care settings, see Howard Brody, *Stories of Sickness* 171–81 (Yale U Press, 1987). A similar problem infects bioethical discussions of the elderly. As Caplan reports, "The paradigmatic bioethics case involving an elderly person is that of a very old man or woman, demented, comatose, or vegetative, who is having one or more major organ systems sustained by a technological intervention in an acute-care setting." Arthur L. Caplan, *Can Autonomy Be Saved?,* in *If I Were a Rich Man Could I Buy a Pancreas? and Other Essays on the Ethics of Health Care* 257 (Indiana U Press, 1992). "But severely impaired, dying persons hardly constitute the average or even a representative sub-sample of the elderly who use health services in the United States. The vast majority of elderly persons who use health-care services . . . are neither demented nor dying . . . ." Idem at 258. Likewise, "the majority of empirical research in ethics concentrates on life and death decisions for terminally ill patients." Robert A. Pearlman, Steven H. Miles, & Robert M. Arnold, *Empirical Research in Medical Ethics,* 14 Theoretical Medicine 197, 198 (1993).

135. Leon R. Kass, *Practicing Ethics: Where's the Action?,* 20 HCR 5, 7 (Jan/Feb 1990) (emphasis in original).

136. Suzanne C. Thompson, Jennifer Pitts, & Lenore Schwankovsky, *Preferences for Involvement in Medical Decision Making: Situational and Demographic Influences,* 22 Patient Education & Counseling 133 (1993).

137. William Martin, *My Prostate and Me: Dealing with Prostate Cancer* 110 (Cadell & Davies, 1994).

138. For example, Jay Katz, *The Silent World of Doctor and Patient* 85–103 (Free Press, 1984).

139. Carolyn Wiener, et al, *Patient Power: Complex Issues Need Complex Answers,* 11 Social Policy 30, 34 (1980).

140. Lee Modjeska, *Keeper of the Night: A Portrait of Life in the Shadow of Death* 95 (LuraMedia, 1995).

141. Jerome P. Kassirer & Stephen G. Pauker, *The Toss-Up,* 305 NEJM 1467, 1467 (1981).

142. Idem at 1468.

143. James L. Johnson, *Coming Back* 13 (Springhouse Publishing, 1979).

144. Joyce L. Dunlop, *Prosthetic Hips,* in Harvey Mandell & Howard Spiro, eds, *When Doctors Get Sick* 80 (Plenum Medical, 1988).

145. Gilda Radner, *It's Always Something* 127–28 (Avon, 1990).

146. Lee Modjeska, *Keeper of the Night: A Portrait of Life in the Shadow of Death* 31 (LuraMedia, 1995).

147. *A Day at the Beach* 150 (Vintage, 1993).

148. For a detailed and engaging example of how a diabetic won and wielded such knowledge, see Mary Cooper Greene, *Living With a Broken String* (no publisher, 1987).

149. Joseph W. Schneider & Peter Conrad, *Having Epilepsy: The Experience and Control of Illness* 181–203 (Temple U Press, 1983).

150. For example, Tim Brookes, *Catching My Breath: An Asthmatic Explores His Illness* (Times Books, 1994).

151. Sandi Gordon, *Parkinson's: A Personal Story of Acceptance* 69–70 (Branden, 1992). More systematically, see Charles W. Lidz, Alan Meisel, & Mark Munetz, *Chronic Disease: The Sick Role and Informed Consent,* 9 Culture, Medicine & Psychiatry 241 (1985).

152. A. Peter Lundin, *Chronic Renal Failure and Hemodialysis,* in Harvey Mandell & Howard Spiro, eds, *When Doctors Get Sick* 364 (Plenum Medical, 1988).

153. William Martin, *My Prostate and Me: Dealing With Prostate Cancer* (Cadell & Davies, 1994).

154. Barbara Creaturo, *Courage: The Testimony of a Cancer Patient* (Pantheon, 1991).

155. Idem at 71.

156. William James, *The Varieties of Religious Experience: A Study in Human Nature* 166 (Modern Library, 1994).

Chapter 5

1. Terrence F. Ackerman, *Why Doctors Should Intervene,* 12 HCR 14, 15 (Aug 1982). Ackerman is unusually aware of the aspects of illness that can impede autonomy. He argues physicians should "intervene" to enhance patients' autonomy.

2. For example, Jay Katz, *The Silent World of Doctor and Patient* 100 (Free Press, 1984); *Canterbury v. Spence,* 464 F2d 772, 782 (DC Cir 1972); *Cobbs v. Grant,* 502 P2d 1, 9 (Cal 1972).

3. Perhaps the most important time for informed consent is not before treatment, but before the patient picks a doctor; and perhaps the most important information is not about the treatment's consequences, but the doctor's qualifications. I have argued at length that many patients will have good reasons to confide their medical decisions to doctors. For

these patients, selecting the right doctor will thus be crucial. This vital and, I suspect, urgently wanted information is (partly for reasonable reasons) unavailable. But what could be more crucial to patients' decisions? As Schuck writes, "Many health services are 'credence' goods, whose evaluation depends on the opinion of experts (usually physicians) who act as gatekeepers to treatment; in contrast, most consumer products are either 'search' goods, whose qualities consumers can ascertain by prepurchase inspection, or 'experience' goods, whose qualities consumers can determine after they have consumed them." Peter H. Schuck, *Rethinking Informed Consent,* 103 Yale L J 899, 929 (1994). But physicians themselves are credence goods. As I suggest later in this chapter, many patients make choices about their doctors. However, these choices are rarely based on the physicians' technical competence, since patients have few reliable ways of evaluating it. The memoirists who tried hardest to find such competence were generally looking for oncologists. The difficulty of that enterprise is suggested by the pilgrimage one patient admiringly describes:

> [U]nlike a lot of patients, the Taylors didn't take anything for granted. The Mayo doctor they flew halfway around the world to see turned out to be "a man of great charm and courtesy and a very compassionate physician," but they were struck by the fact that his name did not appear on any of the most recent articles on the treatment of bone marrow cancer. . . .
>
> With slides and test results in hand, they continued the "journey of discovery" around the U.S.—Chicago, Boston, Dallas, Phoenix, San Francisco, Seattle—looking at other programs at other hospitals, talking to other doctors, other experts, still not taking anybody's word as the last one. To make sure they missed nothing, they recorded all their interviews on tape. . . .
>
> Later, in the solitude of hotel rooms far from home, they reviewed the tapes again and again, writing down unfamiliar words, reading the tea leaves of inflection, struggling to understand what they had heard. Looking for Dr. Right.

Gregory White Smith & Steven Naifeh, *Making Miracles Happen* 39–40 (Little, Brown, 1997). The Taylors finally selected a doctor "who really focused on this particular problem" and who "was doing everything he could to move forward the treatment of what had always been an extremely unresponsive disease." Idem at 40. What were the Taylors looking for? How well could they evaluate it? What did they get? Like many patients, they seemed to feel the best treatment was at the "cutting edge," was the latest experiement. Is this true? When his doctors told Smith they did not know the cause of his condition, Smith himself asked, "How could this be? How could the best minds in medicine not have the answer? I wasn't so much angry at their failure as puzzled." Idem at 42. If a person as sophisticated as Smith had such unrealistic expectations, how well can the average patient judge prospective physicians?

So one dreams about informed consent in the choice of doctors. Facetiously but with feeling, one cancer patient said: "I had never chosen Sheldon Bimberg as my physician. Just as, when buying a car, one cannot get the air-conditioning without purchasing the floor mats, he came as part of the dealer package. . . . Someone should have handed me another informed consent form to read, this time outlining the risks and possible side effects of dealing with Sheldon Bimberg." Evan Handler, *Time on Fire: My Comedy of Terrors* 231 (Little, Brown, 1996). There are proposals to release information about hospitals' procedure and success rates. See, e.g., John E. Wennberg, *Dealing With Medical Practice Variations: A Proposal for Action,* 3 Health Affairs 6 (1984) (although Wennberg would aim this information at providers, not consumers). Information is beginning to be released to the public, although its meaning (and the uses to which it may be put) are currently unclear. See Bradford H. Gray, *The Profit Motive and Patient Care: The Changing Accountability of Doctors and Hospitals* (Harvard U Press, 1991).

4. Eliot Freidson, *Medical Work in America* 36–37 (Yale U Press, 1989).

5. And on demanding grounds:

I didn't go back because I didn't like him. He is widely respected as a physician who keeps up with the latest research and is prepared to champion a treatment, no matter how unfashionable, if good evidence supports it, but he struck me as condescending, aloof, even sneering. He was good enough to take extra time to answer my questions, even to send me extra information by mail, and I know I should overlook his personal manner out of gratitude, let alone self-interest . . . .

Tim Brookes, *Catching My Breath: An Asthmatic Explores His Illness* 136 (Times Books, 1994).

6. Anne Hunsaker Hawkins, *Reconstructing Illness: Studies in Pathography* 191 n. 12 (Purdue U Press, 1993). Two examples of the former kind of shopping are Joie Harrison McGrail, *Fighting Back: One Woman's Struggle Against Cancer* (Harper & Row, 1978), and Laura Chester, *Lupus Novice: Toward Self-Healing* (Station Hill Press, 1987). Two examples of the latter are Cornelius & Kathryn Morgan Ryan, *A Private Battle* (Simon & Schuster, 1979), and William Martin, *My Prostate and Me: Dealing With Prostate Cancer* (Cadell & Davies, 1994).

7. Hawkins, *Reconstructing Illness* at 143 (cited in note 6). Thus Laura Chester sought to choose from the "smorgasbord of therapies" one that "fit my intuitions or needs." *Lupus Novice* at 73 (cited in note 6). For a book which insists that patients shop until they have at least two choices, see Gregory White Smith & Steven Naifeh, *Making Miracles Happen* (Little, Brown, 1997).

8. Josephine Kasteler, et al, *Issues Underlying Prevalence of "Doctor-Shopping" Behavior,* 17 J Health & Social Behavior 328 (1976).

9. Louis Harris & Associates, *Views of Informed Consent and Decisionmaking: Parallel Surveys of Physicians and the Public,* in President's Commission for the Study of Ethical Problems in Medicine and Biomedical and Behavioral Research, *Making Health Care Decisions: The Ethical and Legal Implications of Informed Consent in the Patient-Practitioner Relationship,* Volume Two: Appendices *Empirical Studies of Informed Consent* 21 (U S Gov't Printing Office, 1982). That patients can select doctors in the first place and leave them subsequently may help explain polls that find patients are reasonably content with their own doctors but less content with doctors in general.

10. Marilyn Chase, *Whose Time Is Worth More: Yours Or the Doctor's?,* Wall Street Journal, Oct 24, 1994, at B1.

11. Gayle Feldman, *You Don't Have to be Your Mother* 31–32 (Norton, 1994). For a pronounced version of this pattern, see Barbara Creaturo, *Courage: The Testimony of a Cancer Patient* (Pantheon, 1991).

12. Eileen Radziunas, *Lupus: My Search for a Diagnosis* 39 (Hunter House, 1989).

13. Idem at 33. Even patients who, like Agnes de Mille, resolve to leave decisions to doctors may fire doctors with whom they are dissatisfied. Agnes de Mille, *Reprieve: A Memoir* 53 (Doubleday, 1981).

14. Glenna Wotton Atwood with Lila Green Hunnewell, *Living Well With Parkinson's: An Inspirational, Informative Guide for Parkinsonians and Their Loved Ones* 68 (Wiley, 1991).

15. Peter H. Schuck, *Rethinking Informed Consent,* 103 Yale L J 899, 931 (1994).

16. Idem.

17. Bradford H. Gray, *The Profit Motive and Patient Care: The Changing Accountability of Doctors and Hospitals* 214 (Harvard U Press, 1991).

18. Randall R. Bovbjerg, Philip J. Held, & Louis H. Diamond, *Provider–Patient Relations and Treatment Choice in the Era of Fiscal Incentives: The Case of the End-stage Renal Disease Program,* 65 Milbank Quarterly 177, 198 (1987).

19. Molly Haskell, *Love and Other Infectious Diseases* 29 (Citadel, 1990). Cassell says that some "very manipulative patients" try to control the doctor. "The extent of their success is often amazing, as the doctor finds himself doing things to and for the patient that he would not ordinarily consider doing." Eric J. Cassell, *The Healer's Art* 145 (MIT Press, 1985).

20. One of the two primary reasons patients refuse treatment in hospitals seems to be to extract information from doctors. Paul S. Appelbaum & Loren Roth, *Patients Who Refuse Treatment in Medical Hospitals,* 250 JAMA 1296 (1983).

21. Anselm Strauss, et al, *Social Organization of Medical Work* 208 (U Chicago Press, 1985).

22. For a brief glimpse of this important resource, see idem at 204. For a description of the fellowship that underlies it, see Robert F. Murphy, *The Body Silent* 133–36 (Norton, 1990).

23. For one particularly plain illustration, see William Martin, *My Prostate and Me: Dealing With Prostate Cancer* (Cadell & Davies, 1994).

24. On these programs, see Bradford H. Gray, *The Profit Motive and Patient Care* at 274–320 (cited in note 17). Gray concludes utilization management "has resulted in virtually no well-documented allegations of serious harm to patients," while its results "appear to have been generally acceptable, if not always completely satisfactory to patients and their physicians." Idem at 320.

25. Eric J. Cassell, *The Changing Concept of the Ideal Physician,* 115 Daedalus 185, 195 (Spring 1986).

26. Debra L. Roter & Judith A. Hall, *Studies of Doctor–Patient Interaction,* 10 Annual Rev Public Health 163, 178 (1989). On this trend, see, e.g., Leo G. Reeder, *The Patient–Client as a Consumer: Some Observations on the Changing Professional–Client Relationship,* 13 J Health & Social Behavior 406 (1972); Carolyn Wiener, et al, *Patient Power: Complex Issues Need Complex Answers,* 11 Social Policy 30 (1980); Marie R. Haug & Bebe Lavin, *Practitioner or Patient—Who's in Charge?,* 22 J Health & Social Behavior 212 (1981); Marie Haug & Bebe Lavin, *Consumerism in Medicine: Challenging Physician Authority* (Sage, 1983).

27. Arthur W. Frank, *At the Will of the Body* 102 (Houghton Mifflin, 1991).

28. *Medical Work in America* 8 (Yale U Press, 1989).

29. President's Commission for the Study of Ethical Problems in Medicine and Biomedical and Behavioral Research, *Making Health Care Decisions: The Ethical and Legal Implications of Informed Consent in the Patient–Practitioner Relationship,* Volume One: Report 46 (U S Gov't Printing Office, 1982). To like effect, see, e.g., William M. Strull, Bernard Lo, & Gerald Charles, *Do Patients Want to Participate in Medical Decision Making?,* 252 JAMA 2990, 2993 (1984); Jennifer Susan Mark & Howard Spiro, *Informed Consent for Colonoscopy: A Prospective Study,* 150 Archives of Internal Medicine 777, 778 (1990).

30. Robert Zussman, *Intensive Care: Medical Ethics and the Medical Profession* 153 (U Chicago Press, 1992).

31. Robert M. Kaplan, *Health-Related Quality of Life in Patient Decision Making,* 47 J Social Issues 69, 70 (1991).

32. Idem.

33. An extensive and careful, if now somewhat dated, survey of this research is Alan

Meisel & Loren H. Roth, *Toward an Informed Discussion of Informed Consent: A Review and Critique of the Empirical Studies,* 25 Arizona L Rev 265 (1983).

34. Roter & Hall, 10 Annual Rev Public Health at 167 (cited in note 26). On the other hand, "there is a strong *positive* relation between the amount offered and the absolute amount recalled." Idem (emphasis in original).

35. See Renée R. Anspach, *Notes on the Sociology of Medical Discourse: The Language of Case Presentation,* 29 J Health & Social Behavior 357, 358 (1988).

36. See Meisel & Roth, 25 Arizona L Rev at 265 (cited in note 33).

37. "Autonomy" itself is a problem in rationing, since the information necessary for autonomous decisions takes time, and thus money, to convey. For a brief but effective investigation of this problem, see Peter H. Schuck, *Rethinking Informed Consent,* 103 Yale L J 899, 938–41 (1994). Schuck suspects "policymakers and cost-conscious patients and payors may [come to] view as an insupportable extravagance a doctrine [informed consent] requiring physicians to spend more time engaging in more extensive dialogues with patients about alternatives that are no longer practically available to them, dialogues that are (or may seem) resistant to change, that often occur after the crucial decision has been made, and that seem to have little observable effect on ultimate treatment decisions." Idem at 941.

38. Nonphysicians might provide information, and there have been experiments with video programs.

38a. Gary Klein, *Sources of Power: How People Make Decisions* 31 (MIT Press, 1996).

38b. Idem at 40.

38c. Idem at 31.

38d. Idem at 34.

38e. Idem at 147.

38f. "You rarely get someone to jump a skill level by teaching more facts and rules. . . . [I]n natural settings, perceptual learning takes many cases to develop. . . . We can make training more efficient but cannot radically replace the accumulation of experiences." Idem at 287.

39. Renée Anspach, *Deciding Who Lives: Fateful Choices in the Intensive Care Nursery* 36 (1993).

40. Oliver Sacks, *A Leg to Stand On* 165 (HarperCollins, 1984).

41. Idem at 188.

42. Eric Hodgins, *Episode: Report on the Accident Inside My Skull* 161 (Atheneum, 1964).

43. Barbara Creaturo, *Courage: The Testimony of a Cancer Patient* 10 (Pantheon, 1991).

44. Elaine J. Sobo, *Choosing Unsafe Sex: AIDS-Risk Denial Among Disadvantaged Women* 168 (U Pennsylvania Press, 1995).

45. Reynolds Price, *A Whole New Life: An Illness and Healing* 40–41 (Atheneum, 1994).

46. Philip Roth, *Patrimony: A True Story* 66 (Simon & Schuster, 1991).

47. Idem at 67.

48. Idem at 201.

49. One surgeon comments, "It's so easy for physicians to think we are the masters of our own destinies—potters instead of clay—and this may be even more common among surgeons, who so often function like mini-potters: rebuilding, reworking, rearranging. Surgery is an awesome vocation, but it's just too easy to let success ruin your sense of humility." G. Edward Rozar & David B. Biebel, *Laughing in the Face of AIDS: A Surgeon's Personal Battle* 79 (Baker, 1992).

50. Peter H. Schuck, *Rethinking Informed Consent,* 103 Yale L J 899, 937 (1994).

51. Idem.

52. For a survey of specific suggestions, see Debra L. Roter & Judith A. Hall, *Studies of Doctor–Patient Interaction,* 10 Annual Rev Public Health 163, 175–77 (1989). For an extended and more optimistic argument, see, e.g., Eric J. Cassell, *Talking With Patients: Volume I: The Theory of Doctor–Patient Communication* (MIT Press, 1985).

53. The empirical evidence on this score is slim and equivocal. One study concluded its findings "will provide little sustenance to those who argue that school experiences have little effect on the attitudes that students bring to training." But it also warned, "Only a modest portion of the variance in attitude change" seemed be caused by "the socialization process." Bebe Lavin, et al, *Change in Student Physicians' Views on Authority Relationships With Patients,* 28 J Health & Social Behavior 258, 268 (1987). The most engaging and penetrating empirical investigation of moral ideas in medical education is Charles L. Bosk, *Forgive and Remember: Managing Medical Failure* (U Chicago Press, 1979). But what is its lesson?

54. Judith Shklar, *Legalism: Law, Morals, and Political Trials* 19 (Harvard U Press, 1964). It is suggestive that where practicing physicians might be thought most responsive to educational efforts—improving clinical treatment—"experience with providing feedback to physicians has been uneven . . . ." Bradford H. Gray, *The Profit Motive and Patient Care: The Changing Accountability of Doctors and Hospitals* 227 (Harvard U Press, 1991).

55. Letter from Oliver Wendell Holmes to Frederick Pollock, April 2, 1926, in Mark DeWolfe Howe, ed, 2 *Holmes–Pollock Letters: The Correspondence of Mr Justice Holmes and Sir Frederick Pollock, 1874–1932* 178 (Harvard U Press, 1961).

56. Ezekiel J. Emanuel & Linda L. Emanuel, *Four Models of the Physician–Patient Relationship,* 267 JAMA 2221, 2226 (1992).

57. One great challenge in teaching—gauging how fast and thoroughly students can be expected to learn—must be even harder for doctors, whose patients are more varied than students.

58. 464 F2d 772, 782 n. 27 (1972).

59. Jay Katz, *The Silent World of Doctor and Patient* 92 (Free Press, 1984). Similarly dismissive is David S. Brody, *The Patient's Role in Clinical Decision-Making,* 93 Annals of Internal Medicine 718, 720 (1980): "[H]ealth beliefs, attitudes, and decisions are based on patients' understanding of the seriousness of their illness, the expected benefits of treatments, and the costs (including side effects) of the action . . . . These are relatively straightforward issues that most patients can readily comprehend without too much difficulty within a reasonable time."

60. Robert M. Kaplan, *Health-Related Quality of Life in Patient Decision Making,* 47 J Social Issues 69, 86 (1991) (emphasis in original).

61. Kip Viscusi, *Smoking: Making the Risky Decision* (Oxford U Press, 1992).

62. *Choosing Unsafe Sex: AIDS-Risk Denial Among Disadvantaged Women* 25 (U Pennsylvania Press, 1995).

63. Eric J. Cassell, *The Healer's Art* 140–63 (MIT Press, 1976).

64. Michael Korda, *Man to Man: Surviving Prostate Cancer* 213 (Random House, 1996).

65. Rosalind MacPhee, *Picasso's Woman: A Breast Cancer Story* 61 (Kodansha, 1996).

66. Idem at 63.

67. Howard Latin, *"Good" Warnings, Bad Products, and Cognitive Limitations,* 41 UCLA L Rev 1193, 1221 (1994) (footnotes omitted). Oddly, the reformist tendency in the

law of medicine is to deprecate the problem of providing adequate information while the reformist tendency in product liability law is to find that problem almost insuperable.

68. Idem at 1226.

69. Idem at 1222 (footnote omitted).

70. Idem at 1242 (footnote omitted).

71. Idem at 1243 (footnotes omitted).

72. Oliver Sacks, *A Leg to Stand On* 158 (HarperCollins, 1984).

73. Idem at 159.

74. Lesley Fallowfield with Andrew Clark, *Breast Cancer* 115–16 (Routledge, 1992).

75. Ellen C. Annandale, *Dimensions of Patient Control in a Free-Standing Birth Center,* 25 Social Science Medicine 1235, 1244–45 (1987).

76. Lawrence M. Friedman, *The Republic of Choice: Law, Authority, and Culture* 136 (Harvard U Press, 1990).

77. See generally idem.

78. Marion Deutsche Cohen, *Dirty Details: The Days and Nights of a Well Spouse* 149 (Temple U Press, 1996).

79. Arthur W. Frank, *At the Will of the Body* 112 (Houghton Mifflin, 1991).

80. Ernest A. Hirsch, *Starting Over* 91–92 (Christopher Publishing House, 1977).

81. Betty Johnson, *Change of Heart* 62 (Sayre, 1973).

82. Kenneth A. Shapiro, *Dying and Living: One Man's Life With Cancer* 71 (U Texas Press, 1985).

83. Hirsch, *Starting Over* at 82 (cited in note 80).

84. Charles W. Lidz, Alan Meisel, & Mark Munetz, *Chronic Disease: The Sick Role and Informed Consent,* 9 Culture, Medicine & Psychiatry 11 (1985).

85. Maurice Raskin, *Ulcerative Colitis,* in Harvey Mandell & Howard Spiro, eds, *When Doctors Get Sick* 210 (Plenum Medical, 1988).

86. A. Peter Lundin, *Chronic Renal Failure and Hemodialysis,* in Harvey Mandell & Howard Spiro, eds, *When Doctors Get Sick* 365 (Plenum Medical, 1988).

87. Sandi Gordon, *Parkinson's: A Personal Story of Acceptance* 115 (Branden, 1992).

88. Janet Lee James, *One Particular Harbor* 246 (Nobel Press, 1993).

89. Judith Alexander Brice, *Ulcerative Colitis and Avascular Necrosis of Hips,* in Harvey Mandell & Howard Spiro, eds, *When Doctors Get Sick* 186 (Plenum Medical, 1988).

90. Andrew Potok, *Ordinary Daylight: Portrait of an Artist Going Blind* 48 (Holt, Rinehart & Winston, 1980).

91. Idem at 86.

92. Sobo, *Choosing Unsafe Sex* at 93 (cited in note 44).

93. Rachelle Breslow, *Who Said So?: How Our Thoughts and Beliefs Affect Our Physiology* 88 (Celestial Arts, 1991).

94. "[S]elf-realization tends to pit us against society. The social reality surrounding us is seen as an obstacle to our becoming what we should. . . . The fortress of conscience is always besieged. To protect it, self-realizing people must rely on their own resources, and the social world is seen as soiling . . . ." John Kekes, *Moral Tradition and Individuality* 119 (Princeton U Press, 1989). There will, of course, always be a question in intimate relationships of finding the right balance between independence and dependence. My concern is that the strong view of independence seems to sacrifice too much.

95. Urvashi Vaid, *Foreword,* in Amy Hoffman, *Hospital Time* ix (Duke U Press, 1997).

96. Suzanne E. Berger, *Horizontal Woman: The Story of a Body in Exile* 91–93 (Houghton Mifflin, 1996) (emphasis in original).

97. Idem at 94.

98. Paulette Bates Alden, *Crossing the Moon: A Journey Through Infertility* 18, 45, 278 (Hungry Mind Press, 1996).

99. Idem at 106.

100. Charles Taylor, *The Ethics of Authenticity* 45 (Harvard U Press, 1992).

101. Francesca M. Cancian, *Love In America: Gender and Self-development* 39 (Cambridge U Press, 1987).

102. Idem at 40.

103. Pepper Schwartz, *The Family as a Changed Institution,* 8 J Family Issues 455, 458 (1987).

104. Idem.

105. Rachelle Breslow, *Who Said So?: How Our Thoughts and Beliefs Affect Our Physiology* 56 (Celestial Arts, 1991).

106. On the autonomist view of relationships, see Carl E. Schneider, *Marriage, Morals, and the Law: No-Fault Divorce and Moral Discourse,* Utah L Rev 503 (1994).

107. David A. Tate, *Health, Hope, and Healing* 181 (M. Evans, 1989). One historian believes altruism has come to be seen as foolish or trivial: "The unselfish were people who gave up too much or who had so much that their giving seemed not to count as sacrifice." Peter Clecak, *America's Quest for the Ideal Self: Dissent and Fulfillment in the 60s and 70s* 264 (Oxford U Press, 1983).

108. Musa Mayer, *Examining Myself: One Woman's Story of Breast Cancer Treatment and Recovery* 95 (Faber & Faber, 1993).

109. Idem at 131.

110. Idem at 95.

111. Jill Ireland, *Life Wish* 64 (Jove, 1988).

112. Idem.

113. Rachelle Breslow, *Who Said So?: How Our Thoughts and Beliefs Affect Our Physiology* 66 (Celestial Arts, 1991).

114. Idem at 21.

115. Martha Balshem, *Cancer in the Community: Class and Medical Authority* 115 (Smithsonian Institution, 1993). Balshem observes that this passage casts the family as a threat to the doctor's control of his relationship with his patient. This is part of a larger issue: Because autonomism has conquered the moral high ground, power in medicine is often contested in terms of the patient's right to autonomy. (Just as, when I worked for a teacher's union, we put *all* our arguments in terms of children's interests in a good education.)

116. Sharon H. Imbus & Bruce E. Zawacki, *Autonomy for Burned Patients When Survival Is Unprecedented,* 297 NEJM 308, 308 (1977). They add, "Turning to the family for decision making when death seems imminent for an incompetent patient is rarely satisfactory; guilt-ridden families often find it very difficult to be objective and unselfish in their decision making." Idem at 310.

117. Roberta G. Simmons, Susan Klein Marine, & Richard L. Simmons, *Gift of Life: The Effect of Organ Transplantation on Individual, Family, and Societal Dynamics* 431 (Transaction Books, 1987).

118. Idem at 197, citing Jay Katz & Alexander Morgan Capron, *Catastrophic Diseases: Who Decides What?* (Russell Sage, 1975).

119. Idem at 228.

120. Hilde Lindemann Nelson & James Lindemann Nelson, *The Patient in the Family:*

An Ethics of Medicine and Families 85 (Routledge, 1995). They are referring to Allen E. Buchanan & Dan W. Brock, *Deciding for Others: The Ethics of Surrogate Decision Making* 136–37, 143 (Cambridge U Press, 1989).

121. Arthur W. Frank, *The Wounded Storyteller: Body, Illness, and Ethics* 48–49 (U Chicago Press, 1995). The phrase is Albert Schweitzer's.

122. Idem at 17.

123. See Robert Wuthnow, *Sharing the Journey: Support Groups and America's New Quest for Community* (Free Press, 1994). The enthusiasm is not universal. Suzy Szasz articulates one reason when she says that for her group "[l]ife seemed filled with nothing but disappointment and despair, which the group, as a formal gathering, seemed intent on legitimizing as both involuntary and insurmountable." *Living With It: Why You Don't Have to Be Healthy to Be Happy* 94 (Prometheus, 1991).

124. Wuthnow, *Sharing the Journey* at 176–77 (cited in note 123).

125. Idem at 201.

126. Idem at 175.

127. Idem at 190.

128., Lucy Bregman & Sara Thiermann, *First Person Mortal: Personal Narratives of Dying, Death, and Grief* 104–5 (Paragon House, 1995).

129. Kenneth A. Shapiro, *Dying and Living: One Man's Life With Cancer* 70 (U Texas Press, 1985). Shapiro eventually persuaded his wife to see several psychologists. "One of them even encouraged her to continue her behavior regardless of the effects it had on me because it was a way for her to vent her own feelings and it was up to me to deal with it. I am not sure I follow that logic at all."

130. Ann Swidler, *Love and Adulthood in American Culture,* in Neil J. Smelser & Erik H. Erikson, eds, *Themes of Work and Love in Adulthood* 129 (Harvard U Press, 1980).

131. *Picasso's Woman: A Breast Cancer Story* (Kodansha, 1996).

132. This report comes from an *Afterword* by Kathy LaTour, idem at 275.

133. Idem at 238.

134. Idem at 8.

135. Idem at 11.

136. Idem at 35.

137. Idem at 37.

138. Idem at 43.

139. Idem at 66.

140. Idem at 229.

141. Idem at 231.

142. Stewart Alsop, *Stay of Execution: A Sort of Memoir* 56 (Lippincott, 1973).

143. For example, Jay Katz, *The Silent World of Doctor and Patient* 100–01 (Free Press, 1984):

> It appealed to patients, engulfed by pain and suffering, because surrender to powerful, wise and soothing caretakers was strongly fostered by memories of earlier days when a parent satisfied all discomforting bodily needs. Thus, the regression to more childlike functioning that can result from illness becomes augmented by a patient's wish for caretaking by a parent-physician who, as memory informs, will immediately alleviate all suffering.

144. Eileen Radziunas, *Lupus: My Search for a Diagnosis* 17 (Hunter House, 1989).

145. Mary Cooper Greene, *Living with a Broken String* 67–68 (no publisher, 1987).

146. Betty Johnson, *Change of Heart* 87 (Sayre, 1973).

147. Philip & Joyce Bedsworth, *Fight the Good Fight* 64 (Herald Press, 1991) (emphasis in original).

148. Idem at 49. It is perhaps not coincidental that, while most memoirists of illness are roughly upper-middle class, each of the couples I quote in this paragraph is roughly middle-middle class.

149. Eric Hodgins, *Episode: Report on the Accident Inside My Skull* 191 (Atheneum, 1964) (emphases in original).

150. Arnold R. Beisser, *Flying Without Wings* 41 (Doubleday, 1989).

151. Idem at 43.

152. Gerda Lerner, *A Death of One's Own* 106 (U Wisconsin Press, 1985).

153. Laura Chester, *Lupus Novice: Toward Self-Healing* 53 (Station Hill Press, 1987) (emphasis in original).

154. Mary Alice Geier, *Cancer: What's It Doing in My Life?* 36 (Hope Publishing House, 1985) (emphasis in original).

155. Donald Hall, *Life Work* 123 (Beacon, 1993).

156. Gerda Lerner, *A Death of One's Own* 116 (U Wisconsin Press, 1985).

157. Andrew Potok, *Ordinary Daylight: Portrait of an Artist Going Blind* 86 (Holt, Rinehart & Winston, 1980).

158. Compare Candace Clark, *Misery and Company: Sympathy in Everyday Life* 175 (U Chicago Press, 1997), which notes that someone who never claims sympathy "avoids incurring obligations, prevents others from discharging past obligations, or excludes others from backstage regions where problems and vulnerabilities are apparent." Such people foreclose intimacy.

159. Gillian Rose, *Love's Work; A Reckoning With Life* 60–61 (Schocken Books, 1995).

160. For an angry statement of the claims of the family of a man with multiple sclerosis, see Marion Deutsche Cohen, *Dirty Details: The Days and Nights of a Well Spouse* (Temple U Press, 1996). This book emblematizes how poorly our moral language allows us to express moral ambiguity. Bioethics has few resources for acknowledging families' interests, but here the sick man's entitlement to help decide whether he would go to a nursing home evaporates in the heat of the family's claims.

161. Caren Topliff, *Wrestling Back: A Family's Trial With Paralyzing Injury* 250–51 (DIMI Press, 1996).

162. Hilde Lindemann Nelson & James Lindemann Nelson, *The Patient in the Family: An Ethics of Medicine and Families* 3 (Routledge, 1995).

163. Idem.

164. Joel Solkoff, *Learning to Live Again: My Triumph Over Cancer* 83 (Holt, Rinehart, & Winston, 1983).

165. Robert L. Yocum, *My Adventure With Lupus: Living with a Chronic Illness* 95 (Griffin, 1995).

166. Joanna Baumer Permut, *Embracing the Wolf* 129–30 (Cherokee, 1989).

167. Simone de Beauvoir, *A Very Easy Death* 59 (Pantheon, 1964).

168. Betty Johnson, *Change of Heart* 65 (Sayre, 1973).

169. Mary Alice Geier, *Cancer: What's It Doing in My Life?* 98 (Hope Publishing House, 1985).

170. Kenneth A. Shapiro, *Dying and Living: One Man's Life With Cancer* 122 (U Texas Press, 1985).

171. Marjorie McVicker Sutcliffe, *Grandma Cherry's Spoon: A Story of Tuberculosis* 32 (Geronima Press, 1991).

172. Robert F. Murphy, *The Body Silent* 66 (Norton, 1990).

173. Philip & Joyce Bedsworth, *Fight the Good Fight* 33–34 (Herald Press, 1991).

174. Simone de Beauvoir, *A Very Easy Death* 59 (Pantheon, 1964).

175. *Misery and Company: Sympathy in Everyday Life* 170–74 (U Chicago Press, 1997).

176. *Two-Part Invention: The Story of a Marriage* 146 (Harper & Row, 1989).

177. *Why I Don't Have a Living Will,* 19 Law, Medicine, & Health Care 101, 103 (1991).

178. Robert H. Bellah, et al, *Habits of the Heart: Individualism and Commitment in American Life* 20–21 (U California Press, 1985).

179. Anne Hunsaker Hawkins, *Reconstructing Illness: Studies in Pathography* 129 (Purdue U Press, 1993).

180. Tim Brookes, *Catching My Breath: An Asthmatic Explores His Illness* 278 (Times Books, 1994). On this score, see Susan Sontag, *Illness as Metaphor* (Anchor, 1990).

181. On the cultural and legal expansion of choice in the twentieth century, see Lawrence W. Friedman, *The Republic of Choice: Law, Authority, and Culture* (Harvard U Press, 1990).

182. Emile Durkheim, *The Division of Labor in Society* 398 (Free Press, 1933).

183. "The division of labor itself contributes to this enfranchisement, for individual natures, while specializing, become more complex, and by that are in part freed from collective action and hereditary influences which can only enforce themselves upon simple, general things." Idem at 404.

184. *And There Was Light* 53 (Parabola, 1987).

185. Natalie Davis Spingarn, *Hanging in There* 53–54 (Stein & Day, 1982).

186. Janet Lee James, *One Particular Harbor* 246 (Nobel Press, 1993).

187. *It's Always Something* 181 (Avon, 1990).

188. The problem for patients lies partly in a culture which too warmly embraces the duty of independence. When John Hockenberry was put in a wheelchair by an automobile accident, he encountered "a lot of talk of suicide." People "would ask if I had thought of killing myself" and tell him they did not think they could manage being in his condition. "Many people would make this macabre suggestion to my parents, saying openly that if I found it too difficult to continue my life, they should be ready to accept my wanting to die." What, Hockenberry asks,

> about somebody like my friend Roger, who constantly needed others to take care of his basic needs. How might Roger laugh off the nagging suspicion that the person dressing him believed that suicide would be a more elegant solution to his predicament than going on with his life? Was it the experience of quadriplegia that engendered thoughts of suicide, or did hopelessness come from the experience of being surrounded by people who considered that struggling to live with a disability was, in the end, not worth the effort?

John Hockenberry, *Moving Violations: War Zones, Wheelchairs, and Declarations of Independence* 77 (Hyperion, 1995).

189. Gerda Lerner, *A Death of One's Own* 116 (U Wisconsin Press, 1985). The overvaluation of independence can perversely lead to dependence. Paralyzed by polio, Arnold Beisser realized that "[t]he more a person believes he must rely on himself alone or on just a few others, the more he behaves penuriously. He has all of his eggs in one basket, and so must cling tightly to what he has. His independence is under constant siege, and his brittle self-esteem is continuously on the line if the circle of his dependence is small." Arnold R. Beisser, *Flying Without Wings* 43 (Doubleday, 1989).

190. Ernest A. Hirsch, *Starting Over* 142–43 (Christopher Publishing House, 1977).

191. Lucy Grealy, *Autobiography of a Face* 217 (HarperPerennial, 1995).

192. Lucy Bregman & Sara Thiermann, *First Person Mortal: Personal Narratives of Dying, Death, and Grief* 173 (Paragon House, 1995).

193. Anne Hunsaker Hawkins, *Reconstructing Illness: Studies in Pathography* 151 (Purdue U Press, 1993).

194. *First Person Mortal* at 173 (cited in note 192).

195. "In order for executives, professionals, and others with decision-making responsibilities to avoid the undesirable effects of decisional overload on their efficiency and health, it is probably essential for them to be highly discriminating about the potential challenges they accept and those they reject." Irving L. Janis, *The Patient as Decision Maker*, in W. Doyle Gentry, ed, *Handbook of Behavioral Medicine* 349–50 (Guilford, 1984).

196. Gerda Lerner, *A Death of One's Own* 129 (U Wisconsin Press, 1985).

197. Peter L. Berger, *Facing Up to Modernity: Excursions in Society, Politics, and Religion* 76 (Basic Books, 1977).

198. Idem.

199. Idem at xvi.

200. Idem at xvii.

201. Soren Kierkegaard, *The Sickness Unto Death: A Christian Psychological Exposition for Upbuilding and Awakening* 36 (Princeton U Press, 1980). "What is missing is essentially the power to obey, to submit to the necessity in one's life, to what may be called one's limitations." Idem.

202. Jay Katz, *The Silent World of Doctor and Patient* 121 (Free Press, 1984).

203. Arthur W. Frank, *At the Will of the Body* 58–59 (Houghton Mifflin, 1991).

204. Michael P. Kelly, *Colitis* 34 (Routledge, 1992).

205. See chapter 1.

206. Such a life was most fully institutionalized in monastic orders. As the Rule of St. Benedict says, "We are forbidden to do our own will, since Scripture tells us, *Leave thy own will and desire.*" Saint Benedict, *The Rule of Saint Benedict* 28 (Chatto & Windus, 1909). And thus Ignatius Loyola: "I ought on entering religion, and thereafter, to place myself entirely in the hands of God, and of him who takes His place by His authority. I ought to desire that my Superior should oblige me to give up my own judgment, and conquer my own mind." Quoted in William James, *The Varieties of Religious Experience: A Study in Human Nature* 344 (Modern Library, 1994). Monastic life is made most accessible to secularists by such memoirs and fictional accounts as Monica Baldwin, *I Leap Over the Wall* (Hamish Hamilton, 1951); Katherine Hulme, *The Nun's Story* (Little, Brown, 1956); and Rumer Godden, *In This House of Brede* (Viking, 1969). William James's two lectures on saintliness provide a detached but sympathetic appreciation of the monastic virtues. *The Varieties of Religious Experience* at 285–469 (cited in this note). For a sociological view of monastic life, see Suzanne Campbell-Jones, *In Habit: A Study of Working Nuns* (Pantheon, 1978). For the self-abnegating view applied to illness, see John Donne, *Devotions Upon Emergent Occasions* (U Michigan Press, 1959).

207. Betty Garton Ulrich, *Rooted in the Sky: A Faith to Cope With Cancer* 43 (Judson Press, 1989).

208. "The ideal of a rational plan of life assumes that the individual has a sense of what would constitute a set of the good things in life for her, and that she has looked at her social circumstances and her natural talents and has chosen a path that will maximize her opportunities for acquiring as many of those good things as possible." Howard Brody, *Stories of Sickness* 50 (Yale U Press, 1987). Compare Ronald Dworkin, *Autonomy and the Demented Self,* 64 Milbank Quarterly 4, 10, Supp 2 (1986), which argues that autonomy

requires "the capacity to see and evaluate particular decisions in the structured context of an overall life organized around a coherent conception of character and conviction." The term "life plan" figures in such influential works as John Rawls, *A Theory of Justice* (Harvard U Press, 1971). The phrase "plan of life" goes back at least to Mill. John Stuart Mill, *On Liberty*, in *The Philosophy of John Stuart Mill: Ethical, Political, and Religious* 252 (Modern Library, 1961).

209. James, *The Varieties of Religious Experience* at 8 (cited in note 206).

210. Idem at 371.

211. Carl E. Schneider, *Rights Discourse and Neonatal Euthanasia,* 76 California L Rev 151 (1988); Carl E. Schneider, *State-Interest Analysis in Fourteenth-Amendment "Privacy" Law: An Essay on the Constitutionalization of Social Issues,* 51 Law & Contemporary Problems 79 (1988); Carl E. Schneider, *Making Sausage,* 27 HCR 27 (Jan/Feb 1997).

212. Robert H. Bellah, et al, *Habits of the Heart: Individualism and Commitment in American Life* (U California Press, 1985).

213. Ellen Burstein MacFarlane with Patricia Burstein, *Legwork: An Inspiring Journey Through a Chronic Illness* 4 (Scribner's, 1994).

214. Idem at 14.

215. Idem at xi.

216. Idem at 5.

217. Idem.

218. Idem at 130.

219. Idem at 122–23.

220. Idem at 131.

221. Idem at 134.

222. Idem at 139.

223. Idem at 140.

224. Idem at 156.

225. Idem at 167.

226. Idem at 140.

227. Idem at 168.

Chapter 6

1. Carl E. Schneider, *Marriage, Morals, and the Law: No-Fault Divorce and Moral Discourse,* Utah L Rev 503, 585 (1994). On the drawbacks of legal rules as an instrument of bioethical policy, see Carl E. Schneider, *Bioethics in the Language of the Law,* 24 HCR16 (July/Aug 1994); Carl E. Schneider, *Making Sausage,* 27 HCR 27 (Jan/Feb 1997).

2. This may be what the President's Commission meant in urging "that considerable flexibility should be accorded to patients and professionals to define the terms of their own relationships." President's Commission for the Study of Ethical Problems in Medicine and Biomedical and Behavioral Research, *Making Health Care Decisions: The Ethical and Legal Implications of Informed Consent in the Patient–Practitioner Relationship,* Volume One: Report 38 (U S Gov't Printing Office, 1982).

3. See, e.g., Jack Ende, et al, *Measuring Patients' Desire for Autonomy: Decision Making and Information-Seeking Preferences Among Medical Patients,* 4 J General Internal Medicine 23, 34 (1989). Marc D. Silverstein, et al, *Amyotrophic Lateral Sclerosis and Life-Sustaining Therapy: Patients' Desires for Information, Participation in Decision Making, and Life-Sustaining Therapy,* 66 Mayo Clinic Proceedings 906, 910 (1991), not only reaches the same conclusion, but reports that even the factor most mentioned by other

studies as correlated with a desire to participate in decisions—youth—was not thus associated among their respondents. Bernard Lo, Gary A. McLeod, & Glenn Saika, *Patient Attitudes to Discussing Life-Sustaining Treatment,* 146 Archives of Internal Medicine 1613, 1614 (1986), reports a similar inability to identify "medical, functional, psycho-social, or demographic characteristics" that might identify patients who want to discuss life-sustaining treatment with their doctor. And another study concluded that "[a]ttitudes about appropriate patient role behavior were not effective predictors of observed patient role behavior as exhibited by a patient's comments to the doctor." Analee E. Beisecker, *Aging and the Desire for Information and Input in Medical Decisions: Patient Consumerism in Medical Encounters,* 28 Gerontologist 330, 333 (1988). But see Suzanne C. Thompson, Jennifer Pitts, & Lenore Schwankovsky, *Preferences for Involvement in Medical Decision Making: Situational and Demographic Influences,* 22 Patient Education & Counseling 133 (1993), which reports that age and education level accounted for up to 25% of the variance in a study of desire to make medical decisions.

4. David S. Krantz, Andrew Baum, & Margaret v. Wideman, *Assessment of Preferences for Self-Treatment and Information in Health Care,* 39 J Personality & Social Psychology 977, 988 (1980).

5. Lesley F. Degner & Jeffrey A. Sloan, *Decision Making During Serious Illness: What Role Do Patients Really Want to Play?,* 45 J Clinical Epidemiology 941, 948 (1992).

6. Ashwini Sehgal, et al, *How Strictly Do Dialysis Patients Want Their Advance Directives Followed?,* 267 JAMA 59, 62 (1992).

7. Jack Ende, et al, *Measuring Patients' Desire for Autonomy: Decision Making and Information-Seeking Preferences Among Medical Patients,* 4 J General Internal Medicine 23, 28 (1989). This conclusion accords with the observation that patients' preferences about life-sustaining treatment "do not appear to be strongly correlated with demographic characteristics or health status measures," are "difficult to predict," and are not accurately predicted by doctors. Maria A. Everhart & Robert Pearlman, *Stability of Patient Preferences Regarding Life-Sustaining Treatments,* 97 Chest 159, 162 (1990).

8. Lesley Fallowfield with Andrew Clark, *Breast Cancer* 115 (Routledge, 1992).

9. Suzanne C. Thompson, Paul R. Cheek, & Melody A. Graham, *The Other Side of Perceived Control: Disadvantages and Negative Effects,* in Shirlynn Spacapan & Stuart Oskamp, eds, *The Social Psychology of Health: The Claremont Symposium on Applied Social Psychology* 69, 89 (Sage, 1987).

10. Alan Meisel & Loren H. Roth, *Toward an Informed Discussion of Informed Consent: A Review and Critique of the Empirical Studies,* 25 Arizona L Rev 265, 278 (1983).

11. Eric Hodgins, *Episode: Report on the Accident Inside My Skull* 90 (Atheneum, 1964).

12. Ende, et al, 4 J General Internal Medicine at 28 (cited in note 7).

13. William M. Strull, Bernard Lo, & Gerald Charles, *Do Patients Want to Participate in Medical Decision Making?,* 252 JAMA 2990, 2994 (1984). In another study, doctors "stated correctly whether patients wanted to participate in the decision making or not 27 of 40 times and there was no statistical significance between whether they overestimated or underestimated the amount that the patient wanted to participate." Jennifer Susan Mark & Howard Spiro, *Informed Consent for Colonoscopy: A Prospective Study,* 150 Archives of Internal Medicine 777, 779 (1990). One might attribute these problems to the failure of doctors to talk to patients. But it is sobering that in an analogous situation, "[t]he accuracy of resuscitation predictions . . . was not significantly greater for physicians who discussed resuscitation or CPR with their patients than for those who did not in four of six decisions . . ." and that those who discussed them "were significantly less accurate than

those who did not in the remaining two decisions . . . ." Richard F. Uhlmann, Robert A. Pearlman, & Kevin C. Cain, *Physicians' and Spouses' Predictions of Elderly Patients' Resuscitation Preferences,* 43 J Gerontology M115, M117–18 (1988).

14. David S. Krantz, Andrew Baum, & Margaret v. Wideman, *Assessment of Preferences for Self-Treatment and Information in Health Care,* 39 J Personality & Social Psychology 977, 987 (1980).

15. Barbara Barrie, *Second Act: Life After Colostomy and Other Adventures* 102–3 (Scribner, 1997).

16. Eliot Freidson, *Medical Work in America* 194 (Yale U Press, 1989).

17. E. Haavi Morreim, *Balancing Act: The New Medical Ethics of Medicine's New Economics* 27 (Georgetown U Press, 1995).

18. On these trends, see Eli Ginzburg, *Tomorrow's Hospital: A Look to the Twenty-first Century* (Yale U Press, 1996).

19. See Mark A. Hall, *Making Medical Spending Decisions: The Law, Ethics, and Economics of Rationing Mechanisms* 3-6 (Oxford U Press, 1997).

20. Renée R. Anspach, *Prognostic Conflict in Life-and-Death Decisions: The Organization as an Ecology of Knowledge,* 28 J Health & Social Behavior 215, 215–16 (1987).

21. Marc Berg, *Rationalizing Medical Work: Decision-Support Techniques and Medical Practices* 153 (MIT Press, 1997).

22. Renée Anspach, *Deciding Who Lives: Fateful Choices in the Intensive Care Nursery* (U California Press, 1993).

23. Robert Zussman, *Intensive Care: Medical Ethics and the Medical Profession* 213 (U Chicago Press, 1992).

24. Idem at 214.

25. See Bradford H. Gray, *The Profit Motive and Patient Care: The Changing Accountability of Doctors and Hospitals* (Harvard U Press, 1991).

26. James Q. Wilson, *Capitalism and Morality,* Public Interest 42, 57 (Fall 1995).

27. Eliot Freidson, *Medical Work in America: Essays on Health Care* 198 (Yale U Press, 1989).

28. Idem at 214.

29. Gray, *The Profit Motive and Patient Care* at 324 (cited in note 25).

30. Morreim, *Balancing Act* at 30 (cited in note 17).

31. Freidson, *Medical Work in America* at 221 (cited in note 27). In recent years there has been a debate among sociologists over the extent to which doctors are losing power. Two schools of thought have believed their power is indeed waning. The "deprofessionalization" school (which is particularly associated with Marie Haug) believes that the prestige and confidence a profession needs are slipping away from medicine. The "proletarianization" school (which is particularly associated with John McKinlay) argues that like all workers in capitalist societies, doctors are increasingly employed and subjected by the bureaucracies in which they labor. The principal opponent of these two schools has been Eliot Freidson. Freidson's argument, however, is not that individual doctors retain their power, but rather that medicine as a profession does. This literature is intelligently reviewed in Frederic D. Wolinsky, *The Professional Dominance Perspective, Revisited,* 66 Milbank Quarterly 33 (Supp 2, 1988); Frederic W. Hafferty, *Theories at the Crossroads: A Discussion of Evolving Views on Medicine as a Profession,* 66 Milbank Quarterly 202 (Supp 2, 1988).

32. Eliot Freidson, *Industrialization or Humanization?* in *Medical Work in America: Essays on Health Care* 248, 252 (Yale U Press, 1989).

33. Gray, *The Profit Motive and Patient Care* at 296 (cited in note 25).

34. David M. Eddy, *Clinical Decision Making: From Theory to Practice* 6 (Jones & Bartlett, 1996).

35. Idem at 21.

36. Morreim, *Balancing Act* at 52 (cited in note 17).

37. Daniel F. Chambliss, *Beyond Caring: Hospitals, Nurses, and the Social Organization of Ethics* 51 (U Chicago Press, 1996).

38. Robert Zussman, *Intensive Care: Medical Ethics and the Medical Profession* 57 (U Chicago Press, 1992).

39. Idem.

40. Renée R. Anspach, *Deciding Who Lives: Fateful Choices in the Intensive-Care Nursery* 154 (U California Press, 1993).

41. See Jerry L. Mashaw, *Due Process in the Administrative State* (Yale U Press, 1985).

42. See Carl E. Schneider, *Lawyers and Children: Wisdom and Legitimacy in Family Policy,* 84 Michigan L Rev 919 (1986); Joel F. Handler, *The Conditions of Discretion: Autonomy, Community, Bureaucracy* (Russell Sage, 1986).

43. Zussman, *Intensive Care* at 102 (cited in note 38).

44. Idem at 221.

45. Grant Gilmore, *The Ages of American Law* 111 (Yale U Press, 1977).

46. Similarly, patients' memoirs often say little directly about the competence of doctors. This is largely, I think, because patients can so rarely evaluate it. (The memoirs of doctors mention competence and its absence disproportionately often.) Patients do complain of the kind of incompetence they can detect—principally, a failure to do necessary work, like interpreting a test or reading a chart before a consultation. Overall, patient memoirs are in large part about the struggle to get well and to find skilled help in that struggle.

47. J.W. Money, *To All the Girls I've Loved Before: An AIDS Diary* 58 (Alyson Publications, 1987).

48. James L. Johnson, *Coming Back* 12 (Springhouse Publishing, 1979).

49. Hacib Aoun & Glen Arm, *From the Eye of the Storm, With the Eyes of a Physician,* 116 Annals of Internal Medicine 335, 335 (1992).

50. John Berger & Jean Mohr, *A Fortunate Man: The Story of a Country Doctor* 70 (Holt, Rinehart, & Winston, 1967).

51. Esther Goshen-Gottstein, *Recalled to Life: The Story of a Coma* 179 (Yale U Press, 1988).

52. *Personal History: A Case of the Great Pox,* New Yorker 62, 74 (Sept 18, 1995). Other surveys of patients' memoirs reach similar conclusions. Hawkins observes that recent memoirs express "anger at callous or needlessly depersonalizing medical treatment," Anne Hunsaker Hawkins, *Reconstructing Illness: Studies in Pathography* 5 (Purdue U Press, 1993), and that many patients "are critical of the medical care they have received, often faulting their physicians for being impersonal, detached, and uncaring," idem at 142. Another study of memoirs reports "criticisms made again and again by patient-protagonists." Among these are the accusations that "doctors lie to patients, pretend to possess a knowledge that they do not really have, and are cold-hearted and selfish even when they are factually truthful and medically competent." Lucy Bregman & Sara Thiermann, *First Person Mortal: Personal Narratives of Dying, Death, and Grief* 75 (Paragon House, 1995).

53. Henrietta Aladjem, *The Sun Is My Enemy: One Woman's Victory Over a Mysterious and Dreaded Disease* 67 (Prentice-Hall, 1972).

54. Idem at 51.

55. Linda R. Bell, *The Red Butterfly: Lupus Patients Can Survive* 50 (Branden, 1983).

56. *My Left Foot* 156 (Minerva, 1995) (emphasis in original).

57. Rosalind MacPhee, *Picasso's Woman: A Breast Cancer Story* 36 (Kodansha, 1996).

58. Quoted in William B. Ober, *Boswell's Clap and Other Essays: Medical Analyses of Literary Men's Afflictions* 163 (Harper & Row, 1979).

59. *A Day at the Beach* 143 (Vintage Books, 1993).

60. Robert A. Hahn, *Sickness and Healing: An Anthropological Perspective* 244 (Yale U Press, 1995).

61. Hacib Aoun & Glen Arm, *From the Eye of the Storm, With the Eyes of a Physician,* 116 Annals of Internal Medicine 335, 336 (1992).

62. Seigfried Kra, *The Three-Legged Stallion: And Other Tales From a Doctor's Notebook* 202 (Fawcett Crest, 1990).

63. Hahn, *Sickness and Healing* at 245 (cited in note 60).

64. Fitzhugh Mullan, *Vital Signs: A Young Doctor's Struggle With Cancer* 59 (Farrar, Straus, & Giroux, 1983).

65. Sue Baier & Mary Zimmeth Schomaker, *Bed Number Ten* 186 (CRC Press, 1986).

66. Ilza Veith, *Can You Hear the Clapping of One Hand? Learning to Live With a Stroke* 31 (U California Press, 1988).

67. Tex Maule, *Running Scared: The Odyssey of a Heart-Attack Victim's Jogging Back to Health* 11 (Saturday Review Press, 1972).

68. Gillian Rose, *Love's Work: A Reckoning With Life* 88 (Schocken, 1995).

69. Arnold R. Beisser, *Flying Without Wings* 35 (Doubleday, 1989).

70. Judith Alexander Brice, *Ulcerative Colitis and Avascular Necrosis of Hips,* in Harvey Mandell & Howard Spiro, eds, *When Doctors Get Sick* 179 (Plenum Medical, 1988).

71. Eric Hodgins, *Episode: Report on the Accident Inside My Skull* 37–38 (Atheneum, 1964).

72. *Misery and Company: Sympathy in Everyday Life* 19 (U Chicago Press, 1997).

73. A doctor who became a patient rightly said patients "want to be cared for by people who are gentle, compassionate, and competent. They are not necessarily looking for a 'buddy' who introduces him- or herself by first name, the way your waiter for the evening does at the local Steak and Brew." Charles S. Kleinman, *Hodgkin's Disease,* in Harvey Mandell & Howard Spiro, eds, *When Doctors Get Sick* 314 (Plenum Medical, 1988). Or as Zussman comments in his study of ICUs,

> To say that patients and families prefer to be treated with kindness or that they want basic information is not to say that they want a deep or personal relationship with doctors and nurses. Indeed, some of the high praise for nurses comes precisely from the recognition, as the daughter of one patient put it, that they are "taking care of this person that you love so much, who they obviously don't know from Adam."

Robert Zussman, *Intensive Care: Medical Ethics and the Medical Profession* 93 (U Chicago Press, 1992)

74. Agnes de Mille, *Reprieve: A Memoir* 106–07 (Doubleday, 1981).

75. Robert F. Murphy, *The Body Silent* 21 (W.W. Norton, 1990).

76. Anthony T. Kronman, *Max Weber* 65 (Stanford U Press, 1983).

77. Francis W. Peabody, *The Care of the Patient,* 252 JAMA 813, 817 (1984), reprinted from 88 JAMA 877 (1927).

78. Daniel F. Chambliss, *Beyond Caring: Hospitals, Nurses, and the Social Organization of Ethics* 120 (U Chicago Press, 1996).

79. Eliot Freidson, *Industrialization or Humanization?* in *Medical Work in America: Essays on Health Care* 248, 252 (Yale U Press, 1989). On the tension between rules and discretion, see Carl E. Schneider, *Discretion and Rules: A Lawyer's View,* in Keith Hawkins, ed, *The Uses of Discretion* 47 (Oxford U Press, 1992).

80. Zussman, *Intensive Care* at 87 (cited in note 73).

81. For an elaboration of this point, see Carl E. Schneider, *Marriage, Morals, and the Law: No-Fault Divorce and Moral Discourse,* 1994 Utah L Rev 503, 578–81.

82. Zussman, *Intensive Care* at 40 (cited in note 73).

83. Idem at 59.

84. Peabody, *The Care of the Patient,* 252 JAMA at 818 (cited in note 77).

85. Henry Sumner Maine, *Ancient Law* 165 (Henry Holt, 1906).

86. Bradford H. Gray, *The Profit Motive and Patient Care: The Changing Accountability of Doctors and Hospitals* 325 (Harvard U Press, 1991).

87. Zussman, *Intensive Care* at 30 (cited in note 73).

88. Newsweek 73 (July 28, 1997). The article advises that the "most powerful step you can take is to learn everything you can about your condition or disease."

89. Zussman, *Intensive Care* at 52 (cited in note 73).

90. Idem at 86.

91. Idem at 87.

92. Eliot Freidson, *Industrialization or Humanization?,* in *Medical Work in America: Essays on Health Care* 248, 255 (Yale U Press, 1989).

93. This study has spawned many reports, most usefully SUPPORT Principal Investigators, *A Controlled Trial to Improve Care for Seriously Ill Hospitalized Patients: The Study to Understand Prognoses and Preferences for Outcomes and Risks of Treatments (SUPPORT),* 274 JAMA 1591 (1995). The study was analyzed in *Dying Well in the Hospital: The Lessons of SUPPORT,* a special supplement in HCR (Nov/Dec 1995). Some of what follows grows out of my own contribution to that supplement.

94. Ellen H. Moskowitz & James Lindemann Nelson, *Dying Well in the Hospital: The Lessons of Support,* 25 HCR S4 (Nov/Dec 1995).

95. Reynolds Price, *A Whole New Life* 112–13 (Atheneum, 1994).

96. Paul West, *A Stroke of Genius: Illness and Self-Discovery* 48–49 (Viking, 1995).

97. I am drawing on Sue Fisher, *In the Patient's Best Interest: Women and the Politics of Medical Decisions* (Rutgers U Press, 1986).

98. See, e.g., idem.

99. Alan Wolfe, *Whose Keeper? Social Science and Moral Obligation* 43 (U California Press, 1989).

100. Peter L. Berger & Thomas Luckmann, *The Social Construction of Reality: A Treatise in the Sociology of Knowledge* 51 (Anchor, 1966). For insights into the forces that create such social institutions, see Renée Anspach, *Prognostic Conflict in Life-and-Death Decisions: The Organization as an Ecology of Knowledge,* 28 J Health & Social Behavior 215 (1987).

101. Bernice A. Pescosolido, *Beyond Rational Choice: The Social Dynamics of How People Seek Help,* 97 American J Sociology 1096, 1106–7 (1992).

102. Max Lerner, *Wrestling With the Angel: A Memoir of My Triumph Over Illness* 69 (Simon & Schuster, 1990).

103. *A Preface to Morals* 300 (Macmillan, 1931).

104. Martin Krygier, *Law as Tradition*, 5 Law & Philosophy 237, 258–59 (1986) (emphasis in original).

105. Dan W. Brock, *The Ideal of Shared Decision Making Between Physicians and Patients*, 1 Kennedy Institute of Ethics J 28, 28 (1991).

106. Paul S. Appelbaum & Loren H. Roth, *Patients Who Refuse Treatment in Medical Hospitals*, 250 JAMA 1296, 1301 (1983).

107. Thomas C. Schelling, *Strategic Relationships in Dying*, in *Choice and Consequence* 157 (Harvard U Press 1984).

108. For an illuminating discussion of some of those interests, see David C. Blake, *State Interests in Terminating Medical Treatment*, 19 HCR 5 (May/June 1989).

109. I use "social institution" to mean "a pattern of expected action of individuals or groups enforced by social sanctions, both positive and negative." Robert N. Bellah, et al, *The Good Society* 10 (Knopf, 1991).

110. Schelling, *Strategic Relationships in Dying* at 154 (cited in note 107). To like effect are J. David Velleman, *Against the Right to Die*, 17 J Medicine & Philosophy 664 (1992), and Yale Kamisar, *Are Laws Against Assisted Suicide Unconstitutional?*, 23 HCR 32 (May/June 1993).

111. Robert A. Burt, *The Limits of Law in Regulating Health Care Decisions*, 7 HCR 29, 32 (Dec 1977).

112. Hacib Aoun & Glen Arm, *From the Eye of the Storm, With the Eyes of a Physician*, 116 Annals of Internal Medicine 335, 336 (1992).

113. "When we have seen a sight it ceases to impress us, use is second nature, what is always before our eyes no longer appeals to the imagination, and it is only through the imagination that we can feel the sorrows of others; this is why priests and doctors who are always beholding death and suffering become so hardened." Jean Jacques Rousseau, *Émile* 192 (E.P. Dutton, 1950).

114. See, e.g., Robert A. Scott, et al, *Organizational Aspects of Caring*, 73 Milbank Quarterly 77 (1995).

115. Gayle Feldman, *You Don't Have to Be Your Mother* 116 (W.W. Norton, 1994).

116. Kenneth A. Shapiro, *Dying and Living: One Man's Life With Cancer* 164 (U Texas Press, 1985).

117. Quintus West, *Pulmonary Tuberculosis: A Story of Maturation*, in Max Pinner & Benjamin F. Miller, eds, *When Doctors are Patients* 254 (W.W. Norton, 1952).

118. Eileen Radziunas, *Lupus: My Search for a Diagnosis* 28 (Hunter House, 1989).

119. Roberta G. Simmons, Susan Klein Marine, & Richard L. Simmons, *Gift of Life: The Social and Psychological Impact of Organ Transplantation* 362 (Transaction Books, 1987).

120. Max Lerner, *Wrestling With the Angel: A Memoir of My Triumph Over Illness* 53 (Simon & Schuster, 1990).

121. Candace Clark, *Misery and Company: Sympathy in Everyday Life* 231 (U Chicago Press, 1997).

122. Paulette Bates Alden, *Crossing the Moon: A Journey Through Infertility* 198 (Hungry Mind Press, 1996).

123. Paul West, *A Stroke of Genius: Illness and Self-Discovery* 140 (Viking, 1995).

124. Judith Alexander Brice, *Ulcerative Colitis and Avascular Necrosis of Hips*, in Harvey Mandell & Howard Spiro, eds, *When Doctors Get Sick* 179 (Plenum Medical, 1988).

125. Leon R. Kass, *Practicing Ethics: Where's the Action?*, 20 HCR 5, 9 (Jan/Feb 1990). Kass reports that "a distressed medical student who later complained to her profes-

sor about . . . [the incident] was told that she was too sensitive for the practice of medicine . . . ."

126. Gillian Rose, *Love's Work: A Reckoning with Life* 99 (Schocken, 1995).

127. "Sometimes no more than ten minutes would elapse between my having the soles of my feet scraped roughly for reflexive response by people I might not see more than that single time. It did not occur to me that I could say no. I did not know that often these strangers had nothing to do with my care." Joseph Heller & Speed Vogel, *No Laughing Matter* 84 (Putnam, 1986).

128. Joanna Baumer Permut, *Embracing the Wolf* 14–15 (Cherokee Publishing, 1989).

129. Suzy Szasz, *Living with It: Why You Don't Have to Be Healthy to Be Happy* 14 (Prometheus, 1991).

130. Michael Halberstam & Stephan Lesher, *A Coronary Event* 37 (Popular Library, 1978).

131. Norman Cousins, *Anatomy of an Illness as Perceived by the Patient* 137 (Bantam, 1979).

132. Fanny Gaynes, *How Am I Gonna Find A Man If I'm Dead?* 85 (Morgin Press, 1994).

133. Edward J. Speedling, *Heart Attack: The Family Response at Home and in the Hospital* 70 (Tavistock Publications, 1982).

134. William A. Nolen, *Surgeon Under the Knife* 37 (Dell, 1976).

135. Philip & Joyce Bedsworth, *Fight the Good Fight* 37 (Dell, 1976) (emphases in original).

136. Betty Garton Ulrich, *Rooted in the Sky: A Faith to Cope with Cancer* 33 (Judson Press, 1989).

137. Esther Goshen-Gottstein, *Recalled to Life: The Story of a Coma* 17 (Yale U Press, 1988).

138. Arthur W. Frank, *At the Will of the Body* 27 (Houghton Mifflin, 1991).

139. Lesley Fallowfield with Andrew Clark, *Breast Cancer* 43 (Routledge, 1992).

140. See Howard Spiro, et al, eds, *Empathy and the Practice of Medicine: Beyond Pills and the Scalpel* (Yale U Press, 1993).

141. Joie Harrison McGrail, *Fighting Back: One Woman's Struggle Against Cancer* 32 (Harper & Row, 1978).

142. Charles S. Kleinman, *Hodgkin's Disease,* in Harvey Mandell & Howard Spiro, eds, *When Doctors Get Sick* 311 (Plenum Medical, 1988).

143. Fred Davis, *Passage Through Crisis: Polio Victims and Their Families* 57 (Transaction, 1991).

144. See, e.g., Jody Heymann, *Equal Partner* 83 (Little, Brown, 1995).

145. Natalie Davis Spingarn, *Hanging in There* 37 (Stein & Day, 1982) (emphasis in original).

146. Reynolds Price, *A Whole New Life* 56 (Atheneum, 1994).

147. Arthur W. Frank, *At the Will of the Body* 54 (Houghton Mifflin, 1991).

148. Quintus West, *Pulmonary Tuberculosis: A Story of Maturation,* in Max Pinner & Benjamin F. Miller, eds, *When Doctors are Patients* 253 (W.W. Norton, 1952).

149. Judith Alexander Brice, *Ulcerative Colitis and Avascular Necrosis of Hips,* in Harvey Mandell & Howard Spiro, eds, *When Doctors Get Sick* 182 (Plenum Medical, 1988).

150. Reynolds Price, *A Whole New Life* 145 (Atheneum, 1994).

151. Brice, *Ulcerative Colitis* at 190 (cited in note 149).

152. Paul West, *A Stroke of Genius: Illness and Self-Discovery* 44 (Viking, 1995).

Index

Malpractice liability, xix, 31
Mandatory autonomy
    arguments for, 31–32
    autonomy paradigm, 10–16
    evaluating arguments for, 137–79
    false-consciousness argument, 22–23, 152
    introduction, xii
    moral argument, 23–31, 153–76
    prophylaxis argument, 18, 138–51
    reconsidering, 138, 280–92
    reluctant patient, 48
    therapeutic argument, 18–22, 143–51
    thought processes, 135
    understanding, 17
Manipulative behavior, 120
Mastectomy, 22, 122, 212
Maximizers, autonomy, xvi
Medical decisions
    by doctors, 99–108
    by patients, 38, 92–99
    varieties of, xii, 127–34
Medical disagreements, 142
Medical school, 5
Medication dosage titration by patients, 20–21
Melanoma, 163
Memoirs, patient, 9, 15, 21, 29, 43–45, 57, 71,
    83, 85, 119, 140, 147, 150, 162, 164,
    168, 173, 196–97
Mental retardation, 147
Mercy, 167
Methodological hyper-rationalism, xv–xvi
Mexican Americans, 46
Midwives, 84
Mind-cure movement, 121–22
Mind over body, 121
Modesty, 230
Moral argument for mandatory autonomy,
    23–31, 153–76
Moral issues, xiv, xvii, 46, 117, 126, 129
Multiple sclerosis, 56, 71, 80, 96, 118–19,
    154–55, 172, 178–79
Multivitamin/mineral supplements, 61
Muscle diseases, 38
Muscular dystrophy, 38

National Institutes of Health (NIH), 192
Neonatal intensive care units, 67
"New sick," 27
New times, autonomy in, 181–227
Nonbinding commitments, 174
Noncompliance, 87, 113
Nondirective approach, 15
Nonmedical aspect of medical decisions, 69–74
Nonmedical decisions, 128–30

Normal functioning, 129
"Normal irrationality," 149
"Normal science," 32, 138
Notes
    acknowlegements, 233
    autonomy paradigm, 238–48
    beyond reluctant patient, 292–99
    information, complexity, and control,
        273–80
    introduction, 233–38
    patients' preferences about autonomy,
        248–54
    reconsidering autonomy, 280–92
    reluctant patient, 254–73
Nurses, 58, 66–67, 93, 169, 198–99, 219
Nursing homes, 118

Obligation to know about personal bodily func-
    tions, 29
One-time decisions, 133
Optimism, 120–22
Optional autonomy, 10–13
Orderlies, 219
Organ-donor cards, xviii–xix
Organ donors, 69, 79, 92–94, 98
Ortho-Bionomy, 45
Ovarian cancer, 115, 132–34, 172
Overdramatizing, 52
Overestimation of patients' desire to make med-
    ical decisions, 43

Pain, 21, 51–52, 58, 62–63, 72, 76, 78, 97, 131,
    198, 211
Panic, 63, 121
Pap smears, 211
Paralysis, 120, 147, 152, 166
Paramedic-become-patient, 64, 150
Paraplegia, 124, 168
Parkinson's disease, 125, 132–33, 155
Passivity, patient, 14, 19, 39
Paternalism, physician, xvi, 4, 8, 12, 18, 22, 31,
    84, 86, 91, 193, 230
Patient Advocates for Advanced Cancer Treat-
    ments, 16
Patient-centered physicians, 14
Patient Self-Determination Act, xvi, xviii, 6
Perseverance, 126
Personal relationship between doctor and pa-
    tient, 112, 202, 231
Personal responsibility, 76
Personality types, 39, 59, 115
Phone calls, returning, 226
Physician disbelief of patients' thoughts about
    illness, 273–80

RETURN TO ➤ OPTOMETRY LIBRARY

LOAN PERIOD 1	2 1 MONTH	3
4	5	6

ALL BOOKS MAY BE RECALLED AFTER 7 DAYS.

DUE AS STAMPED BELOW

MAR 9 2000		
AUG 3 1 2000		
OCT 1 8 2000		
FEB 0 4 2005		

FORM NO. DD9

UNIVERSITY OF CALIFORNIA, BERKELEY
BERKELEY, CA 94720-6000